Dentistry with Case Studies

Dentistry with Case Studies

Editor: Jack Baker

AMERICAN
MEDICAL PUBLISHERS
www.americanmedicalpublishers.com

AMERICAN
MEDICAL PUBLISHERS
www.americanmedicalpublishers.com

Cataloging-in-Publication Data

Dentistry with case studies / edited by Jack Baker.
p. cm.
Includes bibliographical references and index.
ISBN 979-8-88740-632-9
1. Dentistry. 2. Oral medicine. 3. Teeth. I. Baker, Jack.
RK51 .D46 2023
617.6--dc23

American Medical Publishers,
41 Flatbush Avenue,
1st Floor, New York,
NY 11217, USA

ISBN 979-8-88740-632-9 (Hardback)

Contents

Preface

The branch of medicine that focuses on the diagnosis, prevention and treatment of oral diseases and disorders is known as dentistry. It involves the maintenance of oral health, the prevention of dental problems, and the diagnosis and treatment of conditions that affect the teeth, gums and other supporting structures of the oral cavity. Dentistry encompasses specialized fields such as orthodontics, endodontics, and periodontics, which focus on the treatment of specific dental problems. It seeks to maintain optimal oral health, prevent dental problems, and restore or enhance the appearance and function of the teeth and surrounding tissues. Some of the treatment methods which are used within this field are dental fillings, root canal therapy, gum treatments, oral surgeries, orthodontics, and prosthetics like dental implants or dentures. This book includes some of the vital pieces of works being conducted across the world, on various topics related to dentistry. Those in search of information to further their knowledge will be greatly assisted by it.

This book is a comprehensive compilation of works of different researchers from varied parts of the world. It includes valuable experiences of the researchers with the sole objective of providing the readers (learners) with a proper knowledge of the concerned field. This book will be beneficial in evoking inspiration and enhancing the knowledge of the interested readers.

In the end, I would like to extend my heartiest thanks to the authors who worked with great determination on their chapters. I also appreciate the publisher's support in the course of the book. I would also like to deeply acknowledge my family who stood by me as a source of inspiration during the project.

Editor

1

Multidisciplinary Approach for Full-Mouth Rehabilitation of a Young Adult Patient with Ameloblastoma

Hung-Yi Liao,[1] May-Show Chen,[1,2] Ya-Fen Yang,[1] Pei-Bang Liao,[1] Sheng-Wei Feng,[1,2] and Po-kai Juan[1,2]

[1]*Division of Prosthodontics, Department of Dentistry, Taipei Medical University Hospital, Taipei, Taiwan*
[2]*School of Dentistry, College of Oral Medicine, Taipei Medical University, Taipei, Taiwan*

Correspondence should be addressed to Sheng-Wei Feng; shengwei@tmu.edu.tw and Po-kai Juan; jordan6412@yahoo.com.tw

Academic Editor: Giuseppe Colella

Ameloblastoma is a benign but locally invasive neoplasm of the odontogenic epithelium that tends to grow slowly in the mandible or maxilla. It can be highly destructive to the surrounding dental anatomy and can cause death by progressive spread to nearby vital structures in rare cases. Marginal resection is the most effective method of eliminating the tumor, but treatment can further contribute to oral and dental deformity and malfunction. This clinical report describes the dental rehabilitation of a young adult patient diagnosed with ameloblastoma and underwent preliminary marsupialization, segmental mandibulectomy, and fibula free flap reconstruction, followed by mandibular dental implant placements. Orthodontic and rapid palatal expansion for maxillary arch correction was also performed. The treatment goal of regaining dental function and a satisfactory appearance was accomplished.

1. Introduction

Ameloblastoma is a benign odontogenic tumor that arises in the jawbone. This tumor occurs in three different variants: multicystic, unicystic, and peripheral, which deserve separate consideration because of differing therapeutic considerations and prognosis [1]. Overall, the tumor is slow growing and locally invasive and has a high recurrence rate. Marsupialization is useful as a preliminary treatment of cystic ameloblastoma.

However, following marsupialization, the tumor still has the potential to infiltrate into the surrounding tissues [2]. Therefore, marginal resection with a safety margin is considered the most effective method of eliminating the tumor. However, it also causes facial deformation and dysfunction, which leads to a decrease in a patient's living quality.

A multidisciplinary approach is needed for the patient's complete rehabilitation, including bone grafting, implant placement, and prosthetic fabrication. Sometimes treatment must combine orthodontic treatment to create an optimum occlusal relationship and gain sufficient space for ideal reconstruction. This report presents the long-term clinical follow-up of a patient with ameloblastoma who successively underwent surgical, orthodontic, and prosthetic treatment for complete oral reconstruction.

2. Case Report

A 26-year-old man came to the Oral and Maxillofacial Surgery Department of Taipei Medical University Hospital (Taipei, Taiwan) in May 2011 due to swelling and pain in the jaw. The intraoral examination revealed a raised mass in the left mandibular buccal vestibular area extending to the labial area without secretory discharge. The color and appearance of the surrounding mucosa were normal. The teeth in this area also have no obvious periodontal pockets (Figure 1(a)). On extraoral examination, the patient's lateral view shows a protruding mandible, and the left and right sides of the face were also slightly asymmetrical. The neurological examination was normal, and there were no swollen and palpable lymph nodes in the neck (Figure 1(b)). A radiographic examination showed a wide range of radiolucent lesions in the mandible from the

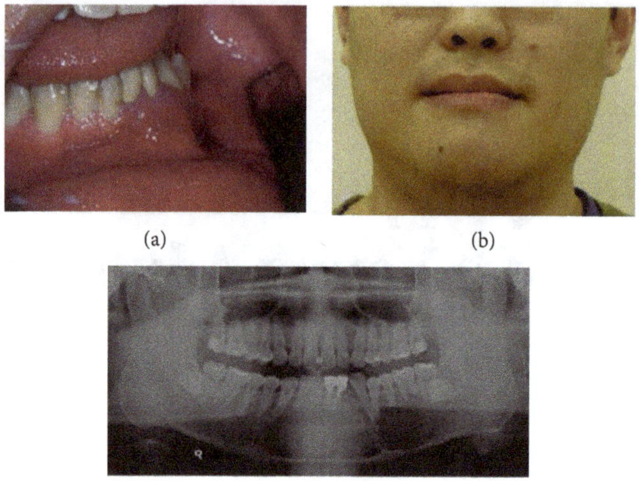

(a) (b)

(c)

FIGURE 1: Initial findings. (a) Intraoral view shows a raised mass over the left buccal vestibular area. (b) Extraoral view shows slight facial asymmetry. (c) Panoramic radiograph reveals multilocular radiolucent lesion over the anterior and left mandible.

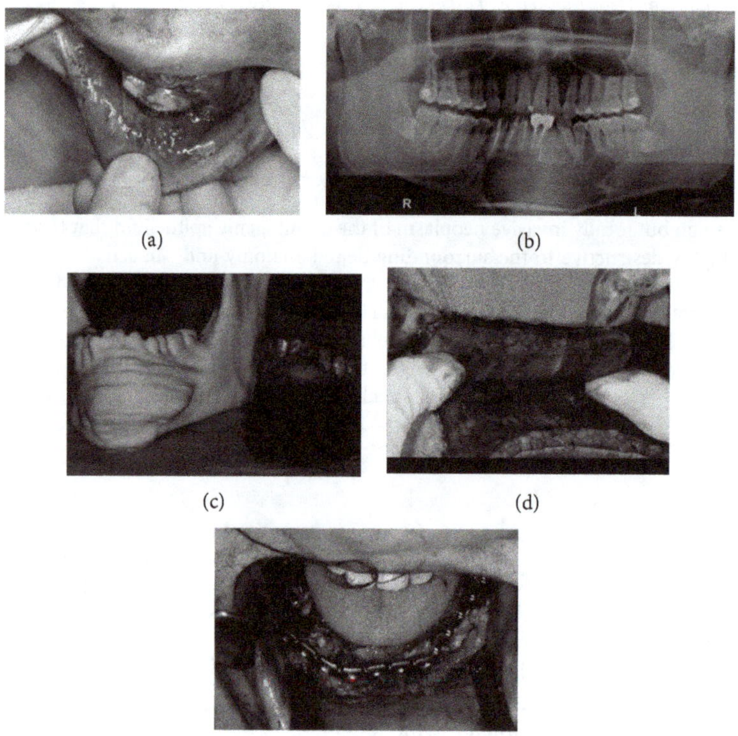

(a) (b) (c) (d) (e)

FIGURE 2: Mandible reconstruction. (a) A soft liner was used as the obturator material after two marsupializations. (b) The tumor size decreased on the left side but remained unchanged in the anterior area. (c) The 3D model was used to simulate the scope of the resection. (d) The free fibular flap was positioned. (e) The flap was fixed with the prebent metal bone band.

canine area on the right to the second molar on the left. The biopsy and pathology reports confirmed that the lesion was consistent with ameloblastoma (Figure 1(c)). The pathology report is presented as follows. Grossly, they are gray and brown and elastic with some bone chips. Microscopically, it shows an ameloblastoma with islands of odontogenic epithelium in plexiform and follicular patterns within a fibrous stroma. The odontogenic epithelium shows peripheral palisading and stellate reticulum. Neither cytological atypia nor increased mitoses is seen.

Marsupialization was performed to reduce the size and destructiveness of the tumor for subsequent resection surgery. The marsupialization was firstly performed in the anterior and left posterior region of the mandible. Soft liner was applied immediately as the obturator materials, and regular visits were arranged to monitor the changes

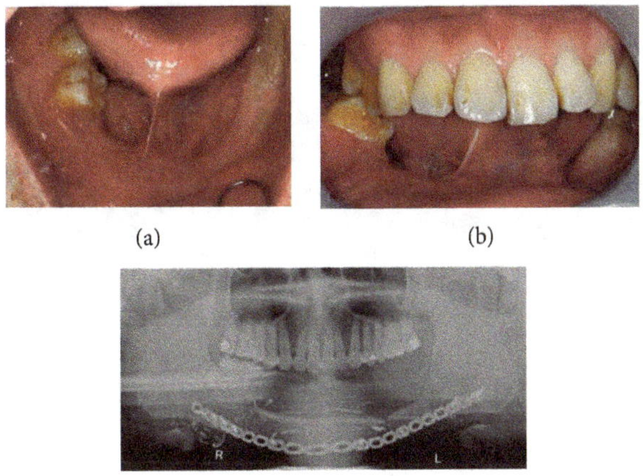

(a) (b) (c)

FIGURE 3: The soft and hard tissues had healed completely and ready for reconstruction. (a, b) Intraoral view. Teeth 46 and 47 were temporarily kept for maintaining vertical support. (c) Panoramic radiograph after segmental mandibulectomy and fibular free flap.

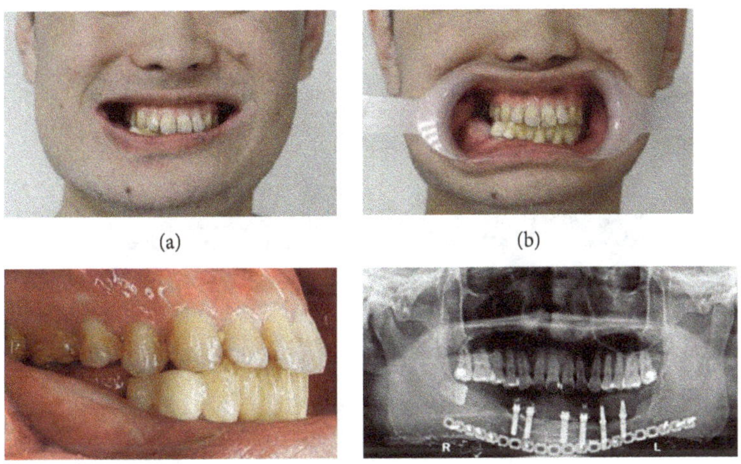

(a) (b) (c) (d)

FIGURE 4: Teeth 46 and 47 were extracted after staged approach implant placement. Cross-bite and lack of restoration space over right side were observed. (a, b) Extraoral view shows narrow maxillary arch and large buccal corridor. (c) Lack of restoration space over lower right posterior area. (d) Panoramic film after staged approach implant placement.

of tumor size and to adjust the obturator (Figure 2(a)). After 4 months, the tumor size was gradually reduced on the left posterior region, but remained unchanged over the anterior region. Thus, the marsupialization was performed again over the anterior region. It took a total of 12 months to reduce the size of the lesion and confirm the scope of the tumor (Figure 2(b)). After that, the segmental mandibulectomy combined with fibula free flap reconstruction was conducted. At that time, three-dimensional (3D) image processing and printing were used to analyze and guide dental implant design and construction. The more precise the reconstruction operation can be, the more the damage can be reduced. Additionally, the entire postoperative period will benefit from precision reconstruction.

Therefore, computed tomography (CT) examination was taken to evaluate the precise extension and region of the tumor. And then, the 3D printing transferred from CT files/images was applied to create a solid model, and the actual scope of the resection could be simulated before surgery (Figure 2(c)). A fibula 3D model was also exported for model surgery, surgical template making, and titanium bone plate bending. During the surgery, the defect was first fixed with a prebent metal bone plate, and then, the fibula part of the removed free flap was divided into three sections according to the surgical template and bent to meet the needs of the defect. Soft tissue defects in the mouth were also reconstructed with free flaps (Figures 2(d) and 2(e)). With the 3D printed models, the surgery can be completed more accurately, and the treatment time can be significantly reduced.

During the healing period, the patient could only use the remaining teeth, 46 and 47, and the opposite tooth. After 9 months, alveoloplasty was performed to correct the uneven and sharp bony edges. The patient was referred to a prosthodontist 3 years after the first visit. At this point, the soft and hard tissues had healed completely and were ready for reconstruction (Figure 3).

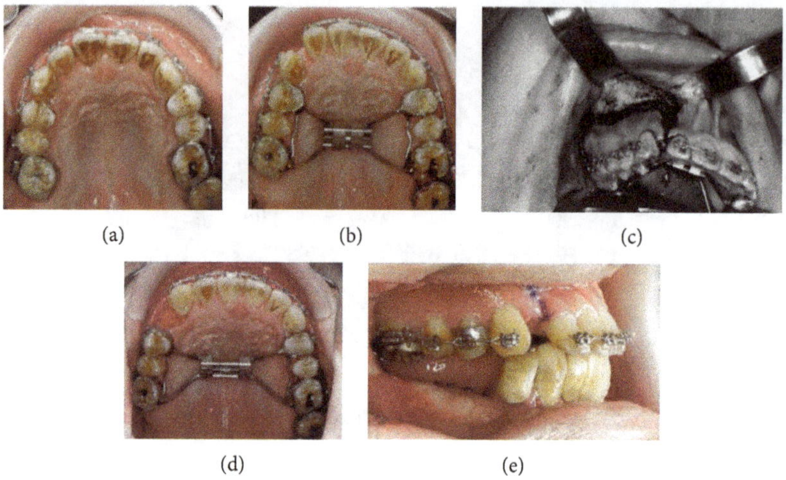

Figure 5: (a) Leveling and alignment after extraction of tooth 17 to create space. (b) Placement of the rapid palatal expander. (c) Posterior segmental osteotomy in the right maxilla. (d) Complete maxillary arch expansion. (e) Correction of the transverse jaw deficiency, with increased restoration space.

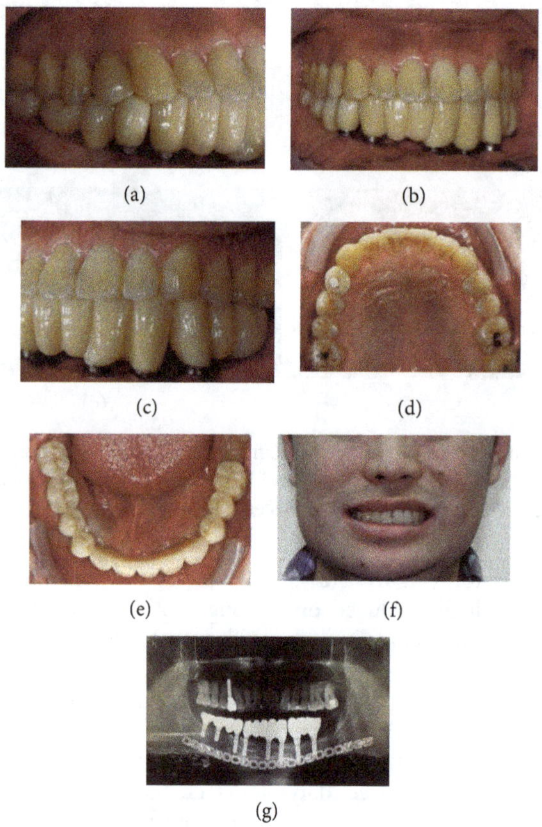

Figure 6: Completed dental reconstruction. (a–c) Final insertion of zirconia implant-supported fixed partial dentures and ideal occlusal plane and occlusion. (d, e) Smooth and symmetrical dental arches. (f) Photograph showing improved asymmetry of face. (g) Radiograph of the final mandible and dental reconstruction.

After a prosthetic evaluation, the problems and preliminary treatment directions were revealed. The patient's treatment program was developed to address the following issues. Full mandible implants were necessary and feasible to meet the physical and psychological needs of the patient. Considering that teeth 46 and 47 were the only two teeth that could be used for chewing, a staged dental implant approach was adopted. The transverse discrepancy in the upper and lower jaws and a deficiency in the right maxilla resulting in asymmetric facial features required resolution but could not be repaired by dentures alone. The cross-bite on the right side required resolution, and the space was limited for restoration on the right side.

A staged approach was conducted. First, four implants in tooth 33, 32, 43, and 44 position were placed in the mandible. After the osseointegration, implant-supported provisional crowns 3332xxx4344 were installed in position. Then, two implants in teeth 34 and 36 were placed on the left mandible and were fitted with 34×36 provisional crowns. Finally, teeth 46 and 47 were extracted (Figure 4). The purpose of the patient's orthodontic treatment was to gain restoration space on the right side and correct the upper jaw deficiency. In the beginning, tooth 17 was extracted and followed by leveling and alignment to create space (Figure 5(a)). After rapid palatal expander (RPE) placement (Figure 5(b)), the right maxillary posterior segmental osteotomy (PSO) (Figure 5(c)), right mandibular alveoloplasty, and extraction of tooth 48 were performed in the same operation to achieve proper interocclusal relationship and gain enough restoration space over right posterior region. Next, the patient was asked to regularly rotate the screw of the conventional Hyrax expander. One rotation per day produces a 0.2 mm lateral expansion, which lasts up to two weeks but varies from individual to individual. After the desired position was achieved, there was no need to continue turning the screw. However, it was still necessary to continue wearing the device for at least three months to stabilize the expansion. PSO and RPE provided the required lateral expansion effect to transform the upper arch into a better shape. Alveoloplasty also increased restoration space (Figures 5(d) and 5(e)). The implant surgery was completed with the implantation of teeth 14, 46, and 47. The provisional teeth were installed after osseointegration. The lower jaw was divided into three groups of cement-retained bridges, and tooth 14 was a screw-retained crown. The prosthesis was made with zirconia-based material. The pontic type was designed to be consistent with the original provisional crowns and appropriate for the patient's extensive mandibular reconstruction. This design did not allow any contact between the pontic bottom and the gums so that the patient could clean the teeth as efficiently as before, and the large-scale bottom hollow was not prone to food impaction. After postoperative treatment was completed, the upper and lower jaws presented smooth and symmetrical dental arches, dental function was restored, and the patient's face showed improved symmetry (Figure 6).

3. Discussion

Ameloblastoma is an odontogenic tumor with highly aggressive and curable features. Nonetheless, a consensus has not been reached on the biologic behavior of this neoplasm and how best to treat it [3]. Because of its highly infiltrative, aggressive nature and to reduce the risk of recurrence, resection of the tumor with 1.0-2.0 cm linear bony margins followed by free autologous grafting is recommended [4]. Hidalgo reported the utility of vascularized fibula flaps for mandibular reconstruction in 1989 [5]. Since then, it has become the first option for mandible reconstruction [6, 7]. A significant advantage is that fibular free flap reconstruction offers adequate bony dimensions and bone quality, allowing for the placement and osseointegration of dental implants and the possibility of restoring masticatory function and aesthetics [8]. The flap operation is difficult to control during conventional surgery and occasionally results in dissatisfying occlusion and appearance. Virtual planning and 3D print modeling using preoperative computed tomographic (CT) data have recently been introduced. The true-to-size models and templates are easy to obtain, and pre-bending of a titanium plate can be done on the model. These techniques permit more accurate and time-saving reconstruction [9].

We encountered several problems throughout the postoperative prosthetic evaluation, including transverse maxillomandibular discrepancy and right maxillary arch deficiency. To correct the malocclusion and make the buccal corridor less obvious, we applied an RPE for orthodontic treatment appropriate for the patient's age and facial structure. Rapid palatal expansion is a technique whereby expansion of 0.5 mm to 1 mm is achieved each day until the posterior cross-bite is relieved. For stability purposes, the RPE usually remains in the patient's mouth for 3–6 months, but this time may vary among patients [10]. In our patient, implant placement was performed via a staged approach for maintaining oral function [11, 12]. The number of implants was increased as much as possible to avoid inappropriate prosthetic design due to a small number of implants.

4. Conclusion

This clinical report illustrated an interdisciplinary treatment approach provided by cooperation between maxillofacial surgeons, prosthodontists, and orthodontists. After eight years of treatment, the patient had no evidence of tumor recurrence, completely reconstructed soft and hard tissues, restored function, improved appearance, and ultimately quality of life. Reconstruction after facial tumor resection remains a challenge. In our patient, a rigorous treatment plan, coupled with a multidisciplinary approach, achieved the treatment goal of restoring the patient's oral and dental function and appearance.

References

[1] O. A. Effiom, O. M. Ogundana, A. O. Akinshipo, and S. O. Akintoye, "Ameloblastoma: current etiopathological concepts and management," *Oral Diseases*, vol. 24, no. 3, pp. 307–316, 2018.

[2] N. Nakamura, Y. Higuchi, H. Tashiro, and M. Ohishi, "Marsupialization of cystic ameloblastoma: a clinical and histopathologic study of the growth characteristics before and after marsupialization," *Journal of Oral and Maxillofacial Surgery*, vol. 53, no. 7, pp. 748–754, 1995.

[3] B. R. Chrcanovic, C. C. Gomes, and R. S. Gomez, "Desmoplastic ameloblastoma: a systematic review of the cases reported in the literature," *International Journal of Oral and Maxillofacial Surgery*, vol. 49, no. 6, pp. 709–716, 2020.

[4] S. E. Feinberg, B. Steinberg, and L. J. Peterson, "Surgical management of ameloblastoma: Currents status of the literature," *Oral Surgery, Oral Medicine, Oral Pathology, Oral Radiology, and Endodontology*, vol. 81, no. 4, pp. 383–388, 1996.

[5] S. Sinno and E. D. Rodriguez, "Nuances and pearls of the free fibula osteoseptocutaneous flap for reconstruction of a high-energy ballistic injury mandible defect," *Plastic and Reconstructive Surgery*, vol. 137, no. 1, pp. 280–284, 2016.

[6] M. Bak, A. S. Jacobson, D. Buchbinder, and M. L. Urken, "Contemporary reconstruction of the mandible," *Oral Oncology.*, vol. 46, no. 2, pp. 71–76, 2010.

[7] D. Okay, A. H. Al Shetawi, S. P. Moubayed, M. Mourad, D. Buchbinder, and M. L. Urken, "Worldwide 10-year systematic review of treatment trends in fibula free flap for mandibular reconstruction," *Journal of Oral and Maxillofacial Surgery*, vol. 74, no. 12, pp. 2526–2531, 2016.

[8] D. Sozzi, G. Novelli, R. Silva, S. T. Connelly, and G. M. Tartaglia, "Implant rehabilitation in fibula-free flap reconstruction: a retrospective study of cases at 1-18 years following surgery," *Journal of Cranio-Maxillofacial Surgery*, vol. 45, no. 10, pp. 1655–1661, 2017.

[9] W. Ren, L. Gao, S. Li et al., "Virtual planning and 3D printing modeling for mandibular reconstruction with fibula free flap," *Medicina Oral, Patología Oral y Cirugía Bucal*, vol. 23, no. 3, pp. e359–e366, 2018.

[10] L. Suri and P. Taneja, "Surgically assisted rapid palatal expansion: a literature review," *American Journal of Orthodontics and Dentofacial Orthopedics*, vol. 133, no. 2, pp. 290–302, 2008.

[11] H. M. Huang, T. J. Chee, W. Z. Lew, and S. W. Feng, "Modified surgical drilling protocols influence osseointegration performance and predict value of implant stability parameters during implant healing process," *Clinical Oral Investigations*, vol. 24, no. 10, pp. 3445–3455, 2020.

[12] Y. H. Su, B. Y. Peng, P. D. Wang, and S. W. Feng, "Evaluation of the implant stability and the marginal bone level changes during the first three months of dental implant healing process: a prospective clinical study," *Journal of the Mechanical Behavior of Biomedical Materials*, vol. 110, article 103899, 2020.

2

Polymorphous Adenocarcinoma: A Rare Case Report with Unique Radiographic Appearance on CBCT

Jagadish Chandra,[1] Junaid Ahmed,[2] K. M. Veena,[3] M. Vijayakumar,[4] Nandita Shenoy,[2] and Nanditha Sujir[2]

[1]*Dept. of Oral Surgery, Yenepoya Dental College, Yenepoya University, Deralakatte, India*
[2]*Dept. of Oral Medicine and Radiology, Manipal College of Dental Sciences, Mangalore, Manipal Academy of Higher Education (MAHE), Manipal, Karnataka 576104, India*
[3]*Dept. of Oral Medicine and Radiology, Yenepoya Dental College, Yenepoya University, Deralakatte, Karnataka, India*
[4]*Department of Surgical Oncology, Yenepoya Medical College, Yenepoya University, Deralakatte, Mangalore, India*

Correspondence should be addressed to Junaid Ahmed; junaid.ahmed@manipal.edu

Academic Editor: Sukumaran Anil

Background. Polymorphous low-grade adenocarcinoma (PLGA) is a slow growing malignant tumor of minor salivary glands and is generally of indolent nature. However, according to the most recent WHO Classification of Salivary Gland Tumors (2017), the cancer is classified as Polymorphous AdenoCarcinoma (PAC). PAC presents as a less aggressive tumor, though it could on rare occasions demonstrate distant metastasis. *Case Presentation.* A 47-year-old man who was referred by a private practitioner for a CBCT scan in reference to a proliferative soft-tissue growth in the hard palate. The growth was mild and tender and there was Grade III mobility in relation to all the maxillary teeth. Panoramic radiograph taken previously had revealed evidence of alveolar bone loss in relation to the maxillary teeth and was inconclusive of any other findings. The CBCT scan revealed evidence of moth-eaten appearance of maxilla with destruction of medial and lateral walls and floor of maxillary sinus. There was also evidence of involvement of right eustachian tube, ethmoidal wall, and nasopalatine canal. An intraosseous malignancy of the palate was suspected, and a total maxillectomy was performed. The tissue sample was sent for histopathological assessment wherein changes diagnostic for polymorphous low-grade adenocarcinoma of the palate were observed. *Conclusion.* PAC is a distinct, yet commonly occurring, minor salivary gland tumor with varied clinical and histologic appearance. This case report highlights the importance of CBCT in diagnosing the intraosseous involvement of such tumors which can help shed some light in enhancing our knowledge about the minor salivary gland malignancies like PAC.

1. Background

Polymorphous low-grade adenocarcinoma (PLGA) is a slow growing malignant tumor of minor salivary glands and is generally of indolent nature. However, according to the most recent WHO Classification of Salivary Gland Tumors (2017), the cancer is classified as Polymorphous AdenoCarcinoma (PAC) [1]. Among all the tumors of oral salivary glands, oral salivary gland carcinomas comprise only 20% of the malignant neoplasms [2]. Lobular carcinoma, terminal duct carcinoma, and low-grade papillary adenocarcinoma were the various names that were used for adenocarcinomas of the minor salivary glands, before Evans and Batsakis [3] categorized them as a separate histologic entity in 1984. The World Health Organization later categorized PAC as a separate category of tumors of minor salivary glands in 1990 [4].

Due to its architecturally diverse structure, clinically indolent behavior, and cytological uniformity, PAC is thought to be a unique entity [5, 6]. Being asymptomatic with a low metastatic potential, it is commonly seen in elder women, with about 24% of primary tumors associated with major salivary glands (i.e., parotid, submandibular, or sublingual gland) and few in locations other than the head and neck, such as the breast and vagina [7, 8].

Although the third most commonly presenting malignant salivary gland tumor, our knowledge about PAC remains restricted to published case reports. Also, the architectural diversity associated with the name can be confusing for histopathological evaluation and can potentially be a diagnostic dilemma. Salivary gland neoplasms can be aggressive, and most of their clinical features often overlap; hence, a detailed examination and clinical investigation should be carried out in order to reach a definitive conclusion. Radiology is an important diagnostic tool for salivary gland pathology. It helps to determine the extent of involvement of bony structures, which can provide foresight into the treatment planning and provide a valuable tool in assessing the clinical picture. Cone Beam Computed Tomography (CBCT) is useful in the assessment of osseous structures and can help the clinician to determine the aggressive nature of the tumor as well as bony involvement due to a clear image of structures that are highly contrasted, and in comparison to most 2-D imaging methods, CBCT can provide a three-dimensional image of structures of the head and neck [9]. The following case report describes a unique case where a patient reported with the complaint of a soft-tissue growth in relation to the maxilla. This case report is aimed at highlighting the importance of CBCT in the detection of malignancies of salivary gland tissues, especially those cases with extensive bony involvement.

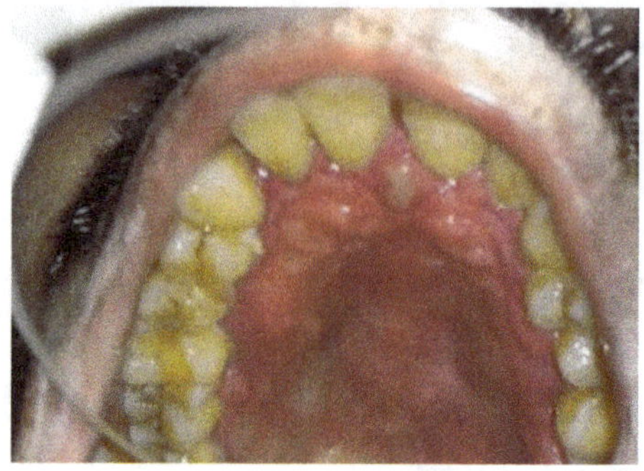

FIGURE 1: Evidence of diffuse, proliferative soft tissue swelling in the region of the hard palate.

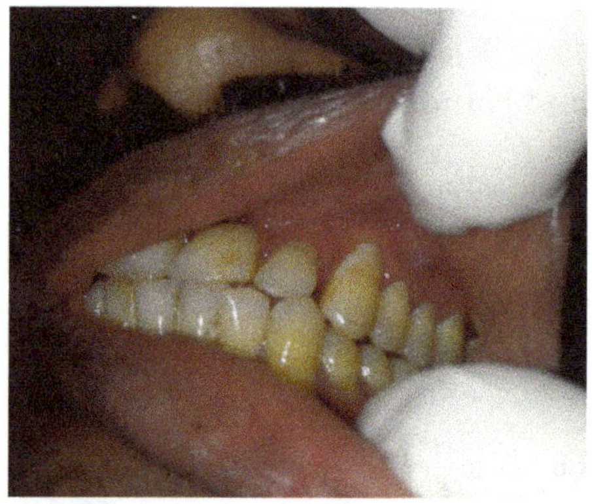

FIGURE 2: Evidence of erythema of the attached gingiva in relation to maxillary posterior teeth. The clinical features resembled a periodontal pathology.

2. Case Presentation

A 47-year-old man was referred to the Department of Oral Medicine & Radiology with a history of soft tissue growth in the palate for the past two months. The growth was sudden in onset, growing rapidly in size over the next two months and localized to the palate. The patient reported no pain during the onset of growth. However, for the past one week, the patient reported mild pain. On clinical examination, there was a diffuse, proliferative soft tissue growth of the maxilla extending from the marginal gingiva in the palatal aspect of the anterior tooth and involving the entire surface of the hard palate up to the level of the hard and soft palate junction along with erythema of attached gingiva in relation to posterior teeth palatally and buccally as well as Grade III mobility of all the anterior and posterior maxillary teeth (Figures 1 and 2). The cervical group of lymph nodes were nonpalpable clinically.

The referring private practitioner had advised a panoramic radiograph earlier which revealed severe bone loss in relation to maxillary teeth suggestive of generalized periodontitis and was inconclusive for any other relevant findings except for a root stump in the lower right quadrant (Figure 3).

The patient was advised for a CBCT scan which revealed a moth-eaten appearance of the palate noticed bilaterally with involvement of nasopalatine canal anteriorly and external resorption of roots in relation to all the maxillary teeth present, with evidence of involvement of anterior and middle ethmoidal sinus, eustachian tube, and nasopharynx on the right side. Based on CBCT and clinical findings, a preliminary diagnosis of intraosseous malignancy involving the palate was suspected (Figures 4–9). The patient was then scheduled for surgery with excision biopsy and total maxillectomy up to the floor of orbit.

The surgical procedure consisted of visualization of hard and soft palate and incision extending laterally around the maxillary tuberosity exposing the posterior border. Following exposure of the maxillary tuberosity, attachment to the soft palate and hard palate was divided. After soft tissue dissection up to the extension of the tumor, the extent of the bone which was tailored to the primary tumor including the lateral wall of the orbit and zygoma to be resected was marked. Following bone guttering, the bony resection was carried out using a chisel and mallet through the frontal process of the maxilla and lacrimal bone. Bleeding encountered during this procedure from the greater palatine artery and the branches of internal maxillary artery was controlled using pressure packing followed by ligation to achieve haemostasis. After mobilizing the segment, final osteotomy was done to separate the maxillary tuberosity from the pterygoid plates. Before removal, thorough clinical examination of the specimen was done to determine the adequacy of the tumor (Figures 10(a) and 10(b) and 11(a) and 11(b)).

The tissue sample was sent for histopathological examination which revealed an unencapsulated tumor within the underlying connective tissue approximating the surface epithelium, with a varied pattern of arrangement of tumor cells that included solid nests, strands, ducts, and tubular and

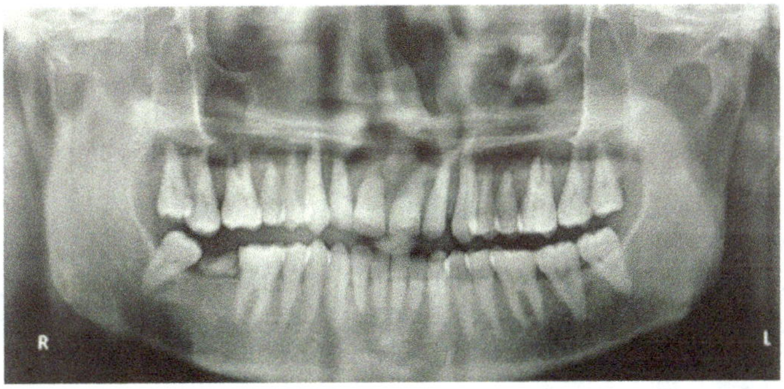

Figure 3: Panoramic radiograph of the patient revealing evidence of interdental bone loss in relation to all the maxillary teeth.

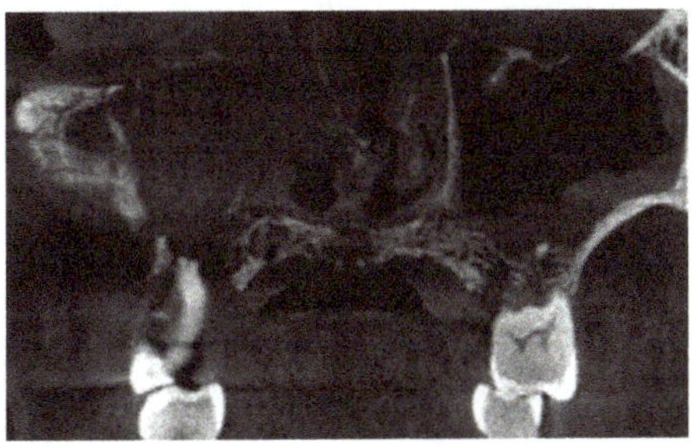

Figure 4: Coronal section of CBCT scan revealing destruction of walls of maxillary sinus along with involvement of nasopalatine canal.

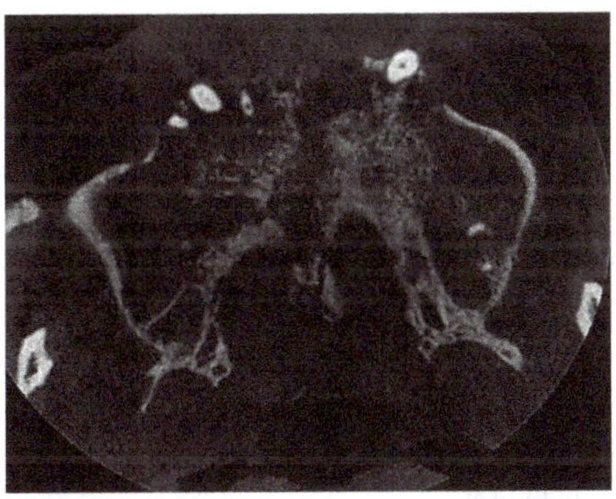

Figure 5: Axial view of CBCT scan revealing moth-eaten appearance of maxilla involving the hard palate and maxillary bone.

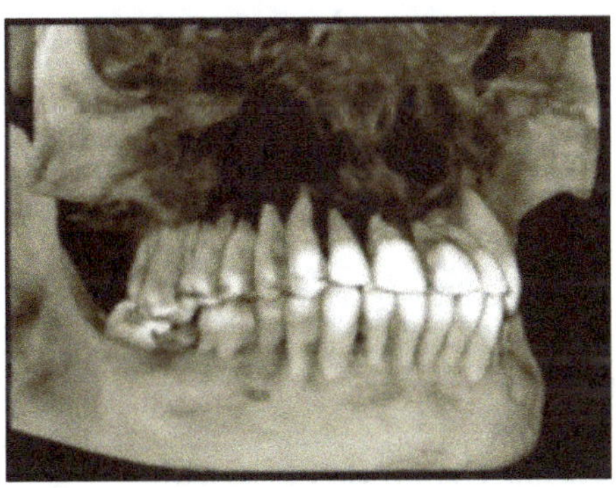

Figure 6: 3D reconstructed CBCT image revealing widespread destruction of maxilla and resorption of all maxillary teeth root apices.

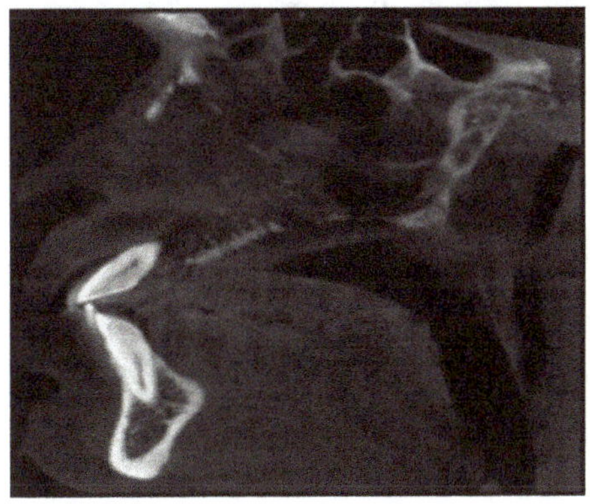

Figure 7: Sagittal section of CBCT revealing destruction of hard palate.

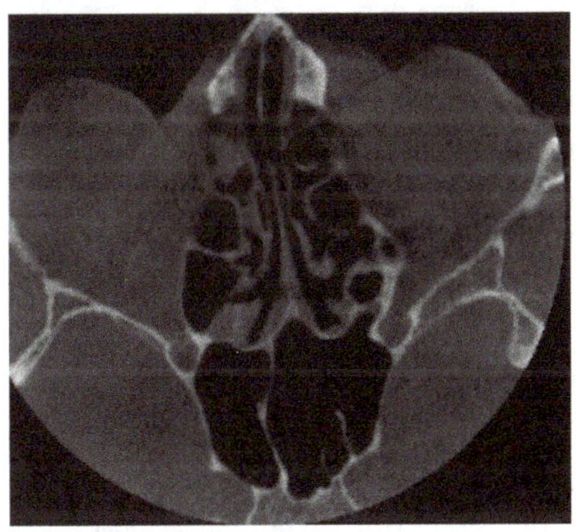

Figure 8: Axial view of CBCT scan revealing involvement of anterior and middle ethmoidal air sinus on the right side.

papillary patterns and was lined by 1-2 layers of oval/cuboidal cells along with a peripheral layer of flat cells suggestive of polymorphous low-grade adenocarcinoma of the palate (Figures 12, 13, and 14). The patient is currently under follow-up for the past six months and is asymptomatic.

3. Discussion and Conclusion

Clinically, PAC presents as a firm, well-circumscribed, painless, and slow growing mass mostly covered by nonulcerated mucosa resembling a benign neoplasm and could be fixed to underlying structures, eroding and infiltrating the underlying

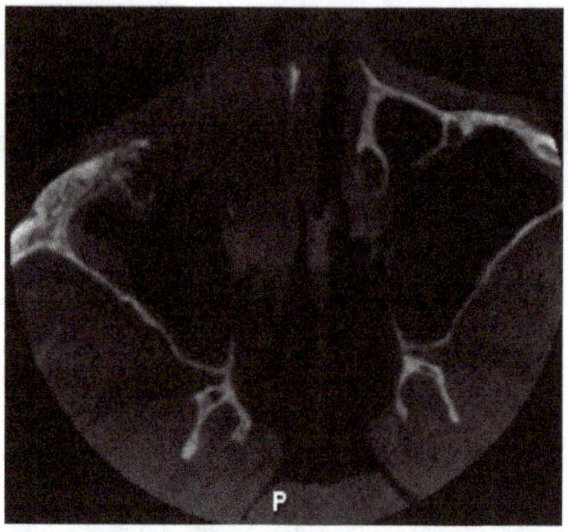

FIGURE 9: Axial view of CBCT scan revealing narrowing and involvement of eustachian tube on the right side.

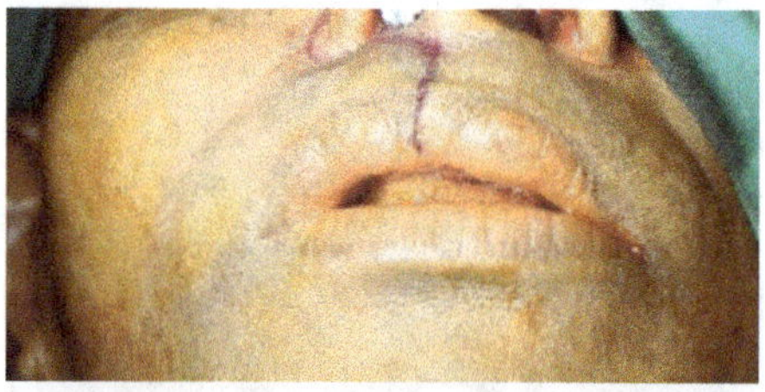

(a)

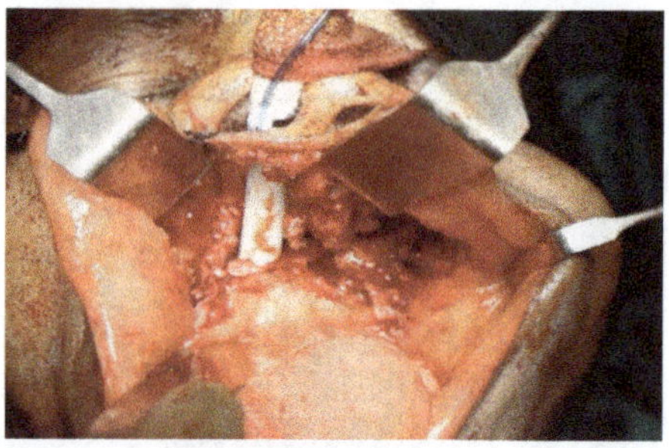

(b)

FIGURE 10: (a, b) Maxillectomy procedure done under local anesthesia.

bone, and is even present with perivascular and perineural invasion. Metastasis when reported is mostly confined to the regional nodes while spread to distant sites is a rarity and so is the transformation of this low-grade entity into a high-grade one [10].

Immunohistochemistry (IHC) has been utilized in a number of case series to distinguish between PAC and ACC, but there is a considerable overlap. Past studies conducted regarding the expression of ki-67 have consistently reported a very low labelling index (LI) in PAC which can assist in differentiating it from adenoid cystic carcinoma (ACC) [11–14]. In a few studies, p40 immunostaining has been demonstrated as a new tool for distinguishing salivary gland tumors with true myoepithelial differentiation from those showing nonspecific p63 expression. When these immunostains are performed in tandem, a discordant p63/p40-immunophenotype can reliably distinguish PAC from both adenoid cystic carcinoma and pleomorphic adenoma, which generally show p63/p40 concordance [15]. Genetic abnormalities may be useful in differential diagnosis of PAC. PACs harbor PRKD1 mutations in >70% cases, and

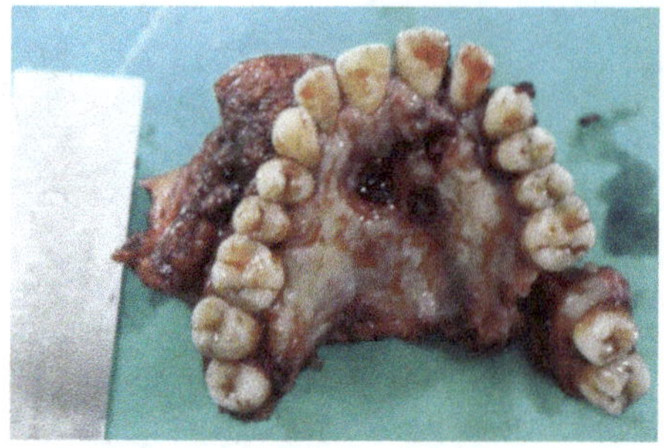

(a)

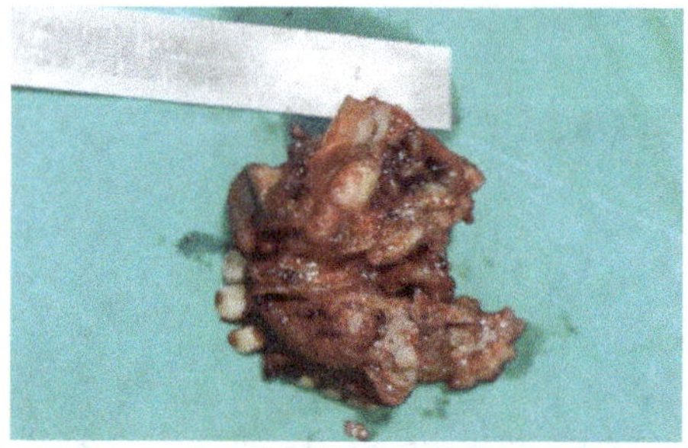

(b)

FIGURE 11: (a, b) Postsurgical maxillectomy specimen.

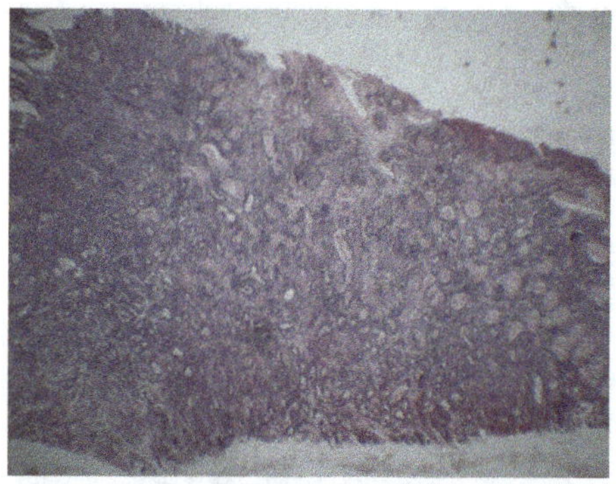

FIGURE 12: H and E section of tissue sample showing unencapsulated tumor close to surface epithelium with tumor cells arranged in solid nests.

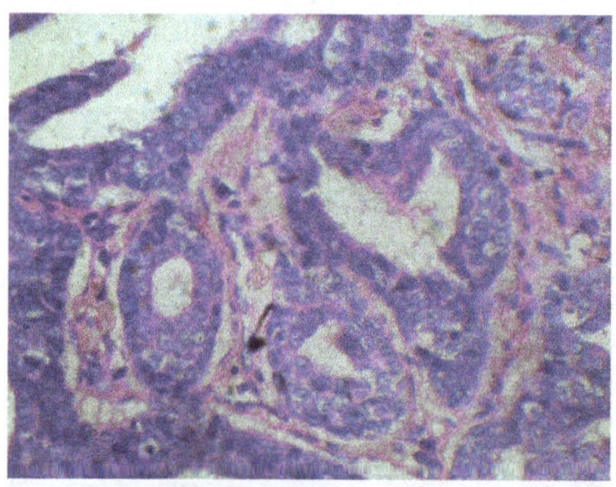

FIGURE 13: H and E sections showing ductal pattern of arrangement of tumor cells with evidence of vesicular nuclei.

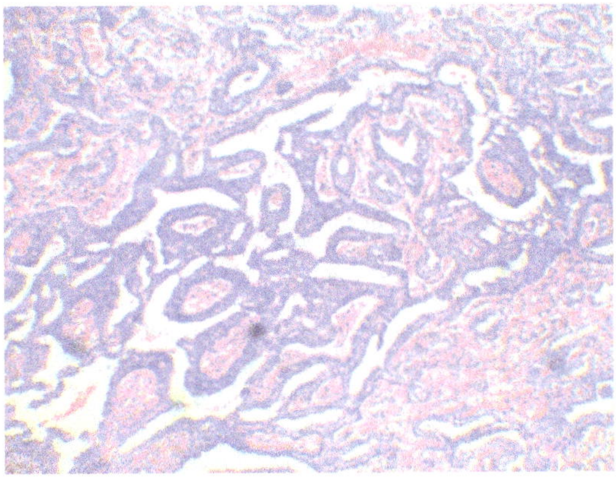

FIGURE 14: H and E sections showing arrangement of tumor cells in tubular pattern in the given tissue specimen.

PRKD1 mutations appear to be pathognomonic for this entity. In contrast, a vast majority of adenoid cystic carcinomas harbor MYB or MYBL1 gene rearrangements. While still not used widely in the clinic, use of these genetic markers may greatly facilitate the correct diagnosis [16].

The differential diagnosis for PAC includes pleomorphic adenoma and adenoid cystic carcinoma. PAC presents with a mucoid to the hyalinized matrix in comparison to pleomorphic adenoma which presents with a chondromyxoid matrix. Also, when compared to pleomorphic adenoma, PAC presents with perineural invasion. Another differentiating feature between the two is that PAC stains positive for S-100 and epithelial membrane antigen (EMA) whereas pleomorphic adenoma stains positive for glial fibrillary acidic protein (GFAP). When compared to adenoid cystic carcinoma, staining is positive for p-53, ki-67, bcl-2, and CD117. Perineural invasion is a feature of both PAC and adenoid cystic carcinoma, but the presence of the targetoid arrangement of perineural invasion is characteristic of PAC [17]. Also, in comparison to PAC, the cells of adenoid cystic carcinoma are smaller with hyperchromatic and angulated nuclei, less cytoplasm, and a coarser nuclear chromatin [18].

In the published literature, radiographic imaging of PAC has been mainly restricted to CT imaging since they provide a better soft-tissue contrast when compared to CBCT [19]. However, according to our knowledge, only a few case reports have highlighted the importance of CBCT in diagnosis of PGLA which describes it as presenting with no evidence of bone scalloping/erosion [20]. The radiographic appearance of PAC in our study resembled that of osteomyelitis and intraosseous malignancy. However, osteomyelitis of jaws is more common in the mandible when compared to the maxilla. Also, osteomyelitis of jaws is preceded most commonly with an identifiable cause of odontogenic infection such as a decayed tooth which was absent in our case. Intraosseous malignancies also present with a poorly defined, moth-eaten appearance. However, they occur more frequently in the mandibular posterior sections compared to the maxilla [21]. Also, these tumors reveal changes suggestive of carcinoma in the microscopic sections as defined by Suei et al. for a definitive diagnosis of intraoral malignancy.

Adjuvant radiotherapy has been indicated in cases where there is metastasis of cervical lymph nodes. A wide excision has been shown to minimize the rate of recurrence in cases of PAC, and radical excision has been suggested for the recurrent cases [22].

3.1. Summary. Minor salivary gland malignancy is an uncommon occurrence in daily practice. However, being the third most common minor salivary gland malignancy, it is necessary for the diagnostician to be well-versed with the clinical, histopathological, and radiographic features of PGLA. Although the knowledge available on this entity is limited, it is necessary to be able to segregate it from the miscellaneous tumors of minor salivary glands in order to provide appropriate treatment for the patient. Due to its tendency for recurrence, it is important to regularly follow-up the patient posttreatment. The importance of radiography especially 3D imaging in the form of CBCT in dental practice is highlighted in this case report as we have noticed that even though salivary gland malignancies usually limit themselves to soft tissue involvement, there are cases wherein extensive involvement of bone with a varied radiological presentation can be observed.

PAC is a distinct, yet commonly occurring, minor salivary gland tumor with varied clinical and histologic appearance. This case report highlights the importance of CBCT in diagnosing the intraosseous involvement of such tumors which can help shed some light in enhancing our knowledge about the minor salivary gland malignancies like PAC.

Abbreviations

PAC: Polymorphous low-grade adenocarcinoma
CT: Computed tomography
CBCT: Cone beam computed tomography
ACC: Adenoid cystic carcinoma
PA: Pleomorphic adenoma
IHC: Immunohistochemistry
LI: Labelling index
EMA: Epithelial membrane antigen
GFAP: Glial fibrillary acidic protein.

Consent

A written consent was obtained from the patient prior to preparation of the case report. The patient's consent has been obtained prior to the submission of the manuscript. The patient has provided written consent to publish this case report.

Authors' Contributions

JH assessed the patient clinically and referred the patient for a CBCT scan. JA assessed the CBCT scan and contributed in the radiographic interpretation of the lesion. The histopathologic assessment of the patient specimen was performed by

VKM. MV along with JH performed total maxillectomy surgery for the patient under general anesthesia. NS helped with the review of this manuscript along with necessary inputs by JA. The CBCT scan for the patient was performed by MN who also majorly contributed to the writing of this manuscript. All authors have read and approved the manuscript.

References

[1] R. R. Seethala, "Update from the 4th edition of the World Health Organization classification of head and neck tumours: preface," *Head and Neck Pathology*, vol. 11, no. 1, pp. 1-2, 2017.

[2] K. Dhanuthai, M. Boonadulyarat, T. Jaengjongdee, and K. Jiruedee, "A clinico-pathologic study of 311 intraoral salivary gland tumors in Thais," *Journal of Oral Pathology & Medicine*, vol. 38, no. 6, pp. 495–500, 2009.

[3] H. L. Evans and J. G. Batsakis, "Polymorphous low-grade adenocarcinoma of minor salivary glands a study of 14 cases of a distinctive neoplasm," *Cancer*, vol. 53, no. 4, pp. 935–942, 1984.

[4] G. Seifert, C. Brocheriou, A. Cardesa, and J. W. Eveson, "WHO International Histological Classification of Tumours Tentative Histological Classification of Salivary Gland Tumours," *Pathology - Research and Practice*, vol. 186, no. 5, pp. 555–581, 1990.

[5] B. A. Moore, B. B. Burkey, J. L. Netterville, R. B. Butcher II, and R. G. Amedee, "Surgical management of minor salivary gland neoplasms of the palate," *Ochsner Journal*, vol. 8, no. 4, pp. 172–180, 2008.

[6] S. Asioli, G. Marucci, G. Ficarra et al., "Polymorphous adenocarcinoma of the breast. Report of three cases," *Virchows Arch*, vol. 448, no. 1, pp. 29–34, 2006.

[7] P. Sukovic, "Cone beam computed tomography in craniofacial imaging," *Orthodontics & Craniofacial Research*, vol. 6, Supplement 1, pp. 31–36, 2003.

[8] W.-Y. Yih, F. J. Kratochvil, and J. C. B. Stewart, "Intraoral minor salivary gland neoplasms: review of 213 cases," *Journal of Oral and Maxillofacial Surgery*, vol. 63, no. 6, pp. 805–810, 2005.

[9] S. D. Vincent, H. L. Hammond, and M. W. Finkelstein, "Clinical and therapeutic features of polymorphous low-grade adenocarcinoma," *Oral Surgery, Oral Medicine, Oral Pathology*, vol. 77, no. 1, pp. 41–47, 1994.

[10] D. Gibbons, M. H. Saboorian, F. Vuitch, S. T. Gokaslan, and R. Ashfaq, "Fine-needle aspiration findings in patients with polymorphous low grade adenocarcinoma of the salivary glands," *Cancer*, vol. 87, no. 1, pp. 31–36, 1999.

[11] D. R. Gnepp, J. C. Chen, and C. Warren, "Polymorphous low-grade adenocarcinoma of minor salivary Gland," *The American Journal of Surgical Pathology*, vol. 12, no. 6, pp. 461–468, 1988.

[12] R. H. W. Simpson, J. S. Reis-Filho, E. M. Pereira, A. C. Ribeiro, and A. Abdulkadir, "Polymorphous low-grade adenocarcinoma of the salivary glands with transformation to high-grade carcinoma," *Histopathology*, vol. 41, no. 3, pp. 250–259, 2002.

[13] C. A. Waldron, S. K. El-Mofty, and D. R. Gnepp, "Tumors of the intraoral minor salivary glands: a demographic and histologic study of 426 cases," *Oral Surgery, Oral Medicine, and Oral Pathology*, vol. 66, no. 3, pp. 323–333, 1988.

[14] D. Beltran, W. C. Faquin, G. Gallagher, and M. August, "Selective immunohistochemical comparison of polymorphous low-grade adenocarcinoma and adenoid cystic carcinoma," *Journal of Oral and Maxillofacial Surgery*, vol. 64, no. 3, pp. 415–423, 2006.

[15] R. Sathyanarayanan, V. Suresh, and B. A. Thomas, "Polymorphous low-grade adenocarcinoma of the palate: a rare case report," *Iranian journal of cancer prevention*, vol. 9, no. 1, 2015.

[16] I. Weinreb, L. Zhang, L. M. S. Tirunagari et al., "Novel PRKD gene rearrangements and variant fusions in cribriform adenocarcinoma of salivary gland origin," *Genes, Chromosomes and Cancer*, vol. 53, no. 10, pp. 845–856, 2014.

[17] V. Surya, J. V. Tupkari, T. Joy, and P. Verma, "Histopathological spectrum of polymorphous low-grade adenocarcinoma," *Journal of oral and maxillofacial pathology*, vol. 19, no. 2, p. 266, 2015.

[18] A. Potluri, J. Prasad, S. Levine, and J. Bastaki, "Polymorphous low-grade adenocarcinoma: a case report," *Dentomaxillofacial Radiology.*, vol. 42, no. 2, p. 14804843, 2013.

[19] E. L. Adekeye and J. Cornah, "Osteomyelitis of the jaws: a review of 141 cases," *British Journal of Oral and Maxillofacial Surgery*, vol. 23, no. 1, 1985.

[20] S. Gupta, C. A. Kumar, and N. Raghav, "Polymorphous low-grade adenocarcinoma of the palate: report of a case and review of literature," *International Journal of Head and Neck Surgery.*, vol. 2, no. 1, pp. 57–60, 2011.

[21] P. Geetha, M. A. Tejasvi, B. B. Babu, H. Bhayya, and D. Pavani, "Primary intraosseous carcinoma of the mandible: a clinicoradiographic view," *Journal of cancer research and therapeutics*, vol. 11, no. 3, 2015.

[22] I. A. El-Naaj, Y. Leiser, A. Wolff, and M. Peled, "Polymorphous low grade adenocarcinoma: case series and review of surgical management," *Journal of Oral and Maxillofacial Surgery*, vol. 69, no. 7, pp. 1967–1972, 2011.

3

Multidisciplinary Approach to Rehabilitation after Tumor Resective Jaw Surgery: A 9-Year Follow-Up

Igor Smojver,[1] Marko Vuletić,[2,3] Spomenka Manojlović,[4] and Dragana Gabrić[2,3]

[1]St. Catherine Specialty Hospital, Zagreb, Croatia
[2]Department of Oral Surgery, School of Dental Medicine, University of Zagreb, Croatia
[3]Croatian Society for Hospital Dentistry / Dentistry of Special Care of the Croatian Medical Association, Zagreb, Croatia
[4]Department of Pathology, School of Medicine, University of Zagreb, Croatia

Correspondence should be addressed to Marko Vuletić; mvuletic@sfzg.hr

Academic Editor: Samir Nammour

A 36-year-old male patient presented at the Department of Maxillofacial Surgery, University Hospital Clinic Zagreb in December 2010 due to a swelling of the left body of the mandible that was noticed 4 months earlier. The patient was referred regarding an atypical clinical and radiological finding in the form of a multicystic appearance in the corpus of the left mandible and teeth mobility in the same region. A probatory biopsy was performed under local anesthesia and sent for histopathologic examination which reported odontogenic myxoma. The tumor was removed with a marginal resection of the mandible from the left first incisor to the left second molar. Two years after surgery, in January 2013, the patient was referred to the oral surgeons for implant-prosthodontic rehabilitation. Two narrow implants were placed at positions 32 and 36, and three months afterwards, implant-retained denture was made using locator connections to compensate lost teeth and to correct the ratio of soft tissues and facial contours. The patient was followed-up for 9 years without any functional and aesthetic problems. Loosing function and aesthetic morbidity, after radical surgical treatment, often have compromised the quality of life of this group of patients. It is important to highlight the need for multidisciplinary collaboration for the complete rehabilitation of the patient after surgical oncology of the maxillofacial region.

1. Introduction

Myxomas are very rare benign tumors of ectomesenchymal origin [1]. These tumors are locally invasive and can occur in various tissues, such as the heart, bones, skin, skeletal muscle, subcutaneous tissue, genitourinary tract, and aponeuroses [2, 3]. Myxomas of the head and neck region occur mainly in the jaw bones, with a very small minority occurring in the pharynx, larynx, paranasal sinuses, and other soft tissues [4]. Odontogenic myxoma, also termed as odontogenic fibromyxoma or myxofibroma, is a subtype of myxoma occurring mainly in the hard, bony tissues of the face, although the lesion may also occur in the surrounding soft tissues [5]. This neoplasm often has infiltrating and locally aggressive character, and according to the WHO, it is the third most frequent odontogenic tumor after odontoma and ameloblastoma [6, 7]. The WHO [6] reports that odontogenic myxoma is up to twice common in females while others report that there is no sex predilection [3, 8]. The tumor may be an incidental finding or may cause symptoms, including pain, paresthesia, and tooth mobility [9]. Thoma and Goldman [10] first described myxomas of odontogenic origin, on the basis of site of occurrence, by association with missing teeth, age at occurrence, and histopathological examination, which showed structural resemblance with dental mesenchyme and the sporadic presence of islands of odontogenic epithelium.

Diagnosis of odontogenic myxomas is based on radiological, histopathological, and clinical findings [11]. Radiographically, a unilocular or multilocular radiolucent image and mixed radiolucency and radio-opacity have been reported [12]. Odontogenic myxoma consisted of spindle shaped to stellate cells in an intercellular matrix rich in mucoid, with no encapsulation and sporadically scattered residual bony trabeculae [13], while the stroma may consist of collagen bundles, hence the designation of myxofibroma [14]. Clinically, it can be characterized by cortical expansion, potential to cause bone destruction, slow growth, soft tissue infiltration, tooth movement, and root resorption [2]. In the differential diagnosis odontogenic keratocyst, follicular cyst, ameloblastoma, aneurysmal bone cyst, central giant cell granuloma, and intraosseous hemangioma [15] may be included. The ideal treatment of this neoplasm has not been fully agreed in the literature. There are different treatment modalities from enucleation and curettage to en bloc resection [7, 9]. If the approach is more radical, there is a lower rate of recurrence but there are more associated morbidities, especially in the aesthetic and functional point of view [9].

The aim of the present research is to describe a case of a 36-year-old man who developed an odontogenic myxoma of the mandible 9 years ago and successful implanto-prosthodontic rehabilitated after resective jaw surgery with a multidisciplinary approach. The purpose of this case report was to highlight the need for multidisciplinary collaboration for the complete rehabilitation of the patient after surgical oncology of the maxillofacial region.

2. Case Presentation

A 36-year-old male patient came to the Department of Maxillofacial Surgery, University Hospital Clinic Zagreb in December 2010 due to a swelling of the left body of the mandible that was noticed 4 months earlier. The patient did not report any other symptoms. After examination, the patient was referred to a maxillofacial surgeon regarding an atypical clinical and radiological finding in the form of a multicystic appearance (bubble-like) in the corpus of the left mandible and pathological teeth mobility in the region of the swelling. There were no enlarged lymph nodes in the neck and head area. Differential diagnosis included keratocystic odontogenic tumor, ameloblastoma, central giant cell granuloma, and odontogenic myxoma.

The patient denied any systemic disease or condition and reported no previous surgeries. A general physical examination was unremarkable. The patient did not have any deleterious habits such as alcohol consumption or smoking and without previous history of swelling or trauma of the mandible. On extraoral examination, the patient displayed some facial asymmetry with an obvious firm and diffuse swelling on the left side of the mandible. The overlying skin was normal in appearance. Intraorally, there was a diffuse swelling in the buccal vestibule. Teeth in the third quadrant were without any pain sensation but with pathological mobility. Lower incisors and canine had mobility grade I and premolars and first molar grade II according to the Miller classification.

The orthopantomogram (OPG) showed a multilocular radiolucency, with fine trabeculation, extending from the left canine, towards the first molar (Figure 1) with no root resorption. A CT scan was made afterwards and revealed the destruction of the buccal cortex of the left body of the mandible. A probatory biopsy was performed under local infiltration anesthesia (4% articaine with epinephrine 1 : 200

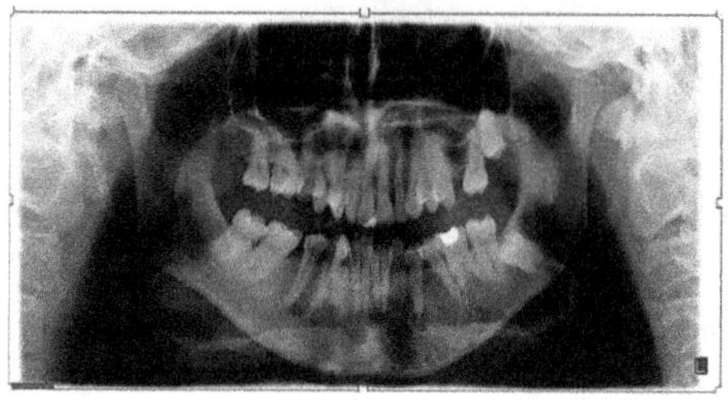

FIGURE 1: First OPG with multicystical lesion in the left mandible surrounding teeth 33 to 36 (2010).

000; 1.8 mL), and the specimen was sent for histopathologic examination which reported odontogenic myxoma.

In accordance with the ethical protocol of the School of Dental Medicine, University of Zagreb, Croatia, written consent was obtained from the patient before surgery in general anesthesia in January 2011. Lower incisors, canine, premolars, and first molar were extracted just before the first incision. A mucoperiosteal flap with full exposition of the buccal aspect of the tumor was performed. The tumor was removed with a marginal resection of the mandible from the left first incisor to the left second molar. The surgical site was examined and precociously cleaned of all myxomatous tissue, and a reconstruction plate was used to reinforce the resected mandible. The surgical specimen was a soft, gelatinous mass measuring approximately 1 cm in diameter, with a mucinous appearance. Histologically, the tumor was composed of randomly oriented spindle-shaped cells with long fine cytoplasmic processes, within an abundant, myxoid ground substance, containing small capillaries and fragments of bone trabecula. Odontogenic epithelium was absent, and clear margins were confirmed (Figures 2 and 3). The patient recovered completely, with no postoperative paresthesia or facial asymmetry.

Two years after surgery, in January 2013, the patient was referred to the Department of Oral Surgery, School of Dental Medicine, University of Zagreb for implant-prosthodontic rehabilitation. A control OPG (Figure 4) and clinical examination (Figures 5 and 6) showed complete recovery with a residual defect in the alveolar extension and left concavity.

Due to the deep bite, orthodontic therapy was started in the upper jaw, and in the lower jaw, implant-prosthodontic rehabilitation was planed with minimally invasive procedures because of the lack of a support zone and defect of soft and bone tissues. Regional nerve block anesthesia (4% articaine with epinephrine 1 : 200 000; 3.6 mL) was administered. After carefully raising the mucoperiosteal flap and isolating the mental nerve, the bone crest was expanded at the planned implant sites, with a piezosurgical bone saw (Piezomed, W&H; Austria: power 90%, cooling 80%, "power" operating mode), and two narrow diameter implants (Straumann, Bone Level Roxolid 3.3 × 10 mm, Basel, Switzerland) were placed at positions 32 and 36 (Figures 7 and 8). After implant placement augmentation was performed with xenogenic bone material (Cerabone, Botiss, Germany) and a resorptive native pericardium membrane (Jason membrane 15 × 20 mm, Botiss, Germany), the sutures were removed on the 10th postoperative day at which time the surgical site was healing as expected.

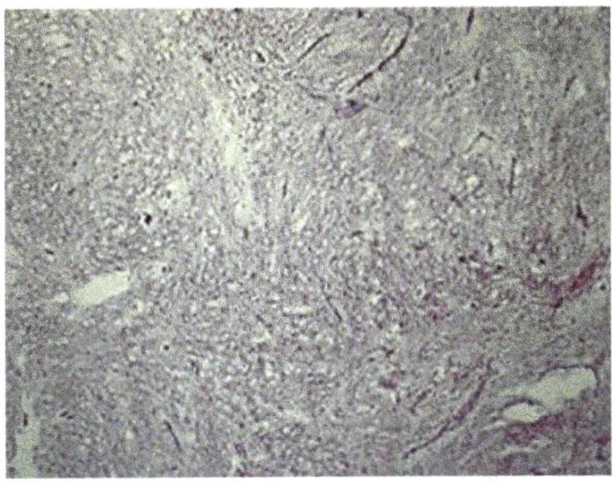

FIGURE 2: Representative photomicrograph of odontogenic myxoma (hematoxylin and eosin, original magnification 100x).

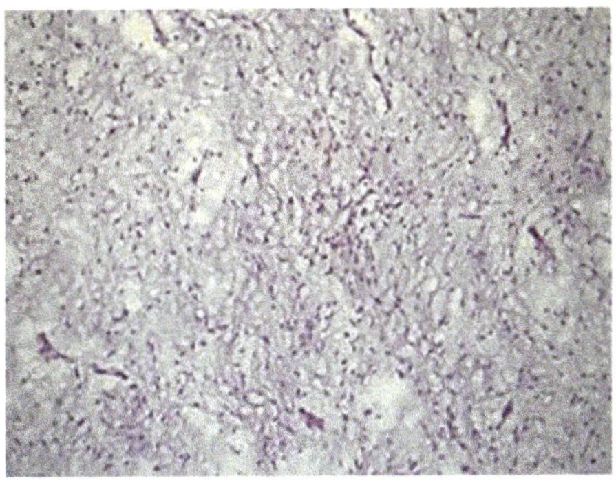

FIGURE 3: Spindle-shaped cells with long fine cytoplasmic processes, within an abundant, myxoid ground substance, containing small capillaries and fragments of bone trabecula (hematoxylin and eosin, original magnification 200x).

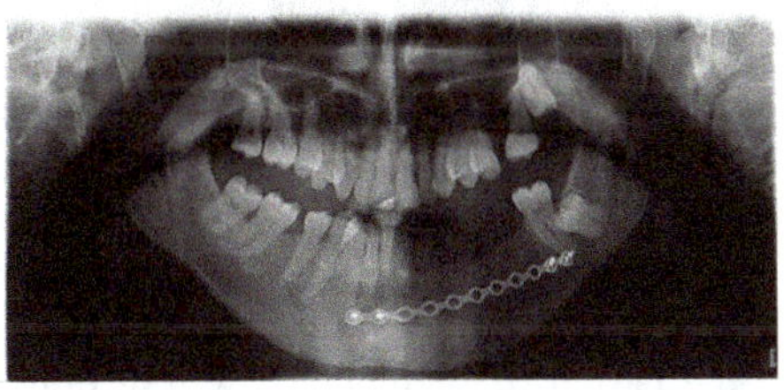

FIGURE 4: OPG 2 years after resective surgery (2013).

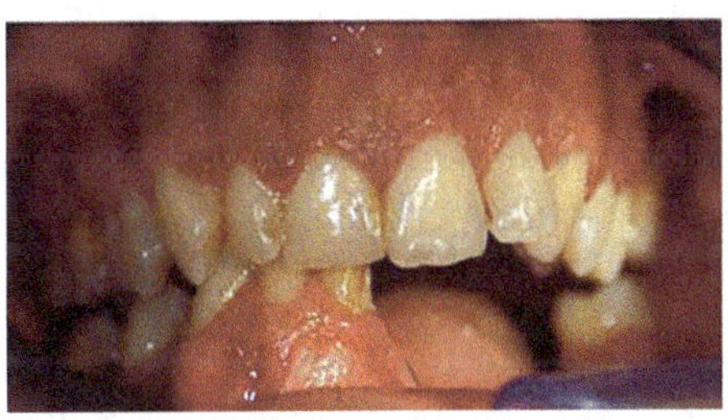

FIGURE 5: Clinical appearance after 2 years postresective surgery-frontal view.

Three months after surgery, a cover denture was made with locator connections to compensate for lost teeth and to correct the ratio of soft tissues and facial contours. No tumor recurrence was found on the follow-up OPG and CBCT for 7 years after implant placement and 9 years post-

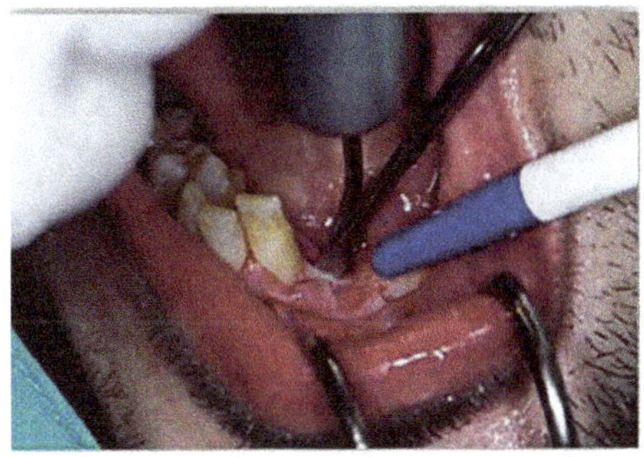

FIGURE 6: Bone splitting with piezo bone saw during implant placement.

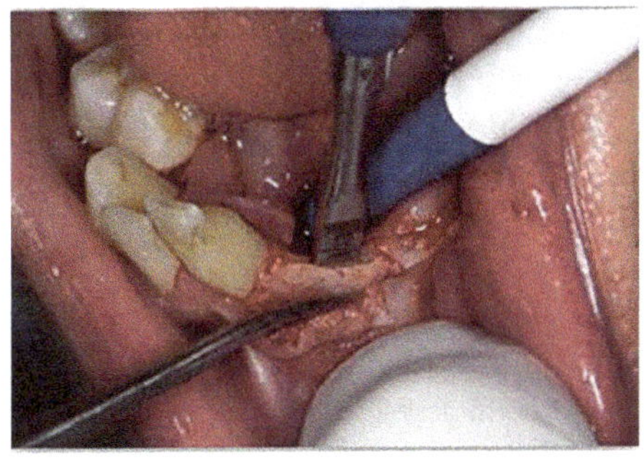

FIGURE 7: Bone splitting with bone mallet and chisel during implant placement.

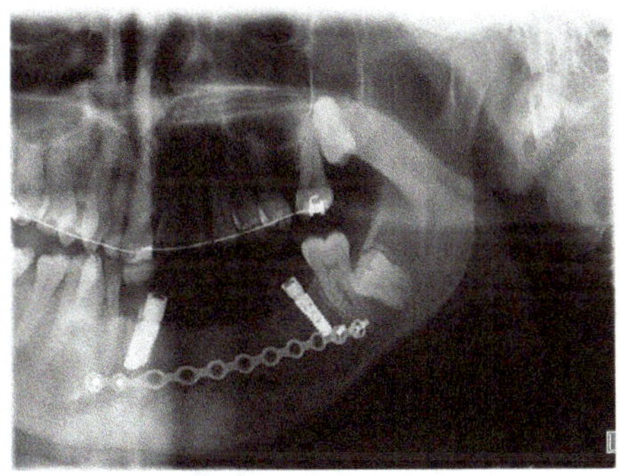

FIGURE 8: Panoramic view after implant placement-2013.

resective surgery (Figures 9–11). The patient was subjectively free from functional and aesthetic problems.

3. Discussion

According to the literature [16], it is reported that odontogenic myxoma is in 0.5-20% of all odontogenic tumors in adults. There is also a regional difference in the prevalence of these tumors, it is more common in the Caucasian and African populations of those from the far east [17]. Rashid and Bashir [18] stated that odontogenic myxoma mainly occurs in the second and third decade of life and is rarely seen in patients younger than 10 years and older than 50 years, while Takahashi et al. [19] reported that the median age in their study of 12 patients was 41.5 years and 5 were over 50 years old. Our patient in this case report was in accordance with this data regarding its age. The exact predilection of

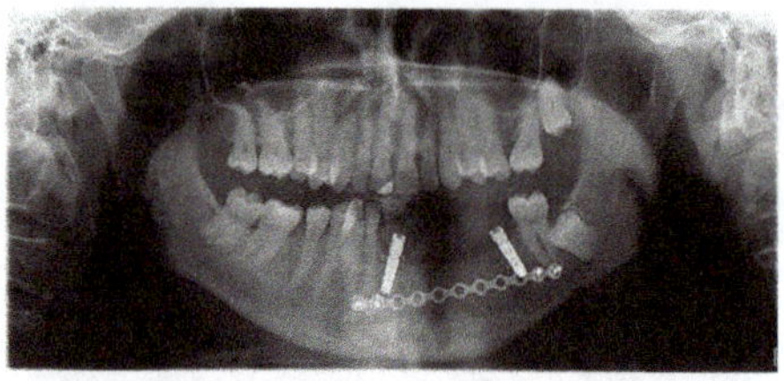

FIGURE 9: OPG (2020)—9-year follow-up.

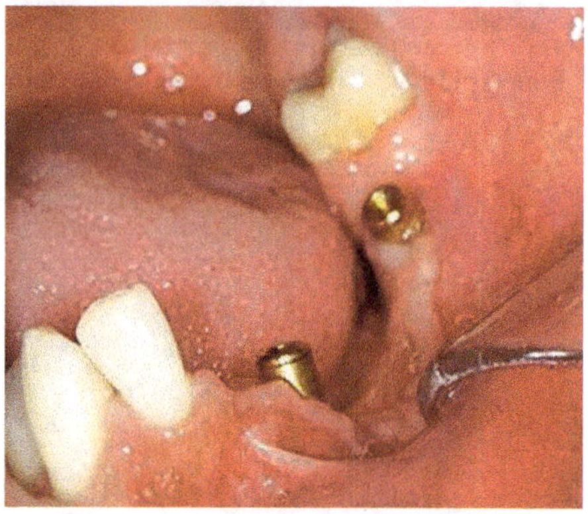

FIGURE 10: Clinical situation with locators (2020).

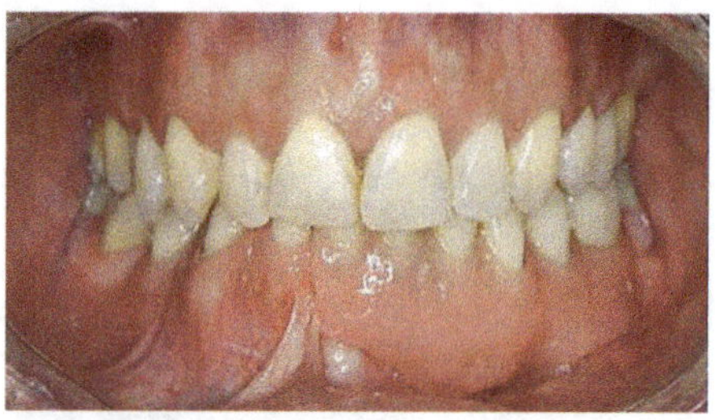

FIGURE 11: Clinical appearance after 9 years postsurgery and 7 years after implanto-prosthodontic rehabilitation.

odontogenic myxoma to either the upper or lower jaw is also a matter of discussion. Most authors [20–22] stated that the lesion is more common in the mandible, especially the molar and ramus region, whereas Subramaniam et al. [16] found equal incidence in both jaws in series of 8 cases. Regardless of the jaw, odontogenic myxoma is usually found in relation to a tooth, typically a premolar or molar [23]. Some researchers reported that the lesion is most often found in the mandibular premolar area in series of 37 cases [24]. In the present case, the lesion was in the region of the mandible involving teeth from the canine to the first molar. Odontogenic myxoma often expands the cortical plates in one or more directions, sometimes perforates the cortical surface, and produces a soft feeling on palpation and impression of fluctuance. Due to its absence of a capsule, it can penetrate into marrow space and be very aggressive [25, 26].

Clinically, the presented case showed symptoms that match all of these mentioned signs but without aggressive behavior and the lingual cortical plate was preserved.

Odontogenic myxomas have been diagnosed with many different imaging features like conventional radiography such as panoramic, occlusal, and periapical, or more accurately like cone beam computed tomography/computed tomography (CBCT/CT) and magnetic resonance imaging (MRI) [27, 28]. Wang et al. [29] stated that involved teeth may have resorption or displacement and a combination of resorption and displacement. The patient in this case report did not have either of these, only highly expressed teeth mobility.

Although benign, odontogenic myxoma is invasive into surrounding normal bone, sometimes breaking through its boundaries [5]. This invasiveness has been attributed to the expression of matrix metalloproteinases (MMP) 2 and 9, which degrade the extracellular matrix (ECM) due to its ability to degrade type IV collagen, the major structural component of the basement membrane. These enzymes purportedly cause tumor cells to penetrate the bony trabeculae by acting on the ECM, thus aiding tumor [30]. On gross examination, odontogenic myxoma resected from the presented patient was a nodular heterogeneous mass, grayish-white color, without demarcation from surrounding tissue. This finding was in concordance with Takahashi et al. [19] which stated that this kind of tumor is uncapsulated and poorly demarcated from surrounding tissues while Li et al. [23] reported that in their 25 cases, most of them had minimal capsule.

Microscopically, the tumor has a mucoid-rich ECM, with scattered stellate cells, connective tissue fibers, irregular calcifications, bony trabeculae, sparse capillaries, and scant blood vessels. Nests of odontogenic epithelium are occasionally seen but not essential for diagnosis [5, 13, 23]. The ECM comprises eosinophilic mucoid tissue, which resembles the connective tissue of the umbilical cord. Spindle-shaped or stellate cells with small hyperchromatic nuclei and cytoplasmic processes are interspersed in collagen or reticulin fibers [31]. Cellular atypia is rare, and the presence of mast cells has been reported while fibers are oriented toward the tumor periphery [2]. All of these classical features were seen in our case.

Surgical treatment of odontogenic myxoma is usually invasive, and it depends on the size of the tumor from conservative, e.g., enucleation and surgical curettage, to radical treatment like partial or segmental jaw resection with free flaps. Smaller lesions can be treated only by curettage, but larger lesions need resection due to their infiltration to the surrounding bone. Large maxillary and mandibular bone defects can be reconstructed by fibular and iliac-crest osteomyocutaneous or osteomuscular free flaps [32]. Free flap helps in dental-prosthetic option even if the placement of implant is a challenge.

Lack of its encapsulation and loose of myxoid composition is the main reason of recurrence, so the method of removal is a crucial determinant [28]. According to the recent literature [6, 33], the recurrence rate is high ranging from 10% to 43% with a mean of 25%. Recurrence following incomplete removal usually occurs within 2 years, but also there are the same cases in which recurrence occurred later [6]. White et al. [28] found, reviewing the literature, 9 cases in the literature that provided length of follow-up period ranged from 3 to 84 months (7 years) with an average of 36 months (3 years) and without recurrences in those patients. Following-up in the presented case report was 9 years, and there was no sign of recurrence. The literature showed no consistent recommendations regarding the ideal treatment of this tumor. Saalim et al. [34] reported that there was no significant difference in recurrence between conservative treatment and resection. They recommend that conservative treatment should be considered wherever possible to provide optimal quality of life for the patient.

The reconstruction of the mandible after radical treatment can be made by fixed or removable prostheses retained by a system attached to the implant. In some cases with reconstructed mandible with free flaps, there might be a problem due to inadequate mechanical retention during mastication so an implant-supported fixed dental prosthesis is the best solution for treatment [35]. Meloni et al. [36] reported the advantages of a protocol for rehabilitation consisting of prosthetic-guided implant insertion, a noninvasive surgical approach, and immediate loading on fixed prosthesis in oncologic patients.

Implant-prosthodontic rehabilitation after marginal resection of the mandible requires filling the edentulous space and compensating the loss of hard and soft tissues, therefore presenting a particular challenge to prosthodontists. Removable dental prosthesis is preferred to an implant-supported fixed dental prosthesis to maintain oral hygiene and recurrent examinations and for long-term maintenance [37]. Elsyad et al. [38] showed that locator attachments were associated with high retention and stability after wear simulation with minimal retention loss compared to a Dolder bar. Overdenture improves chewing efficiency, increases maximum bite force, and clearly improves satisfaction [39]. After consultation with the patient, it was decided that a minimally invasive approach to reconstruct the resulting defect will be made. In order to primarily satisfy the function as well as the aesthetics and due to the above-mentioned advantages of the cover prosthesis in oncology patients, the plan was to make denture worn on two implants retained with locator attachments.

4. Conclusion

Quality of life in patients after radical surgical treatment of odontogenic myxomas is often compromised by loosing function and aesthetic morbidity. A multidisciplinary approach is the basis for complete implanto-prosthodontic rehabilitation of patients after resective surgical oncology.

References

[1] S. C. White and M. Pharoah, *Oral Radiology: Principles and Interpretation*, Elsevier Health Sciences, Amsterdam, 7th edition, 2013.

[2] G. Martínez-Mata, A. Mosqueda-Taylor, R. Carlos-Bregni et al., "Odontogenic myxoma: clinico-pathological, immunohistochemical and ultrastructural findings of a multicentric series," *Oral Oncology*, vol. 44, no. 6, pp. 601–607, 2008.

[3] Y. Leiser, I. Abu-El-Naaj, and M. Peled, "Odontogenic myxoma–a case series and review of thesurgical management," *Journal of Cranio-Maxillo-Facial Surgery*, vol. 37, no. 4, pp. 206–209, 2009.

[4] B. A. Moore, T. Wine, B. B. Burkey, R. G. Amedee, and R. B. Butcher 2nd, "Sphenoid sinus myxoma: case report and literature review," *The Ochsner Journal*, vol. 8, no. 4, pp. 166–171, 2008.

[5] B. R. Chrcanovic, M. B. do Amaral, A. Marigo Hde, and B. Freire-Maia, "An expanded odontogenic myxoma in maxilla," *Stomatologija*, vol. 12, no. 4, pp. 122–128, 2010.

[6] A. K. El-Naggar, J. K. C. Chan, J. R. Grandis, T. Takata, and P. J. Slootweg, Eds., *World Health Organization Classification of Head and Neck Tumours*, IARC Press, Lyon, France, 2017.

[7] B. R. Chrcanovic and R. S. Gomez, "Odontogenic myxoma: an updated analysis of 1692 cases reported in the literature," *Oral Diseases*, vol. 25, no. 3, pp. 676–683, 2019.

[8] R. Gonzalez-Garcia, F. J. Rodriguez-Campo, L. Naval Gias, M. F. Munoz-Guerra, J. Sastre-Perez, and F. J. Diaz-Gonzalez, "Mandibular odontogenic myxoma. Reconstructive considerations by means of the vascularized fibular free flap," *Medicina Oral Patologia Oral y Cirugia Bucal*, vol. 11, pp. 531–535, 2006.

[9] B. W. Neville, D. D. Damm, C. M. Allen, and A. C. Chi, *Oral and Maxillofacial Pathology*, Elsevier Inc., Amsterdam, 4th edition, 2016.

[10] K. H. Thoma and H. M. Goldman, "Central myxoma of the jaw," *Oral Surgery, Oral Medicine, and Oral Pathology*, vol. 33, no. 7, pp. 532–540, 1947.

[11] H. A. Altug, A. Gulses, and M. Sencimen, "Clinico-radiographic examination of odontogenic myxoma with displacement of unerupted upper third molar: review of the literature," *International Journal of Morphology*, vol. 29, no. 3, pp. 930–933, 2011.

[12] C. E. Noffke, E. J. Raubenheimer, N. J. Chabikuli, and M. M. Bouckaert, "Odontogenic myxoma: review of the literature and report of 30 cases from South Africa," *Oral Surgery, Oral Medicine, Oral Pathology, Oral Radiology, and Endodontics*, vol. 104, no. 1, pp. 101–109, 2007.

[13] E. N. Simon, M. A. Merkx, E. Vuhahula, D. Ngassapa, and P. J. Stoelinga, "Odontogenic myxoma: a clinicopathological study of 33 cases," *International Journal of Oral and Maxillofacial Surgery*, vol. 33, no. 4, pp. 333–337, 2004.

[14] Y. Kawase-Koga, H. Saijo, K. Hoshi, T. Takato, and Y. Mori, "Surgical management of odontogenic myxoma: a case report and review of the literature," *BMC Research Notes*, vol. 7, p. 214, 2014.

[15] F. Titinchi, B. A. Hassan, J. A. Morkel, and C. Nortje, "Odontogenic myxoma: a clinicopathological study in a South African population," *Journal of Oral Pathology & Medicine*, vol. 45, no. 8, pp. 599–604, 2016.

[16] H. A. A. SubramaniamSS, R. Kumar, and J. M. Shand, "Odontogenic myxoma in the paediatric patient: a review of eight cases," *International Journal of Oral and Maxillofacial Surgery*, vol. 45, pp. 1614–1617, 2016.

[17] R. E. Friedrich, H. A. Scheuer, and W. Hoeltje, "Recurrent maxillary odontogenic myxoma following partial maxillary resection and consecutive osseous reconstruction including tooth transplantation," *Anticancer Research*, vol. 36, pp. 3155–3160, 2016.

[18] H. Rashid and A. Bashir, "Surgical and prosthetic management of maxillary odontogenic myxoma," *European Journal of Dentistry*, vol. 9, pp. 277–283, 2015.

[19] Y. Takahashi, K. Tanaka, H. Hirai, E. Marukawa, T. Izumo, and H. Harada, "Appropriate surgical margin for odontogenic myxoma: a review of 12 cases," *Oral Surgery, Oral Medicine, Oral Pathology, Oral Radiology*, vol. 126, no. 5, pp. 404–408, 2018.

[20] W. G. Shafer, M. K. Hine, and B. M. Levy, "A Textbook of Oral Pathology," in *Cysts and tumors of odontogenic origin*, pp. 258–317, Elsevier-Saunders, Pennsylvania, 4th edition, 2003.

[21] J. Zhang, H. Wang, X. He, Y. Niu, and X. Li, "Radiographic examination of 41 cases of odontogenic myxomas on the basis of conventional radiographs," *Dentomaxillofacial Radiology*, vol. 36, no. 3, pp. 160–167, 2007.

[22] P. Boffano, C. Gallesio, A. Barreca, F. A. Bianchi, P. Garzino Demo, and F. Roccia, "Surgical treatment of odontogenic myxoma," *Journal of Craniofacial Surgery*, vol. 22, pp. 982–987, 2011.

[23] T. J. Li, L. S. Sun, and H. Y. Luo, "Odontogenic myxoma: a clinicopathologic study of 25 cases," *Archives of Pathology & Laboratory Medicine*, vol. 130, no. 12, pp. 1799–1806, 2006.

[24] B. S. M. S. Siriwardena, H. Crane, N. O'Neill et al., "Odontogenic tumors and lesions treated in a single specialist oral and maxillofacial pathology unit in the United Kingdom in 1992-2016," *Oral Surgery, Oral Medicine, Oral Pathology, Oral Radiology*, vol. 127, no. 2, pp. 151–166, 2019.

[25] M. Tavakoli and R. Williamson, "Odontogenic myxomas: what is the ideal treatment?," *BML Case Reports*, vol. 12, no. 5, article e228540, 2019.

[26] V. Rani, M. K. M. Kadar, A. Babu, L. Sankari, and G. Krishnasamy, "Odontogenic myxoma diagnostic dilemma: a case report and review of literature," *Journal of Cranio-Maxillary Diseases*, vol. 3, p. 163, 2014.

[27] G. Varghese, S. Singh, and L. Sreela, "A rare case of breast carcinoma metastasis to mandible and vertebrae," *National Journal of Maxillofacial Surgery*, vol. 5, no. 2, p. 184, 2014.

[28] J. A. White, N. Ramer, T. R. Wentland, and M. Cohen, "The rare radiographic sunburst appearance of odontogenic myxomas: a case report and review of the literature," *Head and Neck Pathology*, vol. 14, 2020.

[29] K. Wang, W. Guo, M. You, L. Liu, B. Tang, and G. Zheng, "Characteristic features of the odontogenic myxoma on cone beam computed tomography," *Dentomaxillo Facial Radiology*, vol. 46, no. 2, pp. 2016–2032, 2017.

[30] S. P. Miyagi, K. R. Hiraki, M. D. Martins, and M. M. Marques, "Expression of matrix metalloproteinases 2 and 9 in odontogenic myxoma in vivo and in vitro," *Journal of Oral Science*, vol. 50, no. 2, pp. 187–192, 2008.

[31] A. L. N. Francisco, T. C. Chulam, F. O. Silva et al., "Clinicopathologic analysis of 14 cases of odontogenic myxoma and review of the literature," *Journal of Clinical and Experimental Dentistry*, vol. 9, no. 4, pp. 560–563, 2017.

[32] D. A. Hidalgo, "Titanium miniplate fixation in free flap mandible reconstruction," *Annals of Plastic Surgery*, vol. 23, pp. 498-507, 1989.

[33] M. Kauke, A.-F. Safi, M. Kreppel et al., "Size distribution and clinico-radiological signs of aggressiveness in odontogenic myxoma—three-dimensional analysis and systematic review," *Dento Maxillo Facial Radiology*, vol. 47, article 20170262, 2018.

[34] M. Saalim, K. Sansare, F. R. Karjodkar, A. G. Farman, S. N. Goyal, and S. R. Sharma, "Recurrence rate of odontogenic myxoma after different treatments: a systematic," *The British Journal of Oral & Maxillofacial Surgery*, vol. 57, no. 10, pp. 985–991, 2019.

[35] M. Chiapasco, F. Biglioli, L. Autelitano, E. Romeo, and R. Brusati, "Clinical outcome of dental implants placed in fibula-free flaps used for the recon-struction of maxillomandibular defects following ablation for tumors or osteoradionecrosis," *Clinical Oral Implants Research*, vol. 17, pp. 220–228, 2006.

[36] S. Meloni, M. Tallarico, G. Riu et al., "Guided implant surgery after free-flap reconstruction: four-year results from a prospective clinical trial," *Journal of Cranio-Maxillo-Facial Surgery*, vol. 43, no. 8, pp. 1348–1355, 2015.

[37] J. H. Lee, S. H. Kim, H. I. Yoon, I. L. Yeo, and J. S. Han, "Implant-assisted removable prosthetic rehabilitation after distraction osteogenesis in a patient with ameloblastoma recurrence: a case report," *Medicine (Baltimore)*, vol. 98, no. 49, article e18290, 2019.

[38] M. A. Elsyad, M. A. Dayekh, and A. K. Khalifa, "Locator versus bar attachment effect on the retention and stability of implant-retained maxillary overdenture: an in vitro study," *Journal of Prosthodontics*, vol. 28, no. 2, pp. 627–636, 2019.

[39] G. C. Boven, G. M. Raghoebar, A. Vissink, and H. J. Meijer, "Improving masticatory performance, bite force, nutritional state and patient's satisfaction with implant overdentures: a systematic review of the literature," *Journal of Oral Rehabilitation*, vol. 42, no. 3, pp. 220–233, 2015.

4

Case Reports of a New Method for Differential Diagnosis of Calcified Carotid Artery Atheroma

Guilherme Augusto Alves de Oliveira,[1] Cleiterson Rezende de Sá,[2] Omar Ribeiro Santos Junior,[2] Rafael Pereira da Mata Santos,[1] and Flávio Ricardo Manzi[1]

[1]*Department of Dentistry of the Pontifical Catholic University of Minas Gerais (PUC-MG), Belo Horizonte, Minas Gerais, Brazil*
[2]*Preventive Cardiology Department of Núcleo Cardiológico Integrado Ltda., Mateus Leme, Minas Gerais, Brazil*

Correspondence should be addressed to Rafael Pereira da Mata Santos; rpmsantos@sga.pucminas.br

Academic Editor: Jiiang H. Jeng

Introduction. Early diagnosis of calcified atheromas may decrease morbidity and mortality caused by brain and cardiovascular diseases, in which atherosclerosis is the main etiological factor of these pathologies. Dental examinations with the aim of detecting this pathology have been in progress since 1981, such as panoramic radiography, considered the most widely studied method for this diagnosis. However, some limitations of this exam have been reported with reference to inability to visualize the cervical region and difficulty of establishing a precise diagnosis because of many structures and calcifications that have similar radiographic characteristics. *Case Report.* The present study to describe a dental radiographic technique for establishing the differential diagnosis of calcified atheromas regarding other calcifications and reporting 3 clinical cases that demonstrate its effectiveness in different clinical situations. *Discussion.* Manzi Projection can promote a differential diagnosis of calcified atheromas in dental practice and consequently subsidize the clinician for referring the patient to the physician.

1. Introduction

Atherosclerosis may be considered the main cause of the global death rate due to its association with the etiology of cardiovascular and cerebrovascular diseases. Clinically, it is characterized by the formation of atheromatous plaques between the tunica intima and tunica media of the arterial wall [1]. The bifurcation region of the carotid artery represents one of the main sites for the development of atheroma, favored by the presence of a turbulent flow that generates a low intensity yet constant stress on the arterial wall, causing endothelial lesions that will trigger the formation of these lipoprotein plates [2].

These atheromas may undergo a dystrophic calcification process, enabling these plates to be identified in radiographic examinations, e.g., the panoramic radiograph. In this examination, widely used in dental practice, calcified atheroma may be visualized as circled, irregular or heterogeneous, unilateral or bilateral radiopaque masses in the neck soft tissue region, adjacent to the C3-C4 intervertebral space, distinct from the radiopaque structures of this region, next to the hyoid bone [3, 4].

Many other calcifications and structures represented in the cervical region of the panoramic radiograph may make it difficult to diagnose calcified atheromas, as they may present similar radiographic characteristics, such as triticeous cartilage calcification, sialoliths, phleboliths, hyoid bone, calcified lymph nodes, and among others. Thus, complementary examinations are necessary for establishing a differential diagnosis [5, 6].

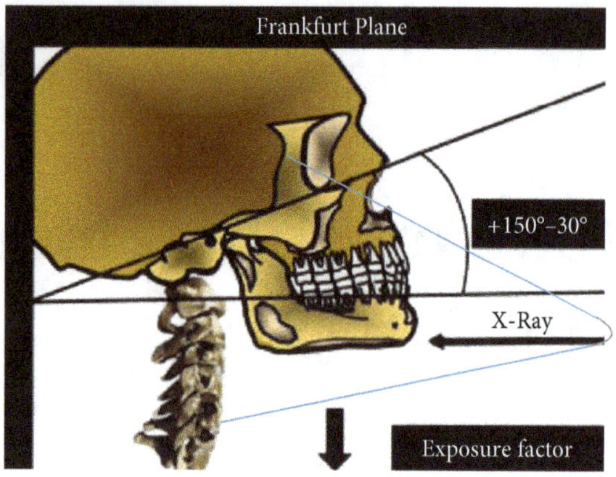

Figure 1: Manzi Projection description.

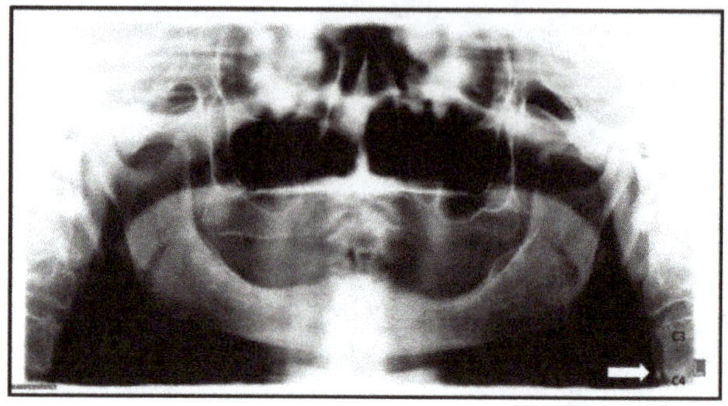

Figure 2: Panoramic radiograph showing radiopaque image circumscribed on the left side of the neck soft tissue region adjacent to the C3 and C4 intervertebral space (arrow).

Notably, Intra-arterial Angiography is the gold standard for the detection of these atheromatous plaques and the stenosis they cause; however, because it is an invasive method with an estimated risk morbidity and mortality of 2%, noninvasive examinations are chosen in clinical practice, in which the Doppler Ultrasound is outstanding, as it has an accuracy rate of up to 90% when compared with Intra-arterial Angiography [7–9].

The purpose of this study is to describe a dental radiographic technique for establishing the differential diagnosis of calcified atheromas relative to other calcifications with similar radiographic characteristics. Furthermore, the intention is to report three clinical cases that demonstrate the diagnostic possibilities of this technique.

2. Technical Report

The Manzi Projection is performed using the cephalometric unit of the panoramic radiographic equipment, in which the technique is described as follows: anteroposterior incidence, Frankfurt plane with vertical inclination between +15 and 30°, angle of the vertical and horizontal X-ray central beam at 0°, and reduction of radiation exposure factors, usually at 50% (Figure 1).

3. Case Reports

3.1. Clinical Case 1. The patient, a 78-year-old woman, systemically presenting the following risk factors related to atheroma formation: diabetes, dyslipidemia, arterial hypertension, and tobacco use. The patient was asked to have a panoramic radiograph taken for dental treatment. The examination was performed with the Kodak Ceph 9000 3D (Carestream Health, Inc.) equipment, in which the presence of radiopaque mass adjacent to the C3-C4 intervertebral space on the left side of the patient was detected, compatible with calcified atheroma (Figure 2).

The Manzi Projection was then performed on the patient to establish a differential diagnosis between calcified atheromas and other calcifications with similar imaginological characteristics. This was performed with the cephalometric unit of the Kodak Ceph 9000 3D (Carestream Health, Inc., Rochester, NY, USA) equipment, by which the presence of bilateral radiopaque masses were detected in the patient, showing that the one on the right side was located adjacent to the C4 vertebra (Figure 3).

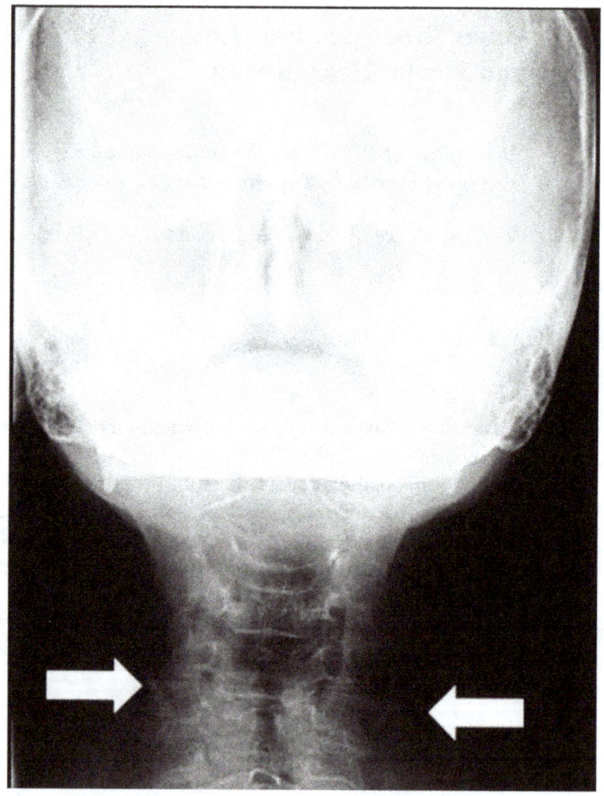

Figure 3: Manzi Projection showing radiopaque image circumscribed on both sides of the neck soft tissue region, in which the left side is adjacent to the C3 and C4 intervertebral space (arrow) and the right side is adjacent to the C4 (arrow).

As these calcifications were also presented in the Manzi Projection, the patient was referred for cardiac monitoring, in which the Doppler Ultrasound was requested to establish the degree of arterial stenosis. The presence of calcified plaque in the carotid bulb (bulbar or medulla oblongata) region of the right and left carotid arteries was detected in this examination, causing between 30 and 49% stenosis.

3.2. Clinical Case 2. The patient, a 56-year-old man, systemically presenting the following risk factors for atherosclerosis: dyslipidemia, arterial hypertension, active periodontal disease, and being a self-declared ex-tobacco user. The panoramic radiograph for dental treatment was requested, in which the presence of bilateral radiopaque masses adjacent to the cervical region was detected (Figure 4).

The patient was asked to undergo the Manzi Projection examination, which demonstrated the presence of radiopaque masses compatible with calcified atheromas on the patient's right side, in which the presence of a second plaque, in a more inferior position than that of the one demonstrated by the panoramic radiograph, and the absence of calcified plaque on the left of the patient were verified (Figure 5).

The patient was referred to the responsible cardiologist, who confirmed, by Doppler Ultrasound, the presence of calcified plaques in the right carotid artery, located in the carotid bulb and common carotid artery region, causing between 30 and 49% stenosis. On the left side, the presence of calcium free plaque was also verified, causing between 30 and 49% stenosis. However, the calcification visualized on the left side of the panoramic radiograph was not a calcified atheroma.

3.3. Clinical Case 3. The patient, a 90-year-old woman, systemically presenting the following risk factors for atherosclerosis: dyslipidemia and arterial hypertension. She was submitted to panoramic radiograph examination for dental treatment in which the presence of a calcified plaque was verified and visualized in the cervical region on the patient's left side (Figure 6).

The Manzi Projection for the differential diagnosis of other calcifications and structures was performed in the dental office, in which the presence of radiopaque masses adjacent to the cervical region was verified, on both sides (bilateral). Relevant to highlight is that the localization of the calcified structure (demonstrated by the panoramic radiograph) was superior position to that of the structures visualized on the Manzi Projection and that these structures did not appear to be prominently in the cervical region, the region of the carotid artery itself (Figure 7).

The patient was referred for cardiac monitoring, in which the Doppler Ultrasound was requested. Thus, on examination, the presence of bilateral calcified plaques in the carotid bulb and common carotid artery regions was verified, causing over 70% stenosis on the right side and between 50 and 69% stenosis on the left side.

4. Discussion

Atherosclerosis is usually asymptomatic, and it is diagnosed by means of medical examinations, such as Doppler Ultrasound, considered the most widely used examination for this purpose, because it is a noninvasive method with excellent accuracy. It differs from Intra-arterial Angiography which, although highly accurate, is an invasive method with an estimated rate of morbidity and mortality of 2% [7–9]

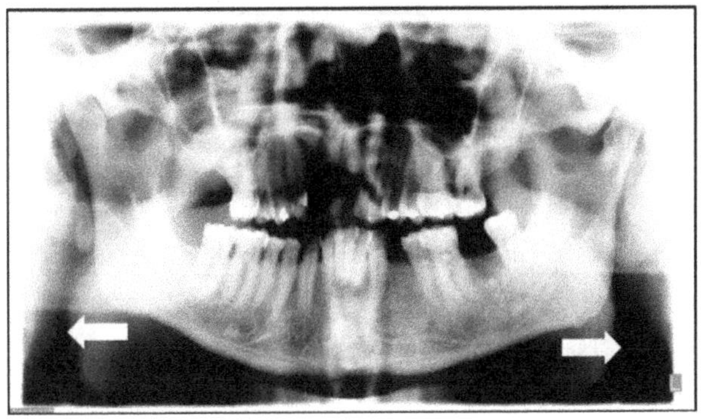

Figure 4: Panoramic radiograph showing the presence of bilateral radiopaque masses (arrows).

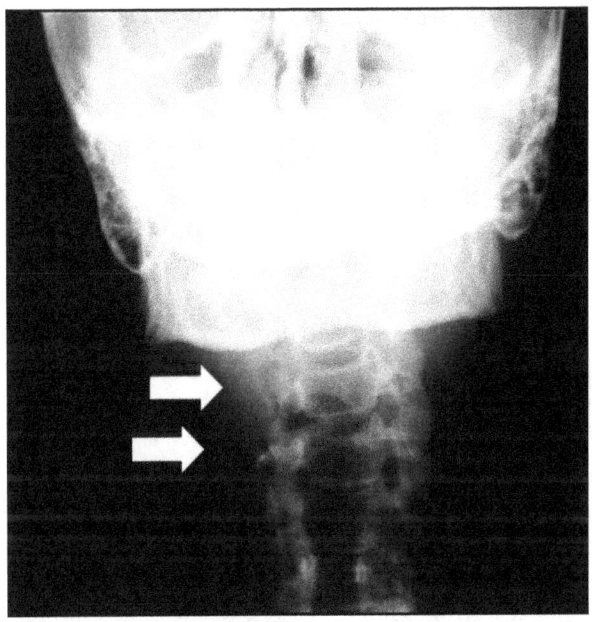

Figure 5: Manzi Projection showing the presence of two calcified plaques adjacent to the cervical region (arrows).

Other calcifications in the soft tissues can be observed radiographically in the cervical region. Carotid atheroma must be distinguished from those other radiopacities that lie in proximity to the artery. Based on the location, the calcified triticeous cartilage is the most likely calcification to be confused with a carotid atheroma. However, as a matter of distinguishing, there are some main features that can be observed. Calcified triticeous cartilages are well delimited and regular radiopacities, while carotid atheroma is visualized as irregular, heterogeneous, verticolinear radiopacities. Also, in a panoramic radiograph, the carotid atheroma appears more laterally than a calcified triticeous cartilage [10, 11].

Intending to provide an early diagnosis of these calcified atheromatous plaques, Friedlander and Lande, as far back as 1981, analyzed the possibility of identifying these calcifications by means of using panoramic radiography. Thirty-five

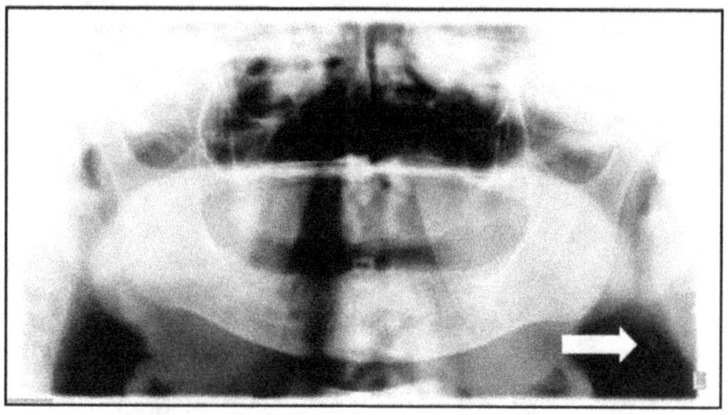

FIGURE 6: Panoramic radiograph showing the presence of radiopaque mass circumscribed on the left side of the cervical region (arrow).

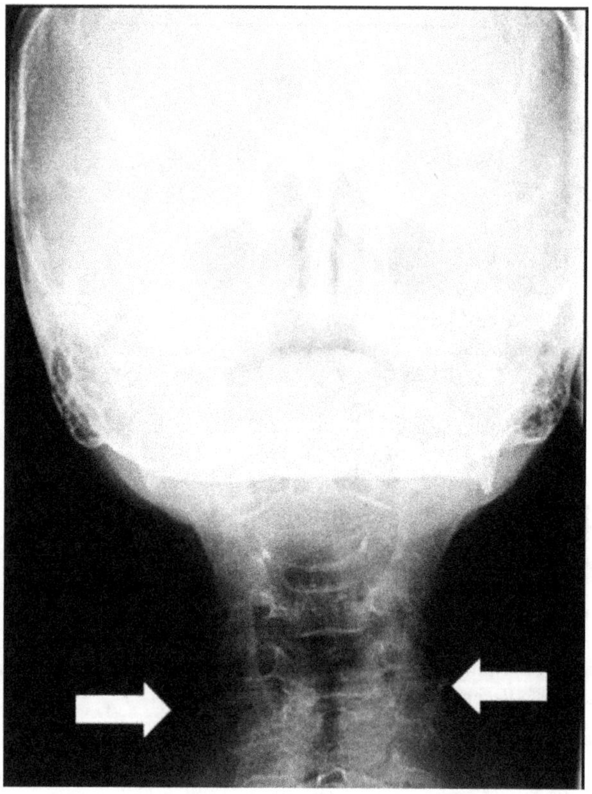

FIGURE 7: Manzi Projection showing the presence of bilateral radiopaque masses, adjacent to the cervical region (arrows). Notice that these structures are inferior to the calcified structure region demonstrated by the panoramic radiograph.

years have passed, and this method is still being studied and compared with other medical examinations for establishing its sensitivity, specificity, and accuracy. Although the panoramic radiograph does not present similar rates when compared with Doppler Ultrasound, its findings must not be disregarded, as the literature infers an association between the presence of calcified plaques in the cervical region (panoramic) and carotid calcifications [10–13].

The Manzi Projection represents a dental radiographic technique that may assist with the differential diagnosis of these calcified atheromatous plaques in the carotid because, in this examination, the course of the carotid artery is displayed without being superimposed by other calcified structures, and enlargement of the vertebral visualization enables an analysis of the cervical region. This is important because around 11% of the carotid bifurcations, the sites most frequently affected by atheromatous plaques are found inferior to the C3-C4 intervertebral space, where visualization in the panoramic radiograph is most unlikely [14]. The patient undergoes the examination with the Frankfurt plane (that starts at the superior portion of the acoustic meatus and is tangential to the infraorbital foramen) leaning slightly in the superior direction (between 15 and 30°), which diminishes the possibility of mandibular superimposition of the cervical region. Because it is an anteroposterior technique, the region of the carotid bifurcation is found closer to the radiographic sensor which, according to the geometric principles of radiological image formation, may clearly distinguish calcified atheromas, in case they exist.

5. Conclusion

The Manzi Projection can promote differential diagnosis of calcified atheroma in relation to other cervical calcifications in dental practice; however, further studies are necessary to establish its accuracy.

Additional Points

Human and Animal Rights. No animals were used in this research. All research procedures followed were in accordance with the ethical standards of the committee responsible for human experimentation (institutional and national) and with the Helsinki Declaration of 1975, as revised in 2008.

Consent

Written and informed consent was obtained from the patient. Informed consent form was submitted to the patients enrolled in this study.

Acknowledgments

The authors would like to thank CAPES (Coordination for the Improvement of Higher Education Personnel) for their financial support.

References

[1] D. Mozaffarian, E. J. Benjamin, A. S. Go et al., "Heart disease and stroke statistics -2015 update: a report from the American Heart Association," *Circulation*, vol. 131, pp. 29–322, 2015.

[2] M. F. Linton, P. G. Yancey, S. S. Davies et al., "The role of lipids and lipoproteins in atherosclerosis," in *Endotext*, L. J. Groot, P. Beck-Peccoz, G. Chrousos, K. Dungan, A. Grossman, and J. M.

Hershman, Eds., pp. 1–174, South Dartmouth (MA): NCBI Bookshelf, 2015.

[3] A. H. Friedlander, "Panoramic radiography: the differential diagnosis of carotid artery atheromas," *Special Care in Dentistry*, vol. 15, no. 6, pp. 223–227, 1995.

[4] A. H. Friedlander and I. K. Friedlander, "Panoramic dental radiography: an aid in detecting individuals prone to stroke," *Brazilian Dental Journal*, vol. 181, no. 1, pp. 23–26, 1996.

[5] L. C. Carter, K. Tsimidis, and J. Fabiano, "Carotid calcifications on panoramic radiography identify an asymptomatic male patient at risk for stroke: a case report," *Oral Surgery, Oral Medicine, Oral Pathology, Oral Radiology, and Endodontics*, vol. 85, no. 1, pp. 119–122, 1998.

[6] F. R. Manzi, F. N. Bóscolo, S. M. de Almeida, and F. H. Neto, "Panoramic radiography as an auxiliary in detecting patients at risk for cerebrovascular accident (CVA): a case report," *Journal of Oral Science*, vol. 45, no. 3, pp. 177–180, 2003.

[7] H. J. M. Barnett, D. W. Taylor, M. Eliasziw et al., "Benefit of carotid endarterectomy in patients with symptomatic moderate or severe stenosis," *The New England Journal of Medicine*, vol. 339, no. 20, pp. 1415–1425, 1998.

[8] European Carotid Surgery Trialists Colaborative Group, "Randomised trial of endarterectomy for recently symptomatic carotid stenosis: final results of the MRC European Carotid Surgery Trial (ECST)," *The Lancet*, vol. 351, no. 9113, pp. 1379–1387, 1998.

[9] E. G. Grant, C. B. Benson, G. L. Moneta et al., "Carotid artery stenosis: gray-scale and Doppler US diagnosis—Society of Radiologists in Ultrasound Consensus Conference," *Radiology*, vol. 229, no. 2, pp. 340–346, 2003.

[10] R. S. Kamikawa, M. F. Pereira, Â. Fernandes, and M. I. Meurer, "Study of the localization of radiopacities similar to calcified carotid atheroma by means of panoramic radiography," *Oral Surgery, Oral Medicine, Oral Pathology, Oral Radiology, and Endodontology*, vol. 101, no. 3, pp. 374–378, 2006.

[11] L. C. Carter, "Discrimination between calcified triticeous cartilage and calcified carotid atheroma on panoramic radiography," *Oral Surgery, Oral Medicine, Oral Pathology, Oral Radiology, and Endodontology*, vol. 90, no. 1, pp. 108–110, 2000.

[12] A. H. Friedlander and A. Lande, "Panoramic radiographic identification of carotid arterial plaques," *Oral Surgery, Oral Medicine, and Oral Pathology*, vol. 52, no. 1, pp. 102–104, 1981.

[13] S. J. Yoon, W. Yoon, O. S. Kim, J. S. Lee, and B. C. Kang, "Diagnostic accuracy of panoramic radiography in the detection of calcified carotid artery," *Dento Maxillo Facial Radiology*, vol. 37, no. 2, pp. 104–107, 2008.

[14] J. Griniatsos, S. Damaskos, N. Tsekouras, C. Klonaris, and S. Georgopoulos, "Correlation of calcified carotid plaques detected by panoramic radiograph with risk factors for stroke development," *Oral Surgery, Oral Medicine, Oral Pathology, Oral Radiology, and Endodontics*, vol. 108, no. 4, pp. 600–603, 2009.

5

The Modified Caldwell-Luc Approach with the use of Collagen Material for Treatment of a Chronic Perforated Maxillary Sinusitis

Ekaterina Diachkova, Elena Morozova, Natalia Blagushina, and Svetlana Tarasenko

Department of Dental Surgery of Borovsky Institute of Dentistry, Sechenov First Moscow State Medical University (Sechenov University), Russia

Correspondence should be addressed to Ekaterina Diachkova; secu2003@mail.ru

Academic Editor: Adrian Kasaj

Oroantral fistula (OAF) often develops after extraction of posterior maxillary teeth and requires surgical closure. If it persists, OAF may result in maxillary sinusitis. This paper reports a case of an oroantral fistula, associated with chronic maxillary sinusitis. A 46-year-old female patient presented with a history of traumatic tooth extraction, which led to OAF formation. Three unsuccessful attempts were made to close it elsewhere. With one operation, we performed Caldwell-Luc surgery and closed OAF with a collagen membrane and plug and a buccal flap. The patient was assessed at 1-, 3-, 6-, and 12-month and 8-year follow-up visits, with no signs of maxillary sinusitis or OAF recurrence being found with the efficient amount of bone and opportunity for further dental rehabilitation like sinus lifting and dental implantation. We believe that this approach may be a viable option in similar cases.

1. Introduction

Oroantral fistula (OAF) is a relatively frequent complication after extraction of posterior maxillary teeth [1]. Therefore, surgeons should be alert to the possibility of its formation, especially when the first and/or the second upper molars are to be extracted [2]. Nevertheless, even gentle extraction does not always guarantee against OAF formation, so a surgeon should be capable of treating this complication.

Immediate postextraction oroantral communications must be closed within 48 hours following surgery. If primary closure has not been achieved within these time limits, the internal surface becomes epithelised and a chronic OAF develops. In such cases, spontaneous closure is impossible [3]. The established communication of the maxillary sinus with the oral cavity is likely to lead to chronic odontogenic maxillary sinusitis. This condition requires a combined approach as treatment of either OAF or sinusitis alone is insufficient [4]. Also, there are no articles that described the treatment of OAF with the maxillary sinusitis when besides the sanitation and covering of communication, authors provided the techniques for stimulation of osteogenesis and creation of good condition for further dental rehabilitation.

In the present case report, we describe a surgical protocol for the treatment of OAF associated with chronic maxillary sinusitis.

2. Clinical Case

A 46-year-old female patient was referred to the Oral and Maxillofacial Surgery Clinic (Sechenov University, Moscow, Russia) with oroantral fistula, associated with left-sided chronic maxillary sinusitis. The patient reported that tooth 2.6 had been extracted elsewhere three years before and afterwards, she noticed leakage of liquids through the nose while drinking. The patient visited a dental surgeon where she was diagnosed with oroantral fistula (OAF). However, an attempt to close it failed and thereafter so did two other attempts. The patient also complained of recurrent episodes of facial pain and pressure.

On examination, OAF and scar tissue at the postextraction site were observed in the projection of absent tooth 2.6.

Besides that, tooth 2.5 was found to be extensively damaged so it could not be restored. The surgical plan included extraction of tooth 2.5, maxillary sinusotomy, and OAF closure with a collagen membrane in one operation. The patient signed the informed consent form for operation and the use of results of treatment for scientific and educational purposes. The patient underwent full preoperative examination (laboratory blood test, biochemical blood test, chest X-ray, coagulogram, and other prescribing for preoperative examination before planned surgery), with no relevant clinical data being found. It was provided orthopantomography for additional investigation and evaluation of the condition of the maxillary sinus.

Surgical treatment included Caldwell-Luc sinusotomy and sinuplasty with the local tissues with our changes: for covering the bone window and oroantral connection and plugging the fistula, we used different forms of bovine collagen ("Collost," BioFarmaHolding, Moscow, Russia) with the 3D orientation of fibrils that can increase the osteoconduction features of material.

Local anaesthesia was obtained with 4% articaine hydrochloride with 1 : 100,000 epinephrine. A 5 cm semilunar incision encompassing OAF was made, and a full-thickness buccal flap was elevated. The oral mucosa adjacent to OAF was excised. Tooth 2.5 was extracted. A round window in the lateral wall of the maxillary sinus was prepared with a cylindrical diamond bur. Special care was taken to leave at least 15 mm of bone between the OAF and the window. The normal mucous membrane was left intact, whereas the diseased sinus membrane was debrided with curettes (Figure 1(a)). The internal surface of the sinus was thoroughly irrigated with 0.05% chlorhexidine gluconate. An inferior meatal nasal antral window was created with a chisel and widened with a rongeur. A deflated balloon of the Foley catheter was placed into the sinus, and a tube was passed through the nasal antral window to the outside.

The balloon was then inflated with 10 ml of sterile saline (Figure 1(b)). The flap was mobilised to ensure full coverage without tension. The extraction socket of tooth 2.5 was filled with a cross-linked bovine collagen matrix. Both the oroantral window and OAF were covered with the collagen membrane (Figure 1(c)). The flap was repositioned and closed with 4/0 polypropylene sutures (Figure 1(d)). The surgical wound was covered with a previously made protective silicon plate, and the patient was instructed to use it when eating.

The patient was prescribed with ceftriaxone 1 g IM twice daily for 7 days, loratadine 10 mg once daily for 7 days, ibuprofen 600 mg thrice daily for 4 days, and oxymetazoline 0.05% nasal spray twice daily for 7 days.

The Foley catheter and the sutures were removed 1 and 7 days after surgery, respectively. No early postoperative complications occurred.

The patient was assessed at 1-, 3-, 6-, and 12-month and 8-year follow-up visits. No signs of chronic maxillary sinusitis or OAF were found during clinical examination and orthopantomography. A significant increase in volume and density of bone at the surgical site is shown in a series of consecutive radiographs (Figure 2).

Two alternatives for further rehabilitation (i.e., dental implantation or placement of a fixed dental prosthesis) were offered to the patient. As the patient refused another surgical intervention, prosthodontic treatment was approved and provided at the fifth month after surgery. Both quality of life and working ability of the patient improved dramatically after completing the treatment.

3. Discussion

As a rule, OAF cannot be closed when sinus infection is present, so complete sinus debridement is mandatory before OAF closure. In this case, the patient required surgical treatment of maxillary sinusitis because the sinus membrane was irreversibly diseased and the patient reported of frequent acute exacerbations of maxillary sinusitis (up to 5 times a year), which occurred regardless of any previous attempts to treat this condition. To prevent reinfection, we decided to perform both sinus debridement and OAF closure in one operation.

To date, surgical techniques tend to be less invasive and radical. This is also true for maxillary sinus surgery, where the traditional Caldwell-Luc approach has been almost completely replaced by functional endoscopic sinus surgery. However, the latter requires high professional skills and special armamentarium, which is not always available. On the other hand, the Caldwell-Luc surgery is a simple, less expensive, and time-tested method, which yields good results [5]. Nevertheless, it is a relatively traumatic procedure, so we decided to place the Foley balloon into the sinus to minimise the risk of postoperative bleeding and swelling. Moreover, it made further membrane placement and suturing easier. Two retrospective studies of 55 cases reported good performance of the Caldwell-Luc surgery with balloon placement, with acute sinusitis being the only and rare complication [2, 6].

Several options for OAF closure are available, all of them having their advantages and disadvantages. The buccal advancement flap technique is the easiest way for closing both immediate and chronic OAFs. Despite some drawbacks, the vestibular depth reduction, and rather limited blood supply being among them, it yields good clinical outcomes [7]. To overcome these limitations, some authors suggested to use a buccal fat pad flap due to its better vascularization [8]. A palatal flap can be considered another option [9]. Nevertheless, a full-thickness flap alone may be insufficient, as the Schneiderian membrane may adhere to the oral mucosa, thereby hindering bone regeneration. This complication can be prevented by placing a collagen membrane to separate the maxillary sinus from the oral cavity. Moreover, some authors advocate placing an autogenous platelet-rich fibrin membrane over the collagen membrane to promote soft tissue healing. Although some promising results have been obtained, it is still unclear whether this approach has greater effectiveness than the collagen membrane used alone [10] or with the collagen plug that creates additional barrier between the oral cavity and maxillary sinus decreasing the migration of microorganism and preventing the recurrence of maxillary sinusitis and OAF.

To make dental implantation possible, bone grafting may be performed when residual bone volume is insufficient or a large bony defect is present. Different types of grafting

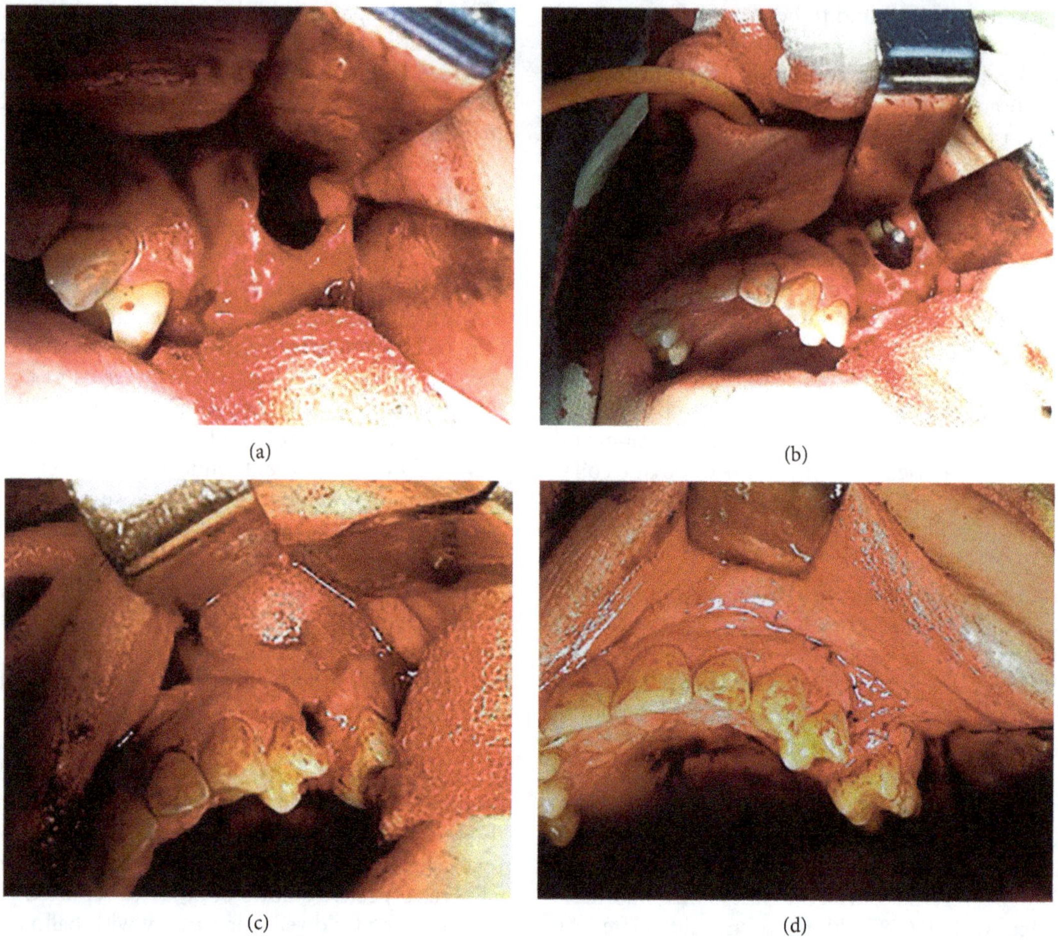

Figure 1: Surgical procedure: (a) sinus debridement through the created window; (b) insertion of the Foley catheter balloon into the sinus; (c) membrane placement over the window and the bony defect; (d) flap placement and suturing.

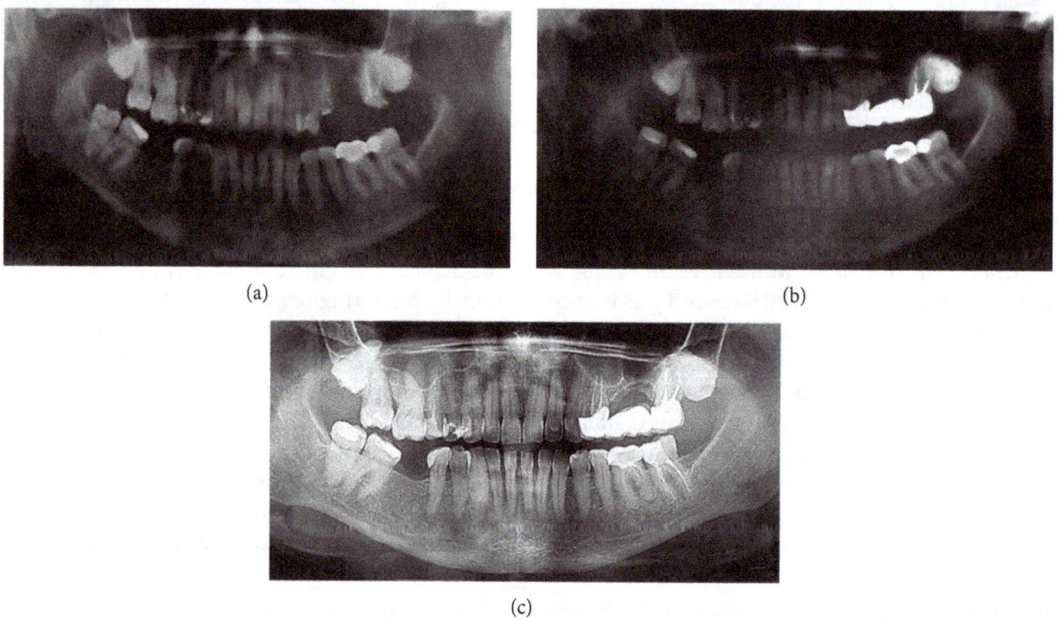

Figure 2: Panoramic radiograph: (a) preoperative radiograph showing bony defect at the postextraction site of tooth 2.6 and failing tooth 2.5; (b) radiograph taken 3 months after surgery showing bone repair; (c) radiograph taken at 8-year follow-up showing the stability of bone volume and absence of any pathological lesions.

materials (e.g., auto-, allo-, and xenografts) have been used for this procedure [4]. The bone plate harvested after creating a window in the lateral wall of the maxillary sinus can be used as an autogenous graft, which allows avoiding additional surgery and reducing total costs [11].

In some cases of OAF, simultaneous sinus floor elevation can make the surgical procedure easier as the area of the defect in the Schneiderian membrane decreases. This approach also facilitates further implant surgery. But it is contraindicated if any signs of sinus infection are present [12]. In our case, the patient had a 3-year history of chronic sinus disease and, furthermore, was unwilling to place a dental implant, so there was no special need for bone grafting. Therefore, this treatment modality was rejected.

Third molar autotransplantation has also been considered a promising treatment for OAF, which has many advantages, some of them being immediate restoring of a missed tooth, low cost, and possibility of orthodontic treatment. However, there is very scarce data of clinical performance in immediate postextraction oroantral communication closure and no data for chronic OAF closure [13]. So, we decided against this treatment in our case.

4. Conclusion

The use of bovine collagen membrane and plug for covering of area of oroantral fistula and bone window during the operation of sanitation of the maxillary sinus helped to get good postoperative results such as the absence of recurrence of inflammatory process (maxillary sinusitis) due to removing the connection with oral cavity, stopping the circulation of microorganisms, and persistent contamination of maxillary sinus, also, with the stimulation of regeneration of bone because of the element of osteoconduction in collagen material and creating the conditions for further dental rehabilitation.

Acknowledgments

This study was supported by the "Russian Academic Excellence Project 5-100".

References

[1] G. B. Cordero, S. M. Ferrer, and L. Fernández, "Odontogenic sinusitis, oro-antral fistula and surgical repair by Bichat's fat pad: literature review," *Acta Otorrinolaringologica (English Edition)*, vol. 67, no. 2, pp. 107–113, 2016.

[2] Y. Anavi, G. Gal, R. Silfen, and S. Calderon, "Palatal rotation-advancement flap for delayed repair of oroantral fistula: a retrospective evaluation of 63 cases," *Oral Surgery, Oral Medicine, Oral Pathology, Oral Radiology, and Endodontology*, vol. 96, no. 5, pp. 527–534, 2003.

[3] P. Parvini, K. Obreja, A. Begic et al., "Decision-making in closure of oroantral communication and fistula," *International Journal of Implant Dentistry*, vol. 5, no. 1, p. 13, 2019.

[4] P. Parvini, K. Obreja, R. Sader, J. Becker, F. Schwarz, and L. Salti, "Surgical options in oroantral fistula management: a narrative review," *International Journal of Implant Dentistry*, vol. 4, no. 1, p. 40, 2018.

[5] J. Hajiioannou, S. Exarchos, V. Lachanas, and J. Bizakis, "In the era of endoscopic sinus surgery, is there still a place for the Caldwell-Luc procedure?," *B-ENT*, vol. 12, no. 2, pp. 99–102, 2016.

[6] Y. K. Kim and S. G. Kim, "A retrospective analysis of the retreatment of failed sinus bone grafts," *Implant Dentistry*, vol. 25, no. 3, pp. 450–454, 2016.

[7] A. Belmehdi and K. El Harti, "Management of oroantral communication using buccal advanced flap," *Pan African Medical Journal*, vol. 34, 2019.

[8] S. P. Sharma, "Three-layered closure of persistent oroantral fistula using chin graft, buccal fat pad, and buccal advancement flap: a case report with review of literature," *Case Reports in Dentistry*, vol. 2019, 5 pages, 2019.

[9] A. Merlini, J. Garibaldi, M. Piazzai, L. Giorgis, and P. Balbi, "Modified double-layered flap technique for closure of an oroantral fistula: surgical procedure and case report," *British Journal of Oral and Maxillofacial Surgery*, vol. 54, no. 8, pp. 959–961, 2016.

[10] M. J. AL-Juboori, M. A. AL-Attas, and L. C. M. Filho, "Treatment of chronic oroantral fistula with platelet-rich fibrin clot and collagen membrane: a case report," *Clinical, Cosmetic and Investigational Dentistry*, vol. 10, pp. 245–249, 2018.

[11] R. J. Weinstock, L. Nikoyan, and H. Dym, "Composite three-layer closure of oral antral communication with 10 months follow-up—a case study," *Journal of Oral and Maxillofacial Surgery*, vol. 72, no. 2, pp. 266.e1–266.e7, 2014.

[12] D. Cortes, R. Martinez-Conde, A. Uribarri, A. Eguia del Valle, J. Lopez, and J. M. Aguirre, "Simultaneous oral antral fistula closure and sinus floor augmentation to facilitate dental implant placement or orthodontics," *Journal of Oral and Maxillofacial Surgery*, vol. 68, no. 5, pp. 1148–1151, 2010.

[13] S. A. Nagori, A. Jose, O. Bhutia, and A. Roychoudhury, "A case of oro-antral communication closed by autotransplantation of third molar," *Journal of Maxillofacial and Oral Surgery*, vol. 14, no. S1, pp. 448–451, 2015.

6

Primary Extra Nodal Diffuse Large B-Cell Lymphoma of the Maxillary Sinus with Symptoms of Acute Pulpitis

Jian-tong Cui, Shao-qing Zhang, and Hui-xia He

Department of Stomatology, The First Medical Center, Chinese PLA General Hospital, Beijing, 100853, China

Correspondence should be addressed to Hui-xia He; hehuixia@plagh.org

Academic Editor: Ricardo Alves Mesquita

Diffuse large B-cell lymphoma not otherwise specified (DLBCL-NOS) is a subtype of large B-cell non-Hodgkin lymphoma with various clinical and pathological manifestations. DLBCL-NOS which primarily arises from maxillary sinus is rare and hard to diagnose due to unique anatomy. Here, we present a case of DLBCL-NOS that developed in the left maxillary sinus of a 72-year-old male, who presented with severe toothache that resembled acute pulpitis. The lesion was diagnosed and treated based on radiographs, histological, immunohistological examinations, and PET-CT analysis. Despite its rare incidence, DLBCL-NOS should still be included in differential diagnoses to rule out malignancy in cases of endodontic disease.

1. Introduction

Diffuse large B-cell Lymphoma (DLBCL) is a group of malignant tumors with great heterogeneity in clinical manifestations, histological morphology, and prognosis. It is the most common type of non-Hodgkin lymphomas (NHL) which accounts for 30-40% of newly reported cases and mainly occurs in elderly men [1, 2]. Similar to NHL, DLBCL is divided into nodal DLBCL and extranodal DLBCL based on primary sites of origin [3]. Nodal DLBCL manifests as painless lymphadenopathy with symptoms of local compression or obstruction in early stage, while extranodal DLBCL has various clinical presentations depending on the extent of local invasion. DLBCL may occur at multiple locations; among which, the gastrointestinal tract is the most commonly affected site, being followed by the head and neck region [2]. Thus, patients with DLBCL have complex clinical manifestations (systemic symptoms involving stomach, lung, skin; B symptoms like fever, weight loss, etc.), histological morphology, and prognosis.

While previous literature has reported cases that occurred at the palate, alveolar ridge, and gingiva, DLBCL at the maxillary sinus has rarely been reported [4–7]. Early diagnosis of DLBCL at maxillary sinus is challenging. Due to its specific anatomy and large air space, a patient can be asymptomatic until the tumor perforates one of the walls. On the other hand, early symptoms resemble those of endodontic diseases, such as spontaneous pain, soft tissue swelling, sinus tract, hypnalgia, and sensitivity to percussion. The lack of unique symptoms and subtle clinical manifestations may obscure proper diagnosis and delay treatment. Due to the disease's aggressive and rapid progression, early diagnosis and treatment would be tremendously beneficial to DLBCL patients. Therefore, dentists should develop a deep understanding of DLBCL and conduct comprehensive examinations for patients with similar symptoms for differential diagnoses and treatments accordingly [2]. Here, we present an unusual case of DLBCL in a 72-year-old male that developed in left maxillary sinus, who initially presented with severe toothache and symptoms similar to those of acute pulpitis.

2. Case Report

A 72-year-old man presented to the Department of Stomatology at the Chinese PLA General Hospital with severe intermittent, spontaneous pain at night in the left maxillary posterior region for a week. Three days before his visit, the patient was diagnosed with apical periodontitis at maxillary left first premolar #12 (Universal Numbering System) and

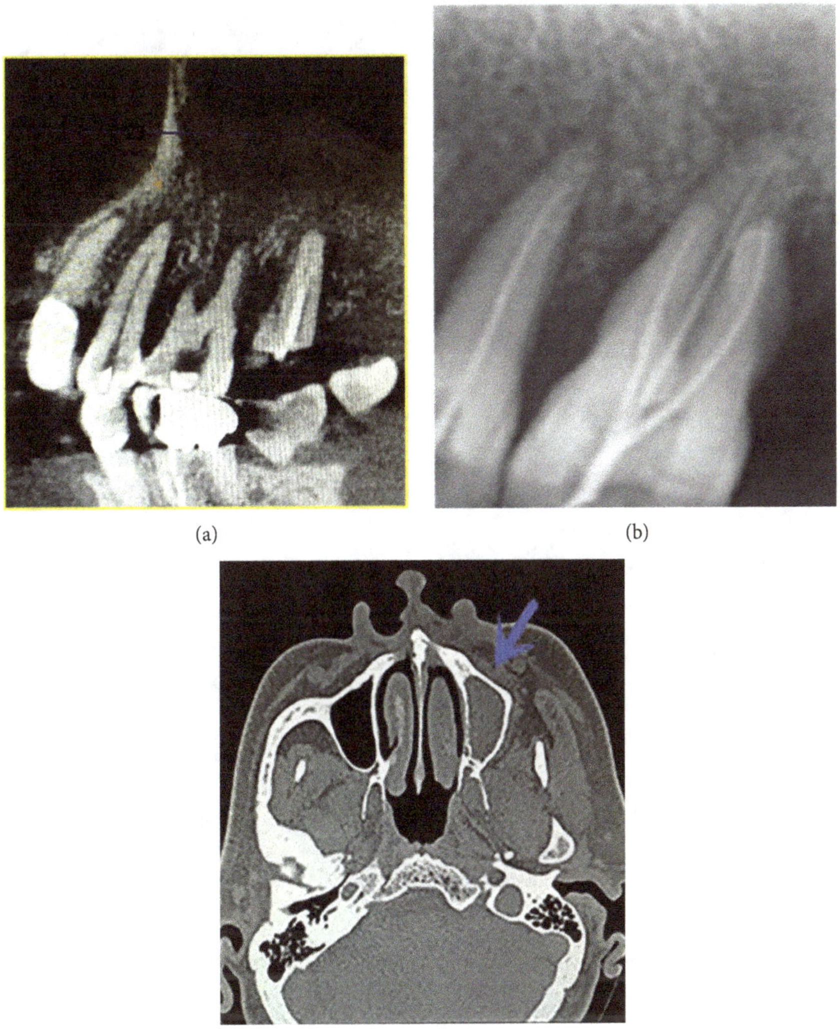

(a) (b) (c)

FIGURE 1: CBCT images showed multiple low-attenuating entities apical to premolars and the first molar. An extensive soft tissue mass was identified in the left maxillary sinus which extended through the medial maxillary sinus wall (a). Dental X-ray image showed appropriate root canal therapy (b). Transverse CT image showed maxillary sinus full of substantial objects which destroyed multiple walls (c).

underwent pulpectomy in a local dental clinic. Since then, he has been taking analgesics and nonsteroidal anti-inflammatory medications, but severe spontaneous pain and hypnalgia were persistent.

No lymphadenopathy and swelling was noticed extraorally, yet intraorally poorly maintained dentition, and generalized edematous and erythematous gingiva were seen. There was extensive coronal structural loss for left maxillary second molar #15, which was endodontically treated 10 years ago, with fracture surface 2-3 mm under gingiva. The inflamed gingival margin was also observed buccally, and probing depth was 5-6 mm. Maxillary left first molar #14 had an exposed pulp cavity with mild mobility and a 5 mm periodontal pocket. The first and second left maxillary premolars, #12-#13, responded positively to percussion, and EPT test suggested necrotic pulps for #12-#14. A cone-beam computed tomography (CBCT) scan was performed instead of an initial Panoramic X-ray (PAN) because of its three-dimensional accuracy and the patient's preference for immediate appointment availability. Multiple well-defined hypo-attenuating entities were seen apical to #12-13 and #15 (Figure 1). Another was seen in the root canal of the residual root of #15, while an extensive soft tissue mass in the left maxillary sinus extending from medial maxillary sinus wall to palate at the left premolar and molar region was identified (Figure 1). As all symptoms suggested the diagnosis of pulpitis of #14 and the diagnosis of periapical periodontitis of teeth #12-13 and #15, root canal therapy was conducted for #12-#14, and residual #15 was removed (Figure 1). Computed tomography (CT) scan was performed, and sections were taken in the axial, coronal, and sagittal planes. Axial section revealed a large soft tissue density lesion almost full of the maxillary sinus, with destruction of multiple walls. It extends medially into the lateral wall of the nasal septum and right nasal cavity involving the inferior and middle turbinates and inferiorly causing destruction of the hard palate and alveolar processes of the left maxilla in the molar region (Figure 1). Left maxillary sinusitis was

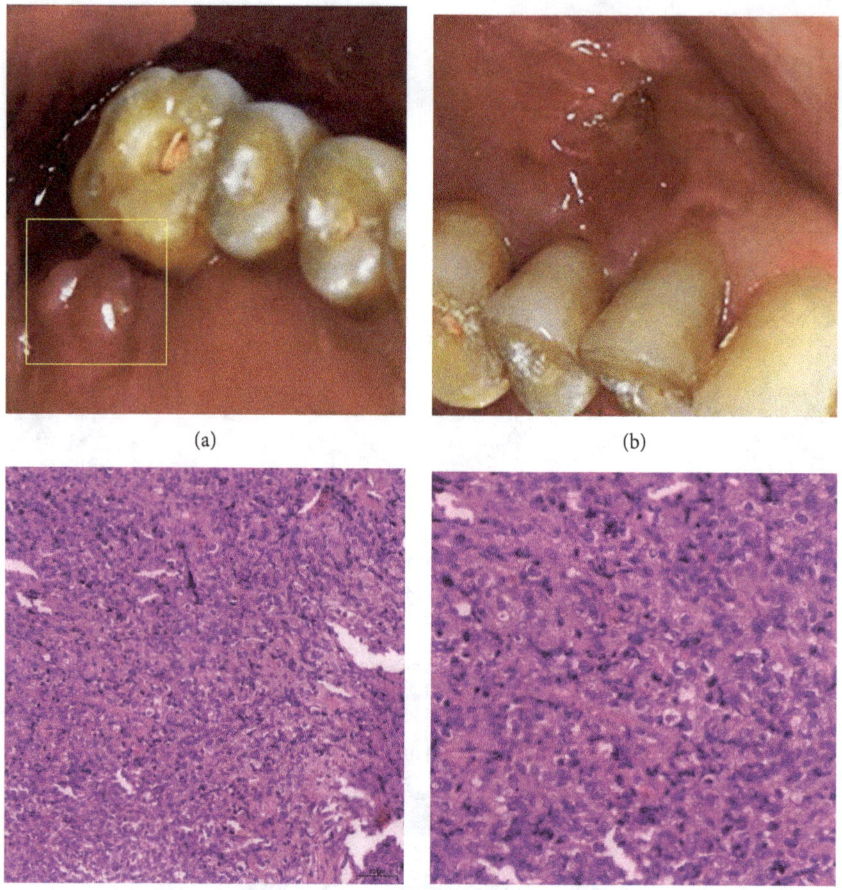

(a) (b) (c) (d)

FIGURE 2: Two weeks after the first visit, intraoral pictures showed the poorly healed extraction socket of #15 with surrounding, localized, conglobate nontender edema (a) and a soft, well-defined, crater-like erythematous ulceration on the buccal gingiva of #13 and #14 (b). Histologic photomicrographs revealed a diffusely infiltrating population of neoplastic lymphoid cells within a fibrotic stroma with vascular channels (c, 200x), and the majority of lymphocytes were large cells (d, 400x).

diagnosed, and the patient was given Ornidazole and Ceftriazone sodium for treatment. The patient reported slight alleviation of pain after the treatment. Yet, 14 days after the first visit, the patient presented to the department again with the chief complaint of recurrent pain at night in the upper molars region and facial paresthesia for 3 days.

Intraorally, the extraction socket of #15 was poorly healed with localized surrounding nontender edema. A soft, well-defined, crater-like erythematous ulceration was also noticed on the buccal gingiva of #13 and #14 (Figure 2). Therefore, NHL, squamous cell carcinoma, sarcoma, plasmacytoma, and malignant melanoma were considered as differential diagnoses. Incisional biopsy for perilesional samples at the margin of the soft tissue mass at #15 revealed diffuse infiltration of neoplastic lymphoid cells within a fibrotic stroma with vascular channels (Figure 2). The majority of lymphocytes were large cells while a few were small ones manifesting as vesicular nuclei with prominent nucleoli. There were a few scattered foamy macrophages among those lymphocytes. Histology suggested the diagnosis of B-cell lymphoma. Positive expressions of CD20, Bcl-2, Bcl-6, and MUM-1 were observed in immunohistochemistry (IHC). Moreover, there was a strong expression of Ki67 (95%), whereas CD10 and CMYC were negatively expressed. Furthermore, CMYC, Bcl-2, and Bcl-6 proto-oncogene rearrangements diagnosed by fluorescence in situ hybridization (FISH) were negative (Figure 3). All of the evidence supported the diagnosis of DLBCL-NOS, cell of origin-post germinal center type, and nondouble expressor. Positron Emission Tomography-Computed Tomography (PET-CT) scan further suggested a hypermetabolic mass of about $2.8 \times 3.3\,\mathrm{cm}^2$ in the left maxillary sinus, indicating the origin of the lymphoma (Figure 3).

The patient was referred to the Department of Oncology and received 6 cycles of standard chemotherapy regimen (R-CHOP, rituximab, cyclophosphamide, doxorubicin, vincristine, and prednisone). Rituximab $375\,\mathrm{mg/m^2}$ dl (day 1) (the first two-cycle), cyclophosphamide $750\,\mathrm{mg/m^2}$ dl, doxorubicin $50\,\mathrm{mg/m^2}$ dl, vincristine $2\,\mathrm{mg/m^2}$ dl, and prednisone 100 mg (days 1-5) were prescribed. Chemotherapy was administered in 3-week cycles, and the patient showed well tolerance to the treatment. The patient's symptoms were eliminated, and no intraoral swelling was identified at the end of the treatment. Imaging analysis of a follow-up PET-CT scan 1 month after the last chemotherapy session showed a negative result for isotope uptake at the left

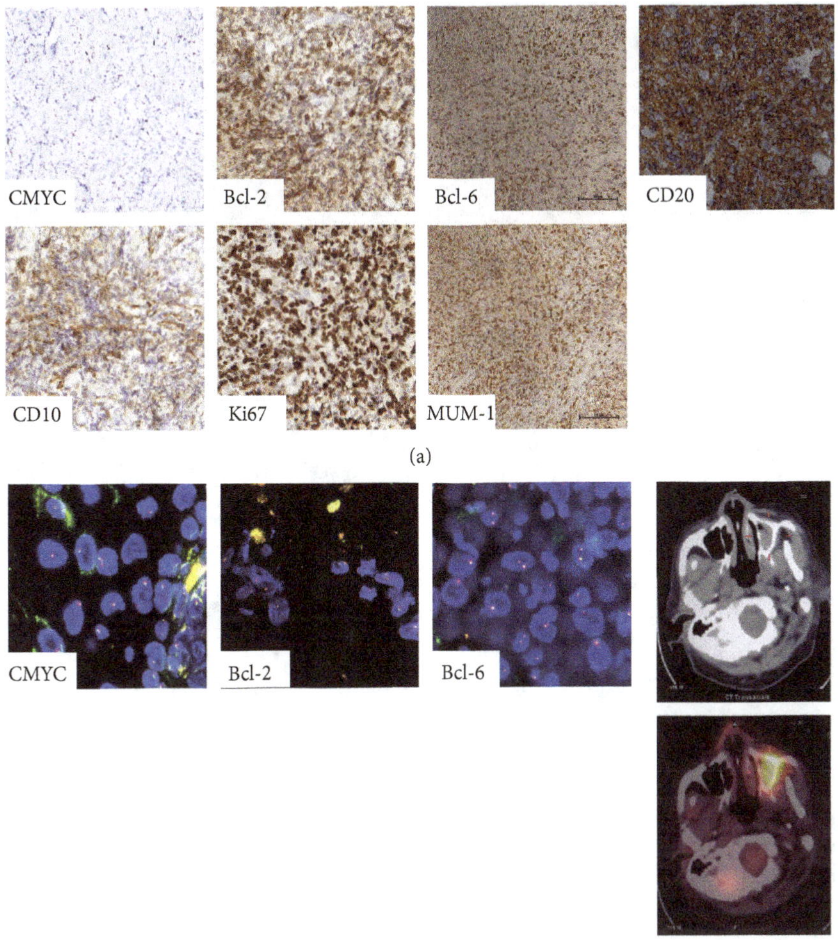

Figure 3: Immunohistochemical analysis showed that CD20, Bcl-2, Bcl-6, and MUM-1 were positively expressed. Ki-67 demonstrated a high (95%) proliferation rate, whereas CD10 and CMYC were negatively expressed (a). Fluorescence in situ hybridization (FISH) is negative for CMYC, Bcl-2, and Bcl-6 proto-oncogene rearrangements (b). Transverse PET-CT images showed about 2.8×3.3 cm hypermetabolic mass in the left maxillary sinus (c).

maxillary posterior region, and the CBCT image showed that substantial object in left maxillary sinus was reduced (Figure 4). The patient was followed up for five-year post-chemotherapy, and no recurrence was seen to date (Figure 4).

3. Discussion

Identifying whether the source of toothache is of odontogenic origin (pulpitis, periapical periodontitis, dentin exposure, cracked tooth, etc.) or nonodontogenic origin (myofascial or neuropathic pain, malignancy, maxillary sinusitis, etc.) is critical yet sometimes challenging. Specifically, the similar symptoms of NHL in the maxillofacial region and those of odontogenic origin may potentially lead to misdiagnoses. The occurrence of DLBCL-NOS in the maxillary sinus, which is often asymptomatic or clinically similar to inflammatory disease, is extremely rare and difficult to be noticed due to its anatomic location and considerable size [3, 8, 9]. In our case, the patient presented with severe spontaneous pain and hypnalgia, while #12-#15 showed obvious tenderness and pulpal necrosis. The CBCT images ruled out the possibility of root fracture and showed diffuse periapical rarefaction associated with the molars and premolars in the left maxillary posterior area. Given that periapical endodontic disease could damage the wall of the maxillary sinus and no systemic symptoms of B-cell lymphoma including fever, weight loss, night sweats, and paresthesia were observed, we extracted the residual root of #15 and conducted endodontic therapy for the symptomatic teeth as usual rather than performing a biopsy.

Yet, the persistent symptoms (pain, unhealed extraction socket) raised our suspicion of pathologies of nonodontogenic sources in the maxillary sinus and led to appropriate workup. It is worthy of the clinician's attention that although periapical lesions are the most commonly encountered radiolucency in the jaws, about 0.65% to 4.22% of clinical cases were misdiagnosed as endodontic periapical pathosis before histopathological diagnoses were made [10]. In this case, further morphological examination showed that large B lymphoma cells were arranged in a spreading pattern with large nuclear and partially or

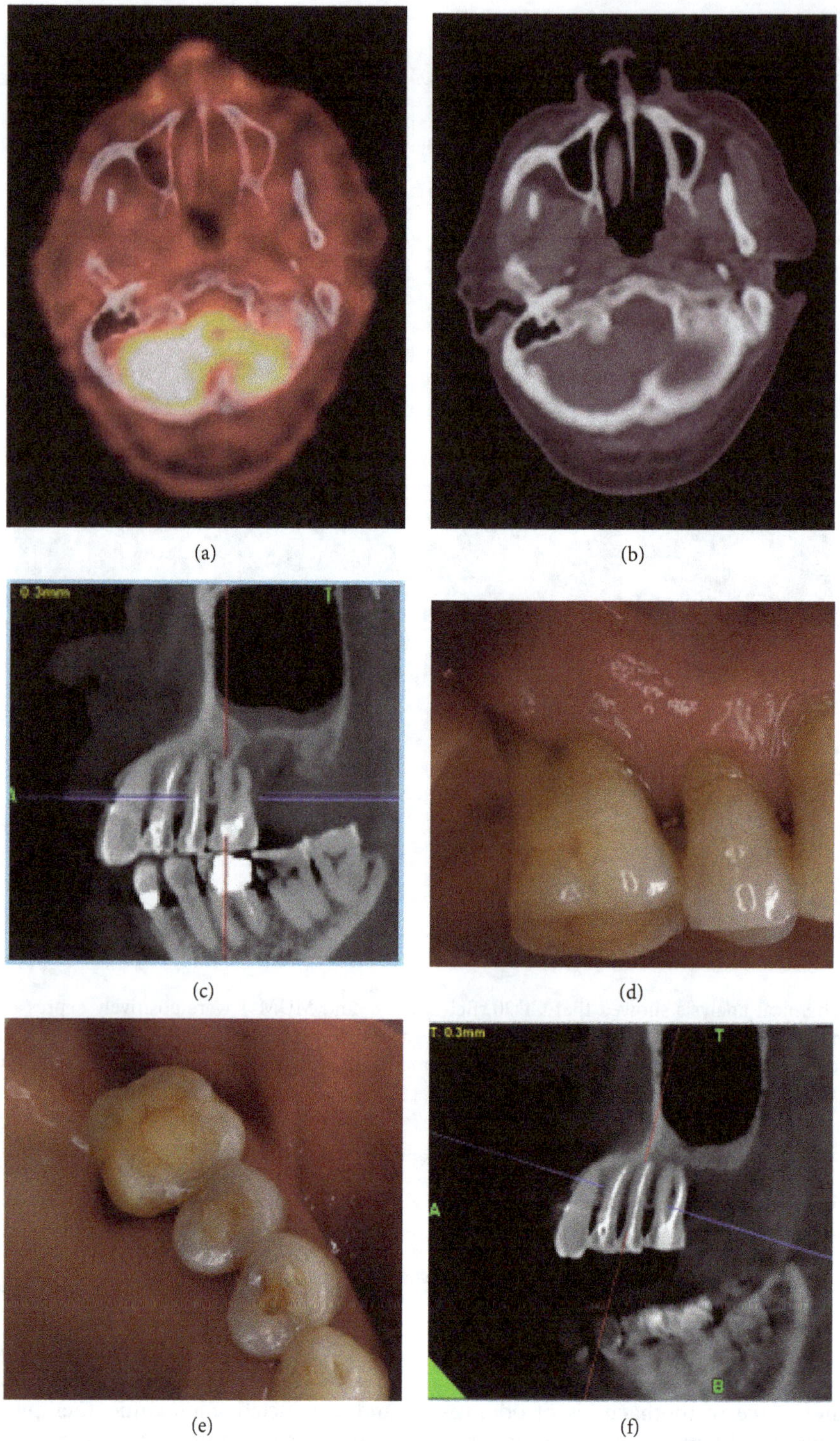

(a) (b) (c) (d) (e) (f)

Figure 4: One month after the end of treatment, no distinct radioactive uptake in the left maxillary sinus was shown in transverse PET-CT images (a, b). CBCT image showed reduced substantial objects in the left maxillary sinus (c). Five years later, intraoral pictures showed healthy gingiva (d, e). CBCT showed that no substantial objects could be found in the left maxillary sinus (f).

completely covered normal lymph nodes or extranode structures. Histopathology result is the gold standard, reaching a definitive diagnosis of DLBCL rather than squamous cell carcinoma, sarcoma, plasmacytoma, or malignant melanoma [7]. Various morphologic variants of DLBCL-NOS have been described with centroblastic, immunoblastic, and anaplastic variants being the most common types [2]. A significant proportion of cases defy assignment into any specific subgroup. Combining with immunohistochemistry, diagnosis and histological grading of lymphoma could be established more accurately [2]. The expressions of CD10, Bcl-6, and MUM-1 are suggested to distinguish between germinal center B-cell-like (GCB) lymphoma and nongerminal center B-cell like (non-GCB). The positive expression of

CD10 or negative expression of CD10 and MUM-1 with Bcl-6 positive expression should lead to identification of GCB tumor which implies a relatively better prognosis. The negative expression of CD10 and positive expression of MUM1 with positive or negative Bcl-6 indicate non-GCB tumor, which is often associated with a relatively poor prognosis [2, 7, 11]. Ki67 is a proliferative marker of neoplastic cells; therefore, the stronger expression of Ki67 is, the worse the prognosis will be. In our case, neoplastic cells were strongly positive for Ki67 (95%), MUM-1, Bcl-6, and Bcl-2 but negative for CD10. Both the histological examination and immunohistochemical analysis suggested the diagnosis of DLBCL NOS and cell of origin-post germinal center type, implying the aggressive characteristics and potentially poor prognosis in this patient if no timely diagnosis and treatment. It is worth noting that patients with a dual rearrangement of MYC and/or BCL2 and/or BCL6 "double-hit" lymphoma have been recognized to have a poor prognosis. In conjunction with FISH and PET-CT diagnosis, all diagnoses proved that it was DLBCL-NOS, cell of origin-post germinal center type, and nondouble expressor, which originated from the maxillary sinus that destroyed the bone plate of the maxillary sinus and the root of the teeth in the left maxillary region, causing pain similar to that of acute pulpitis.

DLBCL-NOS in the oral and maxillofacial regions may have very diverse manifestations including but not limited to local bone invasion, painless soft tissue swelling or ulceration, and toothache similar to that of periapical endodontic disease or pulpitis. Several articles have described delayed definitive diagnosis and relatively poor prognosis due to the atypical manifestation of maxillofacial lymphoma as toothache [4, 6, 12]. Fatahzadeh [4] reported a case of diffuse large B-cell lymphoma of mandible masquerading as toothache, in which etiology was not identified until the clinicopathologic examination was performed. Thus, the importance of proper differential diagnosis for early diagnosis could not be undermined. Comprehensive inspection including clinical evaluation, radiographic examination, histological assessment, and immunophenotypic analysis is necessary for diagnosis and treatment.

To date, the mainstay of the treatment regimen for DLBCL-NOS consists primarily of chemotherapy with the occasional use of radiotherapy. Cyclophosphamide, doxorubicin, vincristine, and prednisone (CHOP) are part of a widely used regimen. Anti-CD20 medication (rituximab) improves complete remission rates in NHL patients while it seems to prolong overall survival, although about 30%-40% of DLBCL patients with CD20 positive are refractory to R-CHOP therapy [2]. For these patients, other treatments such as autologous stem cell transplantation, R-EPOCH (rituximab, etoposide, prednisone, vincristine, cyclophosphamide, and doxorubicin), targeted theories, and novel approaches (chimeric antigen receptor- (CAR-) T cell therapy) could be considered [13]. Recently, many targeted drugs that inhibit signaling pathways in DLBCL cells have entered clinical trials, and many therapeutic agents are available on market. Treatment strategies are also tailored according to DLBCL-NOS patients' risk profiles according to age and age-adapted International Prognostic Index (IPI) [14]. Considering that 6-8 cycles of combined chemotherapy with R-CHOP-21 is the most widely used regimen for patients from 60 to 80 years of age, rituximab was added to the CHOP regimen for the patient in our case, though there is limited experience of the use of anti-CD20 medication during maintenance or consolidation for NHL initial presentation. The average time, reported in previous literature, to arrive at a definitive diagnosis for lymphoma which manifested as a toothache was approximately 5 months [5, 15, 16], while that of our case was about 1 month. With comprehensive inspection and prompt treatment, the patient's symptoms resolved, and no recurrence was seen in the following 5 years.

In summary, we described an unusual case of DLBCL-NOS which initially occurred in the left maxillary sinus and was associated with localized endodontic and periapical disease in a 72-year-old male. This report stresses that dentists should be alert to the possibility of malignancy in the maxillary sinus, especially when the patient presents with persistent maxillofacial pain after involved teeth were managed. Early radiological and histological examinations are encouraged to achieve an accurate diagnosis, precise treatments, and a favorable prognosis.

Acknowledgments

This work was supported by the National High-tech R&D Program (863 Program) (grant number: 2015AA033502).

References

[1] K. E. Grimm and D. P. O'Malley, "Aggressive B cell lymphomas in the 2017 revised WHO classification of tumors of hematopoietic and lymphoid tissues," *Annals of Diagnostic Pathology*, vol. 38, pp. 6–10, 2019.

[2] S. Li, K. H. Young, and L. J. Medeiros, "Diffuse large B-cell lymphoma," *Pathology*, vol. 50, no. 1, pp. 74–87, 2018.

[3] Y. Shi, Y. Han, J. Yang et al., "Clinical features and outcomes of diffuse large B-cell lymphoma based on nodal or extranodal primary sites of origin: analysis of 1,085 WHO classified cases in a single institution in China," *Chinese Journal of Cancer Research*, vol. 31, no. 1, pp. 152–161, 2019.

[4] M. Fatahzadeh, "Primary diffuse large B-cell lymphoma of mandible masquerading as a toothache," *Quintessence International*, vol. 51, no. 1, pp. 50–55, 2020.

[5] F. M. Coskunses, U. Cilasun, P. Celik Topcu, and B. Tokuc, "Primary diffuse large B-cell lymphoma of the mandible: a case report," *Gerodontology*, vol. 37, no. 3, pp. 307–311, 2020.

[6] J. M. Dolan, A. DeGraft-Johnson, N. McDonald, B. B. Ward, T. J. Phillips, and S. M. Munz, "Maxillary and mandibular non-Hodgkin lymphoma with concurrent periapical endodontic disease: diagnosis and management," *Journal of Endodontia*, vol. 43, no. 10, pp. 1744–1749, 2017.

[7] M. R. Abdelwahed Hussein, "Non-Hodgkin's lymphoma of the oral cavity and maxillofacial region: a pathologist

viewpoint," *Expert Review of Hematology*, vol. 11, no. 9, pp. 737–748, 2018.

[8] J. V. Bagan, F. Carbonell, M. J. Gómez et al., "Extra-nodal B-cell non-Hodgkin's lymphomas of the head and neck: A study of 68 cases," *American Journal of Otolaryngology*, vol. 36, no. 1, pp. 57–62, 2015.

[9] N. Martinez-Rodriguez, C. Barona Dorado, J. Cortes-Breton Brinkmann, M. Martin Ares, J. Sanz Alonso, and J. M. Martinez-Gonzalez, "Dental considerations in diagnosis of maxillary sinus carcinoma: a patient series of 24 cases," *Journal of the American Dental Association (1939)*, vol. 149, no. 11, pp. 976–982, 2018.

[10] L. F. Schuch, C. C. Vieira, and A. C. Uchoa Vasconcelos, "Malignant lesions mimicking endodontic pathoses lesion: a systematic review," *Journal of Endodontia*, vol. 47, no. 2, pp. 178–188, 2021.

[11] N. Kusuke, M. Custodio, and S. de Sousa, "Oral lesion as the primary diagnosis of non-Hodgkin's lymphoma: a 20-year experience from an oral pathology service and review of the literature," *European Archives of Oto-Rhino-Laryngology*, vol. 276, no. 10, pp. 2873–2879, 2019.

[12] Y. Hassona, G. Almuhaisen, A. Almansour, and C. Scully, "Lymphoma presenting as a toothache: a wolf in sheep's clothing," *BML Case Reports*, vol. 2017, 2017.

[13] C. Sarkozy and L. H. Sehn, "Management of relapsed/refractory DLBCL," *Best Practice & Research. Clinical Haematology*, vol. 31, no. 3, pp. 209–216, 2018.

[14] B. Kubuschok, G. Held, and M. Pfreundschuh, "Management of diffuse large B-cell lymphoma (DLBCL)," *Cancer Treatment and Research*, vol. 165, pp. 271–288, 2015.

[15] B. Webber, M. Webber, and D. Keinan, "Extranodal large B cell lymphoma of the anterior maxilla. Case report and review of literature," *The New York State Dental Journal*, vol. 81, no. 1, pp. 34–38, 2015.

[16] A. Bugshan, J. Kassolis, and J. Basile, "Primary diffuse large B-cell lymphoma of the mandible: case report and review of the literature," *Case Reports Oncology*, vol. 8, no. 3, pp. 451–455, 2015.

A Noval Method for Surgical Removal of the Impacted Mandibular Third Molar: Sartawi Technique

Hassan Sartawi

Department of Dentistry, Al-Haramain Medical Complex, Riyadh, Ahad Rufaidah, Saudi Arabia

Correspondence should be addressed to Hassan Sartawi; dr.hassan.salah@gmail.com

Academic Editor: Darko Macan

Background. The goal of this article is to present and evaluate the clinical effectiveness of a new surgical approach using a triangular flap with slight modification and a 3-0 black braided silk surgical suture as flap retractor which is later used after the surgical procedure as a normal suture, aiming to decrease procedure time, soft tissue retraction, and tools for removal of impacted mandibular third molar. *Methods.* Patients requiring removal of fully impacted or semi-impacted lower third molars are treated with a new approach using minimal steps and tools, a simple triangular flap, slight mucoperiosteum elevation, as the flap sides are secured and reflected with a silk suture by an assistant holding both sides of the suture from behind the patient. *Results.* The surgical area at the procedure was efficiently exposed, and the separation of the crown from the roots was easily done using a surgical handpiece, separation and removal of the crown, removal of the roots with a straight elevator, without the need of flap retractor or overexposure of the surgical side with a conventional triangular flap or others. After the treatment, the two sides of suture are tied together with double overhand knots, and the surgical site was fully repositioned and closed without any complications. 5- and 7-day follow-up was done on the patients, and no complications were reported. *Conclusions.* This preliminary study presents a new surgical approach (Sartawi technique) which can be used during extraction of impacted and semi-impacted lower third molars, the results showed that the operation time was noticeably reduced, the size of exposed mucoperiosteum tissue was minimized compared to the conventional method, the use of the mucoperiosteum elevator was eliminated, and number of suture knots and suture used to close the surgical site reduced to a single stitch.

1. Introduction

Impaction is defined as the inability of a specific tooth to maintain its right position in the jaw due to malposition, lack of space, or other impediments [1]. Another definition is tooth that fails to erupt into the dental arch within the expected time [2]. In 2004, another definition was introduced by Farman: teeth that prevented from eruption due to a physical barrier with the path of eruption [3].

Despite major advances in the practice of dentistry, extraction of impacted third molars still carries risks of intra- and postsurgical complications. The compilation rate of 4.6-30.9% following the extraction of third molars is reported in the literature [4–8], which may occur intraoperatively or develop during the postoperative period.

An understanding of anatomical features of the surrounding structures and causes of extraction complications of the impacted tooth is important for the performance of proper extraction with minimal risk of complications. Extraction techniques using proper surgical protocols and correct technical approach permit efficient extraction procedures and decrease intraoperative complications which may include bleeding, damage to adjacent teeth, injury to surrounding tissues, displacement of teeth into adjacent spaces, fracture of the root, maxillary tuberosity, or the mandible. Postoperative complications may include swelling, pain, trismus, prolonged bleeding, dry socket, infection, and sensory alteration of the inferior alveolar nerve or lingual nerve.

The extractions of impacted mandibular third molars are one of the most common complaints that require surgical intervention [9, 10]. The aim of this preliminary study is to present a simplified version compared to the traditional techniques atraumatic as possible in minimal amount of time, which could lead to a significant impact on intra- and post-surgical complications.

2. Material and Methods

Study samples: a total of two patients suffering from mesioangular impacted left mandibular third molars were treated using this technique.

The patients' cases were recorded and reported in this case study as follows. A 24 years old male patient (case 1) and 26-year-old male patient (case 2) presented to the clinic suffering from continuous pain in the mandibular left region, none of them reported any past medical history or systemic diseases, conventional X-ray examination (panoramic and periapical) showed mesioangular impaction of the left mandibular third molar with slight resorption in the distal root of the second molar (Figures 1 and 2), and both cases were indicated for surgical removal of the impacted third molar.

Signed consent forms were taken from the two patients, and the method was performed in accordance with the relevant guidelines and regulations.

Ethical approval was obtained from the Ethics Committee of Al-Haramain Medical Complex, Ahd Rofidah, Saudia Arabia.

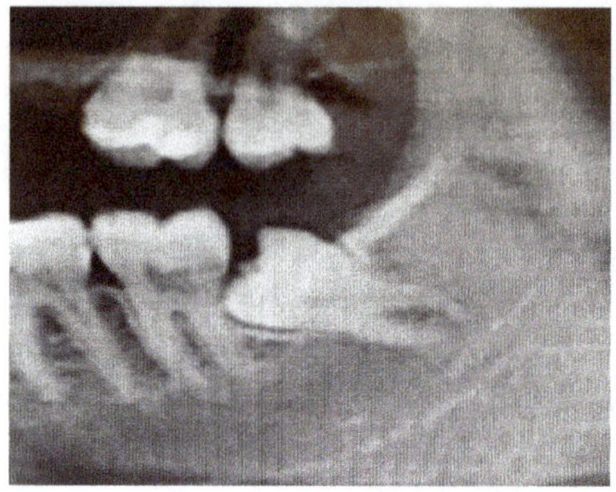

Figure 1: X-ray case 1.

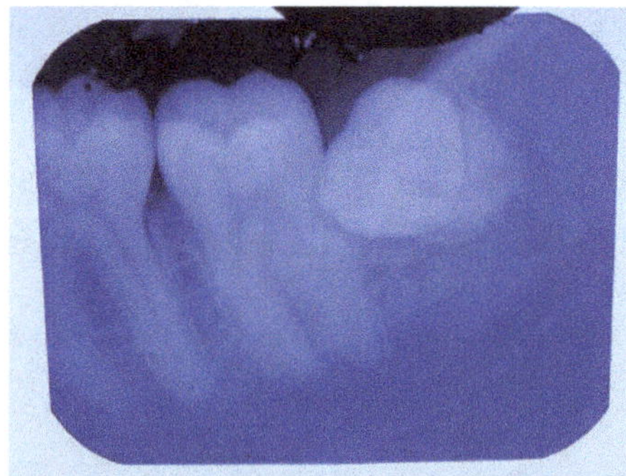

Figure 2: X-ray case 2.

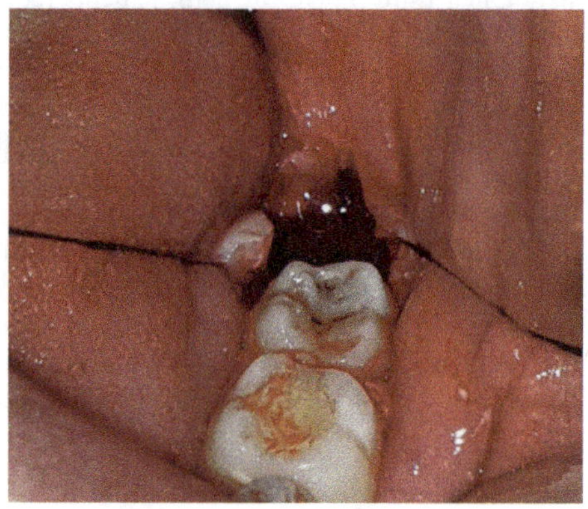

Figure 3: Intraoperative case 1.

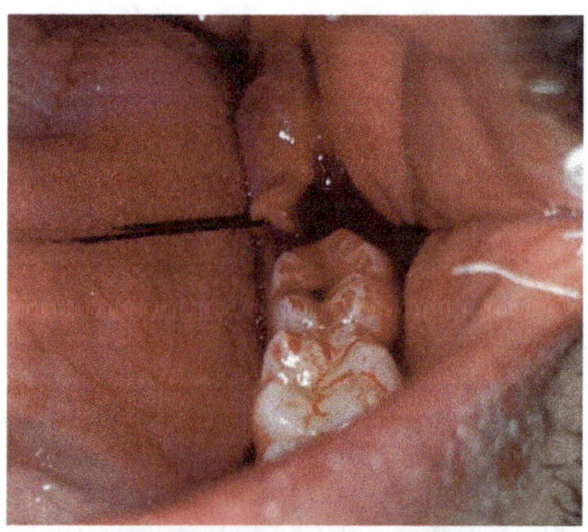

Figure 4: Intraoperative case 2.

2.1. Surgical Method. Step 1: anesthesia: inferior alveolar nerve block, buccal nerve block, lingual nerve block, and local infiltration for homeostasis in the surgical field with 2% lidocaine hydrochloride were administered (1 : 200000 epinephrine).

Step 2: gaining access to the impacted tooth: incision for a triangular flap extending to the middle buccal gingival sulcus of the mandibular second molar with surgical blade and slightly reflected from both incision sites enough to expose the crown using mucoperiosteum elevator.

Step 3: Sartawi's technique part 1: two 30 cm 3/0 silk surgical threads were used. One was inserted into the buccal side of the flap in the middle point of the flap line distally to the second molar and passed outside the mouth to the left side of the patient; meanwhile, the other was inserted into the lingual side of the flap in the middle point of the flap line and passed outside the mouth to the right side of the patient (Figures 3 and 4).

Step 4: Sartawi's technique part 2: two weaves of gauze were placed at both corners of the mouth to protect it from the pulling friction of the silk thread from behind the patient. The assistant pulled the threads from both sides to compensate for a flap retractor (Figure 5).

Step 5: bone Removal and tooth sectioning using surgical drill and a straight elevator used to luxate and remove the roots, the teeth were extracted (Figures 6 and 7), and the socket was irrigated with normal saline, and bony irregularities were corrected.

Step 6: Sartawi's technique part 3: both surgical threads mentioned in step 3 were tied in a double overhand knot

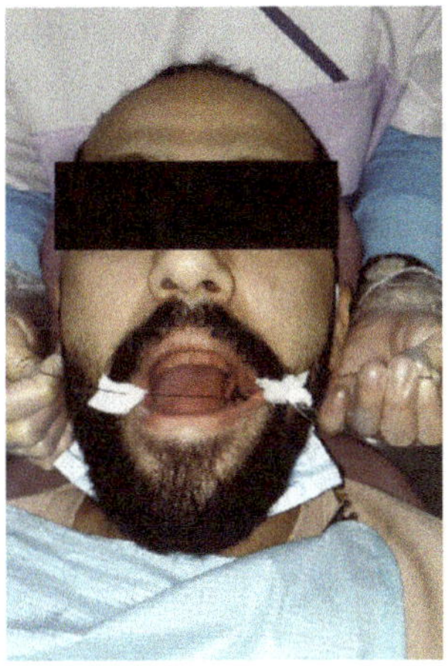

FIGURE 5: Intraoperative.

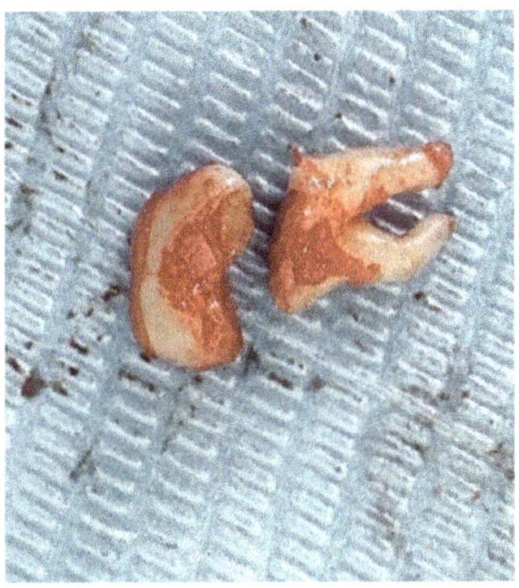

FIGURE 6: Extracted tooth case 1.

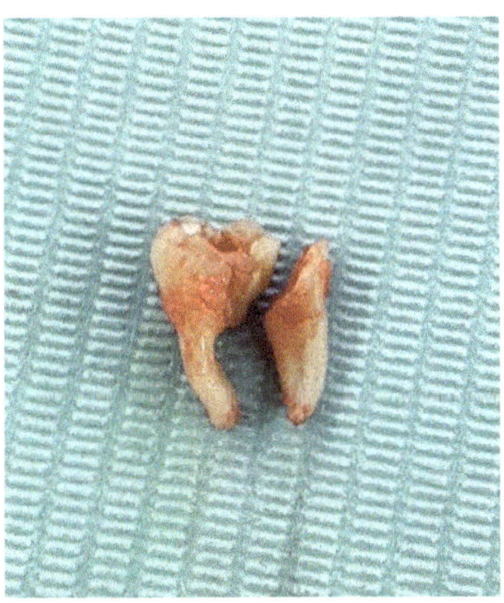

FIGURE 7: Extracted tooth case 2.

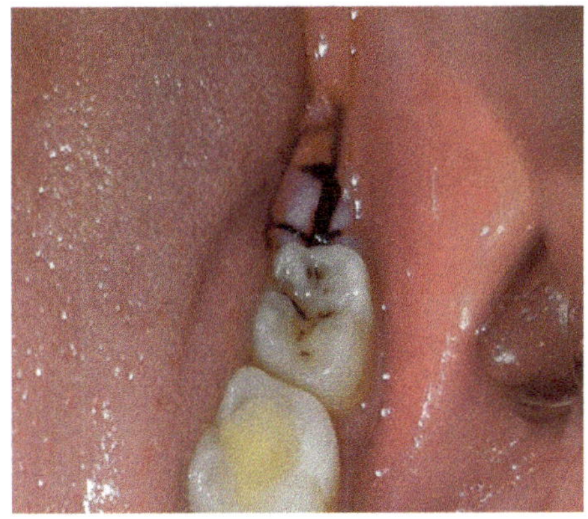

FIGURE 8: Postoperative case 1.

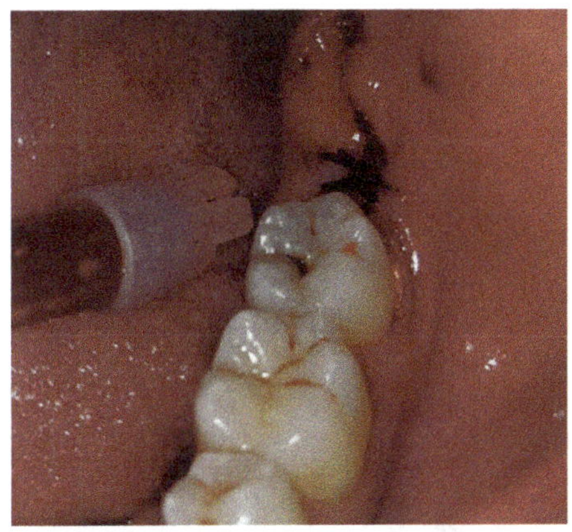

FIGURE 9: Postoperative case 2.

causing complete closure of the surgical site, not requiring any further stitches (Figures 8 and 9).

Following the procedure, detailed postoperative instructions were given to the patients, and suitable antibiotics and analgesics were prescribed.

Slight postoperative bleeding was noticed immediately after the procedure was completed, which was managed with pressure packs.

2.2. Postoperative Follow-Up. Both patients presented to the clinic 5 days after the surgical procedure for the follow-up process. and none of them reported any complications; except in case one, patient reported white discoloration at the surgical site and was found to be a slight food particle stagnation (Figures 10 and 11).

at 7 days which both patients presented for removal of the stitches, and complete tissue healing was noticed.

3. Discussion

There are several intraoperative and postoperative complications that might occur during and after the extraction of the impacted mandibular third molar which can be reduced by understanding the possible causes and how to prevent each of these complications; the Sartawi technique focused on four major causes and ways to prevent it, and those four major causes are instruments, flap design, suture stitches, and time.

Less the number of oral surgical instruments, such as flap retractor, used in oral cavity operations would decrease the possibility of tissue trauma and buccal and lingual nerve damage [11, 12] as well as decreasing the possibility of

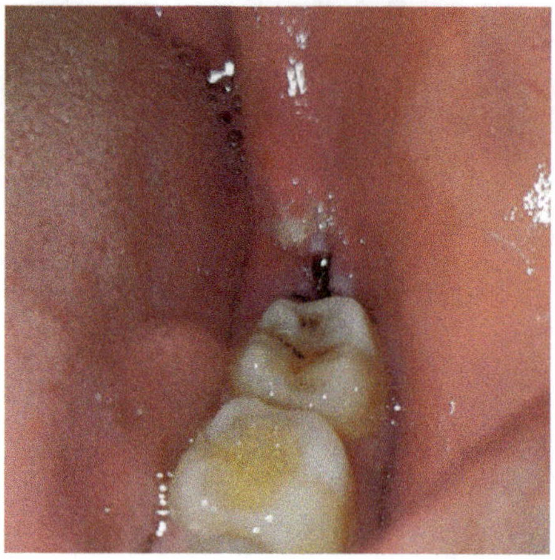

FIGURE 10: 5 days follow-up case 1.

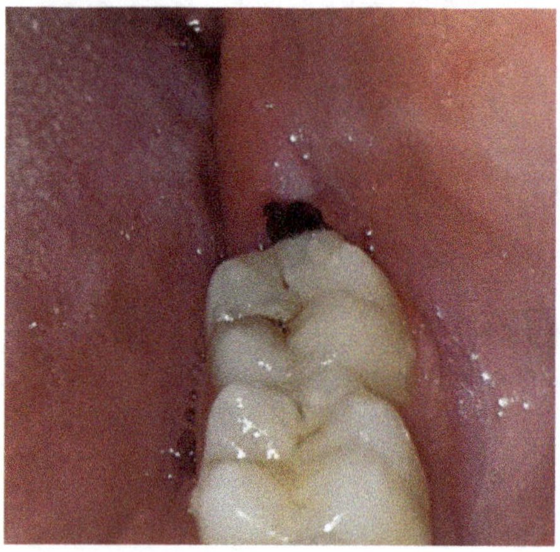

FIGURE 11: 5 days follow-up case 2.

infection caused by the instruments used, and the Sartawi technique limits the abovementioned risks as the flap retractor is totally eliminated from the surgical procedure.

There are variable styles of flap design used in the removal of the impacted mandibular third molar, mainly envelop and triangular flaps, and their modification has been developed to minimize those complications; the triangular flap design is associated with patients consuming the least pain killer [13]; therefore, in the Sartawi technique, the flap used was a triangular flap with a slight modification that leads to minimize mucoperiosteum elevation.

Number of stitches has a significant effect on the postsurgical complications, where more stitches can lead to accumulation of food, causing infections and halitosis. There are no specific data available on the correlation between the number of stitches/knots and their effect on wound healing; however, barbed suture (knotless) is considered a safe and efficient alternative to conventional stitches for the suturing of free flaps to the local tissue [14], thereby it can be quoted that using lesser knots leads to better healing and consecutively lesser complications; in the Sartawi technique after the suture is used as a flap retractor, the two sides are brought together in a double overhand knot and cause complete closure of the surgical flap with a single double knot stitch.

The time of the operation and postsurgical complications have a direct correlation, where increasing the operating time is associated with more postoperative morbidity [15], and the duration of surgery affected the acute postoperative symptoms and signs after the lower third molar extraction [16], and in the Sartawi technique, the time of the surgical operation is reduced dramatically which leads to less intra- and postsurgical complications.

Nevertheless, there are some limitations and drawbacks for the Sartawi technique, mainly the need for a second assistant as the first one's hands are full holding the threads retracting the flap. The operating field is smaller compared to the conventional method and causes less control for the surgeons performing it and can only mastered if the surgeon is well experienced with the conventional methods. The study samples were limited to 2 patients with mesioangular impaction and was not performed on patients with other types of anatomical impaction positions.

4. Conclusion

According to this preliminary study, the use of this technique was tolerated by the two patients, and they did not have any intra- or postoperative complications; the steps are easily done by an experienced oral surgeon familiar with the conventional surgical protocols of impacted mandibular third molar surgery; however. larger studies are needed to evaluate significance and the quality of this technique as this technique is worthy of clinical promotions.

Acknowledgments

Thanks are due to Al-Haramain Medical Group owners, doctors, and staff for their support and encouragement to record this study and publish it and all the nurses who assisted in the surgical procedures and special thanks are due to Dr. Marwan Mohammed for his academic guidance throughout the publication process and Dr. Mahdiah Sartawi who did the proofreading of this article.

References

[1] W. H. Archer, *Oral Surgery: A Step-by-Step Atlas of Operative Techniques*, W.B. Saunders Company, Philadelphia, PA, USA, 4th edition, 1966.

[2] L. J. Peterson, "Principles of Management of Impacted Teeth," in *Contemporary Oral and Maxillofacial Surgery*, L. J. Peterson, E. Ellis III, J. R. Hupp, and M. R. Tuker, Eds., pp. 215–248, Mosby, St. Louis, MO, USA, 3rd edition, 1998.

[3] K. N. Agarwal, R. Gupta, M. M. Faridi, and N. Kalra, "Permanent dentition in Delhi boys of age 5-14 years," *Indian Pediatrics*, vol. 41, no. 10, pp. 1031–1035, 2004.

[4] G. F. Bouloux, M. B. Steed, and V. J. Perciaccante, "Complications of third molar surgery," *Oral and Maxillofacial Surgery Clinics of North America*, vol. 19, no. 1, pp. 117–128, 2007.

[5] C. H. Bui, E. B. Seldin, and T. B. Dodson, "Types, frequencies, and risk factors for complications after third molar extraction," *Journal of Oral and Maxillofacial Surgery*, vol. 61, no. 12, pp. 1379–1389, 2003.

[6] M. Chiapasco, L. De Cicco, and G. Marrone, "Side effects and complications associated with third molar surgery," *Oral Surgery, Oral Medicine, and Oral Pathology*, vol. 76, no. 4, pp. 412–420, 1993.

[7] R. H. Haug, D. H. Perrott, M. L. Gonzalez, and R. M. Talwar, "The American Association of Oral and Maxillofacial Surgeons age-related third molar study," *Journal of Oral and Maxillofacial Surgery*, vol. 63, no. 8, pp. 1106–1114, 2005.

[8] A. L. Sisk, W. B. Hammer, D. W. Shelton, and E. D. Joy, "complications following removal of impacted third molars: the role of the experience of the surgeon," *Journal of Oral and Maxillofacial Surgery*, vol. 44, no. 11, pp. 855–859, 1986.

[9] O. Breik and D. Grubor, "The incidence of mandibular third molar impactions in different skeletal face types," *Australian Dental Journal*, vol. 53, no. 4, pp. 320–324, 2008.

[10] S. Šečić, S. Prohić, S. Komšić, and A. Vuković, "Incidence of impacted mandibular third molars in population of Bosnia and Herzegovina: a retrospective radiographic study," *Journal of Health Science*, vol. 3, no. 2, pp. 151–158, 2013.

[11] E. Valmaseda-Castellón, L. Berini-Aytés, and C. Gay-Escoda, "Lingual nerve damage after third lower molar surgical extraction," *Oral Surgery, Oral Medicine, Oral Pathology, Oral Radiology, and Endodontics*, vol. 90, no. 5, pp. 567–573, 2000.

[12] J. W. Pichler and O. R. Beirne, "Lingual flap retraction and prevention of lingual nerve damage associated with third molar surgery: a systematic review of the literature," *Oral Surgery, Oral Medicine, Oral Pathology, Oral Radiology, and Endodontics*, vol. 91, no. 4, pp. 395–401, 2001.

[13] G. B. Grossi, C. Maiorana, R. A. Garramone, A. Borgonovo, L. Creminelli, and F. Santoro, "Assessing postoperative discomfort after third molar surgery: a prospective study," *Journal of Oral and Maxillofacial Surgery*, vol. 65, no. 5, pp. 901–917, 2007.

[14] E. Crosetti, A. Caracciolo, G. Arrigoni, E. Delmastro, and G. Succo, "Barbed suture in oral cavity reconstruction: preliminary results," *Acta Otorhinolaryngologica Italica*, vol. 39, no. 5, pp. 308–315, 2019.

[15] S. A. Bello, W. L. Adeyemo, B. O. Bamgbose, E. V. Obi, and A. A. Adeyinka, "Effect of age, impaction types and operative time on inflammatory tissue reactions following lower third molar surgery," *Head & Face Medicine*, vol. 7, no. 1, p. 8, 2011.

[16] N. Mobilio, R. Vecchiatini, M. Vasquez, G. Calura, and S. Catapano, "Effect of flap design and duration of surgery on acute postoperative symptoms and signs after extraction of lower third molars: a randomized prospective study," *Journal of Dental Research, Dental Clinics, Dental Prospects*, vol. 11, no. 3, pp. 156–160, 2017.

8

Periostitis Ossificans: Report of Two Cases Resolved with Endodontic Treatment

Hana Bougatef, [1,2] **Eya Moussaoui**, [1,2] **Ines Kallel**, [1,2] **Mahmoud Smaoui**, [1,2] **Lamia Oualha**, [1,2] **and Nabiha Douki** [1,2]

[1]*Department of Dental Medicine, EPS Sahloul, Sousse, Tunisia*
[2]*Faculty of Dental Medicine, Oral Health and Oro-Facial Rehabilitation Laboratory Research (LR12ES11), University of Monastir, 5019 Monastir, Tunisia*

Correspondence should be addressed to Hana Bougatef; bougatef.hana@hotmail.com

Academic Editor: Darko Macan

Periostitis ossificans is a chronic disease characterized by an ossifying periostitis, occurring in children and young adults, commonly as a reaction to a mild infection or irritation. It is also characterized by the presence of lamellae of newly formed periosteal bone outside the cortex, giving the characteristic radiographic appearance of "onion skin." *Aim.* The aim of this paper was to present the clinical and radiographic findings, as well as the postoperative follow-up of two cases diagnosed with periostitis ossificans of dental origin, and to discuss the differential diagnosis and treatment modalities. *Case Reports.* In the first case, a 16-year-old adolescent was referred for a persistent mandibular swelling. Intraoral examination showed two sinus tracts in relation to the carious necrotic left mandibular first molar. The periapical radiograph showed a periapical lesion in relation to the two root canals of the left mandibular first molar. Occlusal radiographs revealed the "onion skin" bone formation aspect. In the second case, a 10-year-old girl presented to our department with a slightly painful mandibular swelling. The periapical radiograph showed a periapical lesion in relation to both the mesial and distal roots of the carious necrotic right mandibular first molar. Cone beam computed tomography (CBCT) showed a subperiosteal bone formation with an "onion skin" aspect. Diagnosis of periostitis ossificans in the two cases was confirmed and the lesion was resolved by simply an endodontic treatment. *Conclusion.* Specific attention should be given to clinical and radiographic exploration in case of children with mandibular swelling. As osteosarcoma can be misdiagnosed, additional examinations, such as computed tomography, can be useful in differential diagnosis and in searching malignancy signs.

1. Introduction

Periostitis ossificans is a specific type of chronic sclerotic osteomyelitis, primarily affecting children and adolescents. It is characterized by a rigid bony swelling at the periphery of the jaw following a low-grade chronic odontogenic infection [1–4].

It is also known as Garre's osteomyelitis and chronic osteomyelitis with proliferative periostitis [5].

This pathological entity was first described by Carl Garré in 1893 as an irritation-inducing focal thickening of the periosteum and the cortical bone of the tibia [6].

Periostitis ossificans generally affects children and young adults. It is commonly associated with an infection of low virulence, such as odontogenic infection resulting from dental caries, mild periodontitis, dental eruption, or complication due to dental extraction [4, 7]. It affects the mandible much more commonly than the maxilla.

During the early period, a thin crust-like convex layer appears over the cortex. It is considered as a pathognomonic feature [4, 8, 9].

In this work, the clinical and radiographic findings of two cases diagnosed with periostitis ossificans of dental infection origin are presented. The differential diagnosis and treatment modalities are also discussed.

2. Case Reports

2.1. Case No. 1. A 16-year-old adolescent was referred to our department for a mandibular swelling persisting for two months. The patient had received an antibiotherapy for 7 days (Augmentin®). The patient's medical history was not contributing.

Extraoral inspection showed facial asymmetry due to firm, nontender 1.0 × 1.5 cm mass over the lateral aspect of the left mandibular region. The overlying skin was unremarkable, and no fluctuance or discharge was noted (Figure 1).

There was no lymphadenopathy, and the patient was afebrile.

Intraoral examination showed two sinus tracts in relation to the carious left mandibular first molar, which was painful at axial and transversal percussions, with no mobility (Figures 2(a) and 2(b)).

The tooth was necrotic with sista 2.4 classified carious lesion. The periapical radiograph showed a periapical lesion in relation to the two root canals of the left mandibular first molar (Figure 3(a)).

The sinus tract was traced with a gutta-percha point, leading to the left mandibular first molar as shown in the periapical radiograph (Figure 3(a)).

Occlusal radiographs revealed an "onion skin" bone formation aspect (Figure 3(b)).

CBCT was not possible due to the patient's limited financial means.

Diagnosis of periostitis ossificans was confirmed by the clinical and radiographic features, as well as the causal relationship with endodontic infection.

A complete endodontic treatment was performed in only one session without further antibiotherapy.

The sinus tract disappeared in only one week (Figure 4).

Regular follow-up, during 8 months, revealed clinical healing after 4 months with disappearance of mandibular swelling (Figure 5(a)), periapical lesion regression after 8 months (Figure 5(b)), and disappearance of periosteal reaction after 4 months (Figure 5(c)).

2.2. Case No. 2. A 10-year-old girl presented with a painful swelling of the right lateral and posterior mandibular region. As described by the patient's parents, swelling was progressive over five months.

Extraoral inspection showed facial asymmetry due to hard, nontender swelling in the right mandibular region.

Intraoral examination showed swelling and redness at the bottom of the vestibule in relation to the right mandibular first molar.

A temporary coronal filling was present on the tooth. It was painful at axial and transversal percussions.

The periapical radiograph showed an open pulp chamber with temporary coronal filling and a well-limited radiolucent periapical image unilocular in relation to both the mesial and distal root of the right mandibular first molar (Figure 6).

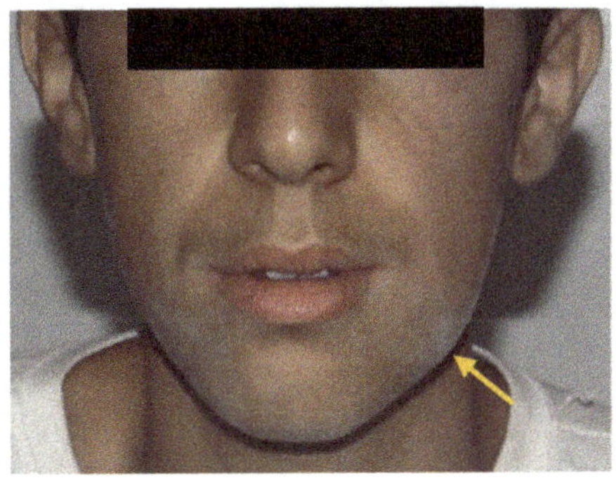

FIGURE 1: Extraoral examination revealed a left mandibular swelling.

The axial section in CBCT examination revealed the presence of about 3 lamellae of newly formed periosteal bone in the lateral and medial cortices, giving the characteristic of an "onion skin" appearance with cortical rupture in relation to the distal root (Figures 7(a)–7(c)).

This was also confirmed by 3D reconstruction (Figure 8). This pathognomonic sign confirmed the diagnosis of periostitis ossificans associated with an odontogenic infection of the right mandibular first molar.

In the first appointment, a pulp stone was found in the access cavity center, arguing in favor of a chronic and slow irritative phenomenon: silent necrosis. In fact, the patient did not report any pain history (Figure 9(a)). It was eliminated with ultrasonic tips (Figure 9(b)).

Root canal shaping with abundant sodium hypochlorite irrigation was carried out and endodontic medication using calcium hydroxide was placed for two weeks.

In the second and last appointment, root canal filling with gutta percha and zinc oxide eugenol as an endodontic sealer using the lateral condensation method was carried out.

The treatment was followed by clinical and radiographic monitoring after 2, 4, 8, and 12 months.

At the 4-month follow-up, the periapical radiograph showed signs of bone healing in the periapical region (Figure 10(a)).

The occlusal radiograph showed partial disappearance of external and internal bone formation (Figure 10(b)).

At the 8-month follow-up, the periapical radiograph showed a reduction of more than half of the primary periapical lesion size (Figure 11(a)). The occlusal radiograph revealed total healing of the periostal reaction (Figure 11(b)).

Complete bone healing was seen in the periapical radiographs with total disappearance of periapical radiolucency at the 12-month follow-up (Figure 11(c)).

After 20 months, complete bone healing was still observed in the periapical radiograph, and the tooth was asymptomatic and functional (Figure 12).

3. Discussion

Periostitis ossificans refers to the diagnosis of periostitis with subperiosteal bone formation. It is also known as proliferative periostitis, characterized by reactive bone expansion as

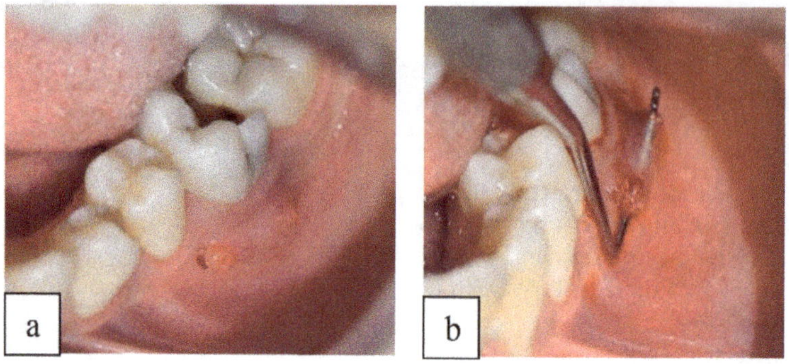

(a) (b)

Figure 2: (a) A penetrating carious lesion in the first left mandibular molar. (b) Two sinus tract in relation with the first left mandibular molar.

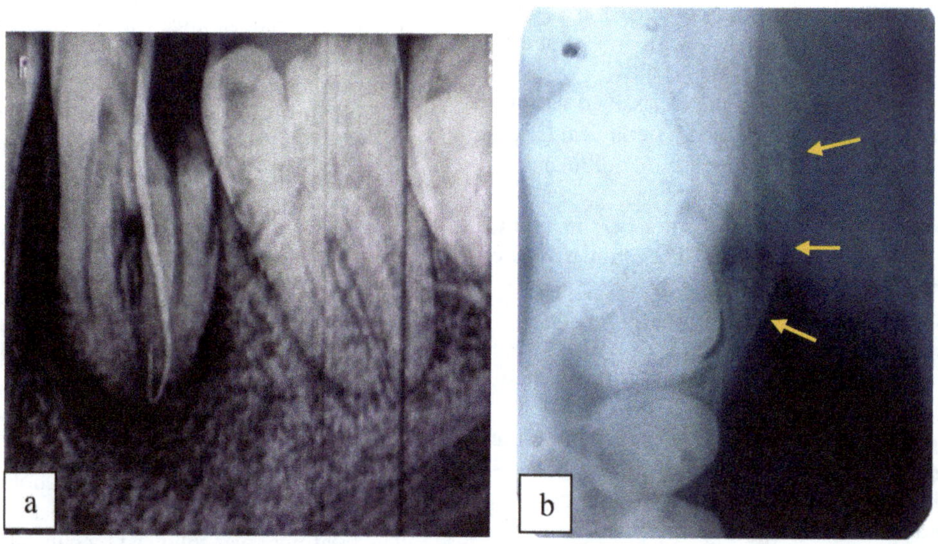

(a) (b)

Figure 3: (a) Periapical radiograph revealed a not limited periapical lesion. (b) Occlusal radiograph revealed a periostitis reaction in relation with the external cortex.

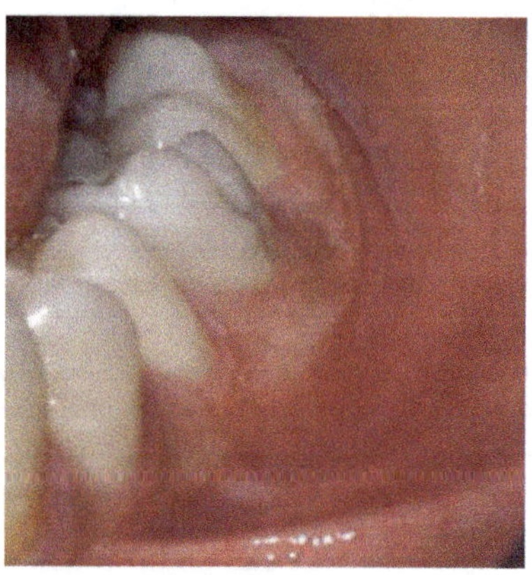

Figure 4: Sinus tract disappearance after 1 week.

a result of rigid bony swelling at the periphery of the jaw following a chronic low-grade infection [1, 10].

It commonly occurs in children and young adults when the osteoblastic activity of the periosteum is at its peak [10]. It more often affects the mandible than the maxilla [4].

3.1. Ethiopathogeny and Diagnosis. In our cases, the causative agent was a pulp necrosis of the lower first molar associated with a chronic periapical infection in the two young patients.

It may be speculated that the following steps took place. A carious lesion in the mandibular first molar infected the pulp, and then it progressed to the periapical region. It extended through the cancellous bone and then through the cortical bone on the lateral aspect of the mandible. Later, the inflammatory process spread and applied pressure to the periosteum, being irritated by noxious stimuli. The periosteal osteoblasts were stimulated to form the initial bone.

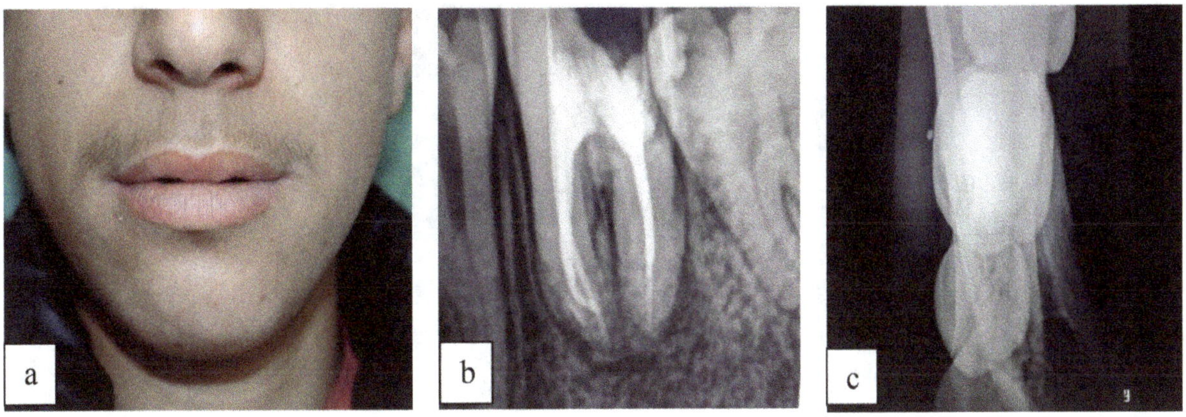

(a) (b) (b)

FIGURE 5: (a) Clinical healing after 4 months with extraoral swelling disappearance. (b) Periapical radiographic control after 8 months showed periapical lesion regression. (c) Occlusal radiograph showed periostitis disappearance after 4 months.

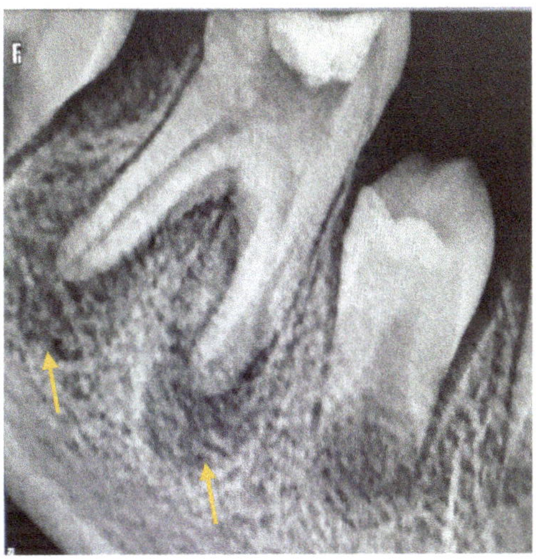

FIGURE 6: First mandibular molar with periapical lesions appended to the two root apices.

With episodic stimuli, bone formation continued in the form of successive layers of new bone [1, 11].

The swelling size may vary from 1 to 2 cm to reach the entire length of the jaw on the affected side. The thickness of the newly formed bone can reach 2-3 cm [7].

Gradually, the cortex thickens as a result of successive new bone deposits. This lamellar structure is referred to as an "onion skin" aspect on radiographs [4, 8, 9].

The number of laminations varies from 1 to 12. Radiolucent separation is present between the new bone and the original cortex. Within the new bone, areas of small sequestra or osteolytic radiolucencies may also be found [3, 12].

The patient's medical history usually reveals an episodic pain with dormant periods and progressive swelling. Those may be the only symptoms, but subjective signs may be variable.

The degree and duration of the symptoms depend on various factors, such as the virulence of the causative organisms, the presence of underlying diseases, and the immune status of the host [13].

This progressive evolution reveals the benign nature of this pathology, being unlike the malignant one, often characterized with a fast evolution of symptoms [14].

In our cases, the two patients presented a history of intermittent dental pain. The first patient was referred for persistent mandibular swelling, evolving for two months. The second one presented with a localized swelling, evolving for five months, according to his parents.

Clinically, this is usually manifested by facial asymmetry caused by localized unilateral mandibular hard swelling, which can be seen and it is palpable both in the extraoral and intraoral examination.

The overlying skin appears normal. Trismus and lymphadenopathy can be observed [15].

Attention should be given to the objective symptoms that are not associated with signs of malignancy, such as dental mobility, hypoesthesia, dental displacement, and severe trismus [14].

At the clinical examination, our patients presented with a small and well-limited mandibular swelling in the posterior region with neither trismus nor lymphadenopathy. The intraoral examination revealed hard swelling in the bottom of the vestibule related to the first mandibular molar. The mucosa was erythematous.

In the first case, two sinus tracts were present. The left mandibular first molar presented a carious lesion sista 2.4 and was painful at axial and transversal percussions. In the second case, the right mandibular first molar presented an incomplete endodontic treatment with occlusal temporary coronal filling.

The patients' age as well as the clinical aspect led to the diagnosis of periostitis ossificans. Ewing sarcoma and osteosarcoma, occurring at the same age, were also possible diagnoses. So, radiographic examinations were necessary to confirm the right diagnosis.

Periapical radiograph can confirm a dental low-grade infection with the presence of apical radiolucency, bone loss, marginal cyst, or extraction site.

Occlusal radiograph can explore the horizontal dimension of the jaws. Thus, if well-performed, it shows the thickened bone with lateral and/or internal periostal reaction [15].

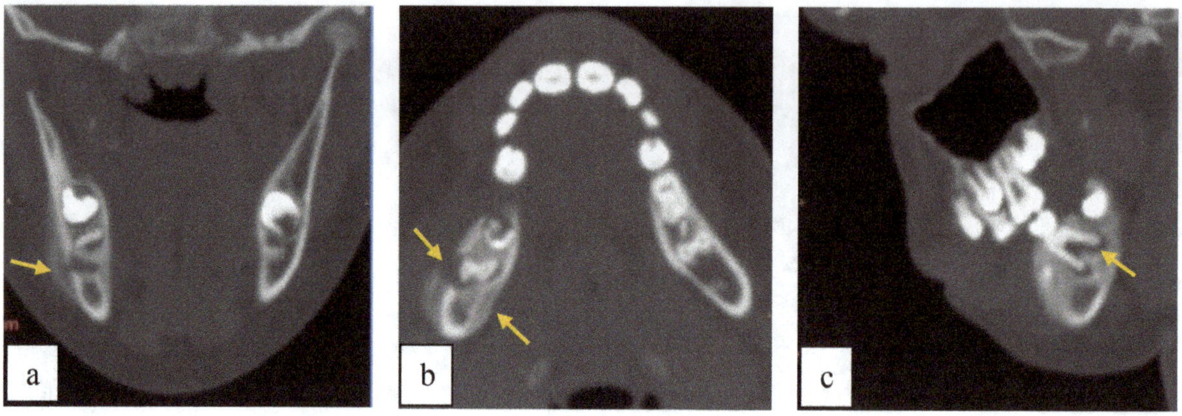

(a) (b) (c)

FIGURE 7: Computed tomography exam: (a) Coronal section showing "onion skin" aspect of lateral periostitis and the radiolucency in relation with first molar's roots. (b) Axial section showing periostitis in both external and internal mandibular cortex with lateral rupture of the cortical. (c) Sagittal section showing radiolucency in relation with first molar's roots.

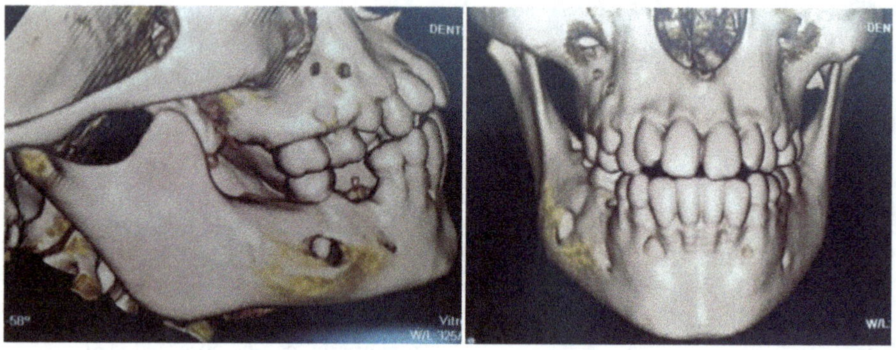

FIGURE 8: 3D reconstruction showing the bone formation associated with cortical's rupture.

In fact, occlusal radiographs are necessary and they may aid in establishing a diagnosis. In case of periostitis ossificans, this radiograph clearly shows the periostal reaction, characterized by a number of lamellae blowing the external jaw cortical. This is a pathognomonic radiological feature, known as the "onion skin" aspect.

However, 3D radiographic examinations is highly indicated to explore the local extension of the disease, its relationship to the anatomic structures, and its exact characteristic like density, limits, and size.

Maxillary CT scan can distinguish between the two types of periostitis: the "onion skin" aspect as a sign of benignity and the "sun ray" aspect as a sign of malignancy [16].

CBCT, being less expensive with lower dose of radiation, is also useful to show the "onion skin" aspect of the periosteal reaction on the axial and coronal sections [16].

In the first case, preoperative radiographs showed a deep carious lesion penetrating in the pulp chamber in relation to the left mandibular first molar with a well-limited radiolucent periapical image unilocular in relation to both the mesial and distal tooth root.

Due to the patient's limited financial conditions, only an occlusal radiograph was performed to confirm our diagnosis, and it showed the "onion skin" aspect of the periosteal reaction.

In the second case, preoperative radiographs showed an opened access cavity having temporary coronal filling with a periapical lesion.

As the patient had already performed a CBCT imaging, occlusal radiographs were only useful for follow-up and monitoring. They were used to see the external cortical aspect, the regression of bone formation, the healing sign, and the favorable evolution.

In the CT scan, the axial and coronal sections showed a localized bone formation with an "onion skin" aspect, a sign of benignity, and a pathognomonic feature of periostitis ossificans.

3.2. Differential Diagnosis. Periostitis ossificans should be distinguished from benign and malignant pathologies causing bone formation. Most of them usually develop in the same age range [4, 8, 17].

Ewing's sarcoma and osteosarcoma occur in the same age presenting with hard swelling, similar to periostitis ossificans. However, they can be distinguished from periostitis ossificans by the clinical complications (dental mobility, facial neuralgia, and lip paresthesia) and the radiological "sun

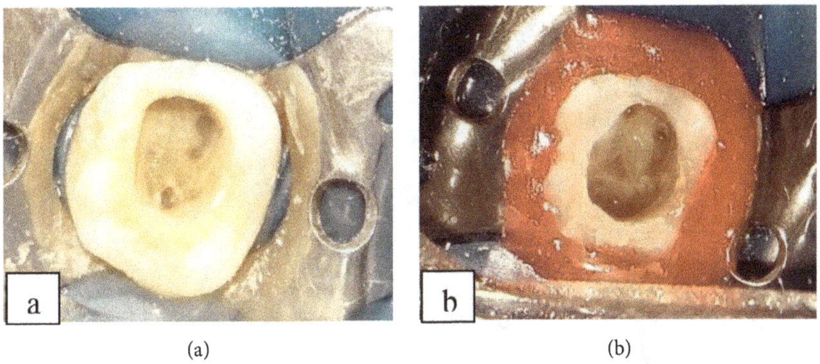

FIGURE 9: (a) Pulp stone in the chamber obliterating canal orifices. (b) Widen the canal orifices with ultrasonic tips.

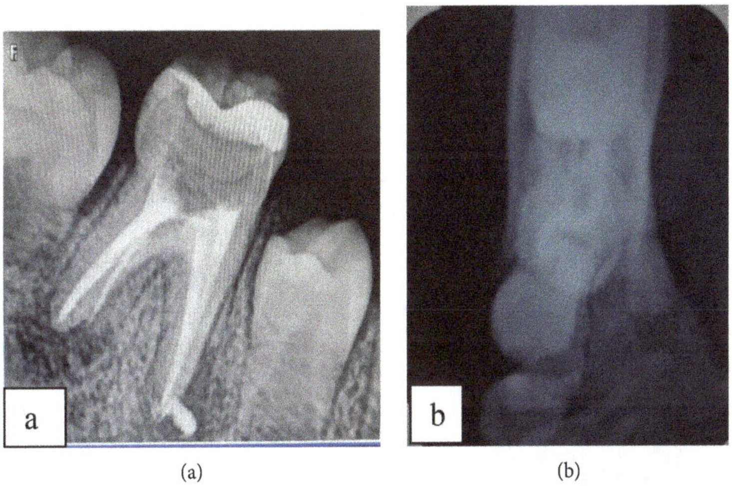

FIGURE 10: (a) Postoperative periapical radiograph after 4 months with signs of bone healing. (b) Occlusal radiograph after 4 months: partial disappearance of the periostitis.

ray" aspect, causing very rapid bone enlargement and more osteolytic reactions in the bone [2, 18].

Fibrous dysplasia should have been included in the differential diagnosis. It is classified as bone-related lesions [19].

The symptoms of fibrous dysplasia and periostitis ossificans may be clinically indistinguishable [8, 20].

It can be seen at an early age, and the bone proliferation is similar to periostitis in both shape and volume. However, fibrous dysplasia is distinguished by the radiographic aspect of "ground glass appearance" as well as the cortex thinning [2, 4, 8].

Caffey disease is a genetic bone disorder that could have the same appearance of an "onion skin" as periostitis ossificans. However, it is distinguished from periostitis ossificans by the early age of onset (prior to two years of age). It is more common in the ramus and the mandiblar angulus region with bilateral involvement and occurrence in multiple bones [2].

Primary chronic osteomyelitis (PCO) is an uncommon nonbacterial chronic inflammatory disease of unknown etiology. It can be associated with other conditions, such as autoimmune diseases and syndromes, including Majeed syndrome, cherubism, and "SAPHO (Synovitis, Acne, Pustulosis, Hyperostosis, and Osteitis) syndrome" [21].

PCO of the jaw has been reported in children. The mandible is the most affected site in the maxillofacial region. Clinically, it is characterized by acute pain and aseptic swelling.

Radiological examination reveals the presence of radiolucent areas combined with progressive osteosclerosis and laminations of the periosteum, without the presence of a dental origin [22].

Primary tuberculous osteomyelitis is a rare form of osteomyelitis caused by tuberculosis. In children, the mandibular region is very unlikely to have higher frequency compared to the maxilla.

Clinically, it is characterized by pain, swelling, and discharge through the intra or extraoral sinus tract. Radiographically, it appears as blur radiolucency with erosion of the cortex. The bone is gradually replaced by granulomatous tissue.

Pathologically, diagnosis can be confirmed by the presence of tuberculous granulomas [23, 24].

In our cases, mild odontogenic infection was a proven cause. The clinical examination (slow evolution, absence of dental mobility, and hypoesthesia) and the radiographic aspects, especially the "onion skin" aspect, were sufficient to establish the diagnosis. It was then confirmed by the favorable evolution following treatment.

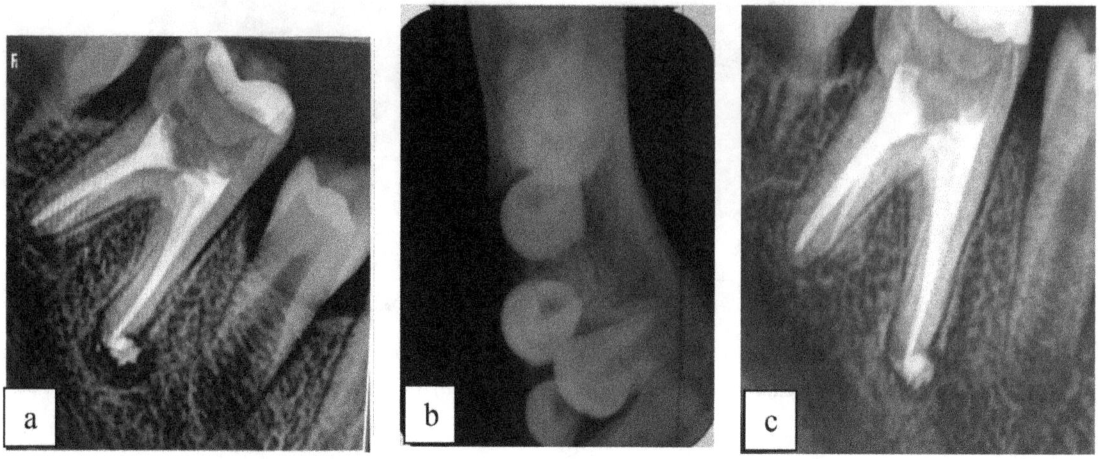

(a) (b) (c)

Figure 11: (a) Reduction of the periapical lesion size on the periapical radiograph after 8 months. (b) Occlusal radiograph showed total resolution of the periostitis after 8 months. (c) Periapical radiograph after 12 months: total regression of the apical radiolucency.

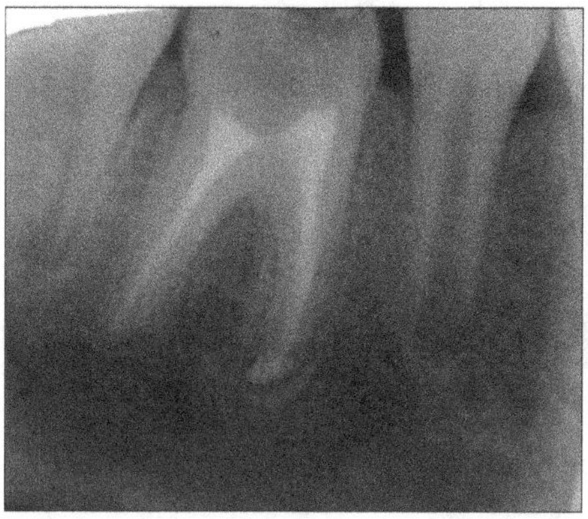

Figure 12: Periapical radiograph after 20 months: total regression of the apical radiolucency.

Often, clinical and radiologic findings are sufficient to establish diagnosis. Yet, histological examinations are sometimes necessary to confirm diagnosis [25–27].

When performed, they reveal a benign fibro-osseous tissue with peripheral osteoblastic activity due to a reactive new bone deposition. New periosteal deposits are parallel to each other with respect to the bone cortex.

Central osteoblasts and osteoclasts are evident. Lymphocytes and plasma cells are found in the marrow space [15].

3.3. Treatment and Evolution. There has always been a dilemma in planning the treatment strategies for periostitis ossificans because of some update in the classification of mandibular osteomyelitis [4].

Periostitis ossificans has long been considered like other types of osteitis that can arise from either local extension or hematogenous spread. For this reason, the treatment plan has been radical for many years, and it has been based on extraction with long term antibiotherapy [28].

With the evolution of diagnostic terms over the years, different opinions appeared regarding the most suitable treatment plan for periostitis ossificans [9].

The treatment plan can be conservative or radical, with or without associated antibiotic therapy [9].

The role of endodontic therapy in the management of periostitis ossificans has been questionable. Batcheldor et al. suggested the possible efficacy of tooth conservation and endodontic intervention [8, 29].

Tooth conservation with an early adequate root canal treatment with or without antibiotherapy has been highlighted in the last few years. In fact, it was proven through some reported cases that endodontic treatment alone is sufficient and able to resolve this pathology.

Even more, hyperbaric oxygen therapy and endodontic treatment have proven to be successful [1, 30, 31].

In the present case reports, endodontic treatment was the treatment of choice due to the patients' young age, the possibility of maintaining the tooth, and the positive attitude of the patients and their parents toward this treatment plan.

The primary challenges of root canal treatment are to eliminate infection, secure healing of the bone lesion, and therefore conserve the tooth [32–34]. Indeed, optimal prognosis depends on the ability to create favorable conditions for adequate healing.

To improve the success rate of endodontic treatment, especially for necrotic teeth, more focus should be put on the chemo-mechanical preparation.

In fact, disinfection of the root canal space is the key to eradicate bacteria within the root canal, leading to periapical healing. This is ensured by both root canal shaping and irrigation [35].

Because of its complexity, the root canal system of a necrotic tooth harbors thousands of microorganisms. They are found especially within a biofilm form, adhering firmly to the dentinal walls and resisting to the irrigation solutions [35].

The strategies recommended for improving disinfection after chemo-mechanical preparation include the use of an interappointment endodontic medication or an optimized one-visit endodontic treatment [36].

Many studies, using microbial culture, have confirmed the advantage of using endodontic medication based on calcium hydroxide to complete root canal disinfection [37].

However, many other studies have proven that the 2-visit protocol involving an interappointment medication together with calcium hydroxide results in an improved microbiological status of the root canal system when compared to the 1-visit protocol. They suggested that residual surviving microorganisms are entombed by root space obturation, and they die due to the absence of nutrients [37].

Yet, this topic is still a subject of debate and some studies have shown controversial conclusions.

In the first case, endodontic treatment was performed in one visit. Root canal filling was carried out using bioceramic sealers for their antibacterial proprieties. Fortunately, the result was satisfying with periapical healing.

In the second case, as the patient did not support long sessions, root canal dressing was placed based on calcium hydroxide during two weeks. This was intended to enhance disinfection.

Concerning the antibiotherapy, according to the literature, there is no consensus about its use as well as the treatment duration, varying from six, eight weeks to twelve months [38].

In our cases, the patients received antibiotherapy (Augmentin®) for seven days. It was given by the child's parents in the first case and by the dentist in the second case. The prescription was not renewed.

The efficacy of nonsteroidal anti-inflammatory drugs (NSAIDs) with regard to Garré's sclerosing osteomyelitis of the jaw bone is not clear. Few reports have focused on this treatment strategy because most of the cases were resolved with certain dental managements [39].

For better management, regular follow-up is crucial until complete healing is achieved [1].

In fact, when endodontic treatment is performed, long-term follow-up should be conducted. Biopsy is indicated if the lesion continues to increase in size after an apparently successful treatment [8, 29].

For lesions of limited size, we usually obtain good therapeutic effects and favorable prognosis within few months.

After the elimination of the infection source, the bone gradually remodels itself and the original facial symmetry will be restored. This bone remodeling may be improved by the overlying muscle pull, which is attached to it [9].

In the two cases reported, our therapeutic attitude was successful. At the 12-month follow-up, bone healing was noted without any other complications.

The first patient was followed-up for 11 months. Periosteal reaction healing was observed at 4 months with mandibular swelling disappearance. Then, complete periapical healing was seen at 11 months.

The second patient was followed-up for 20 months. Periosteal reaction healing was observed at 4 months. Regression of periapical radiolucency was seen at 12 months.

Thus, for the two cases, there was no need for surgery as response to conventional endodontic treatment was favorable.

It is known that periostitis ossificans is curable if adequate treatment is given. However, if the correct diagnosis is delayed by more than 6 months, it may progress into a persistent and deforming form [9].

Surgical remodeling can be performed if no spontaneous regression is present, especially when adequate diagnosis and management are perfectly achieved [8].

4. Conclusion

Periostitis ossificans is a pathology coexisting with some conditions, including chronic infection in young patients with an energetic osteoblastic activity in the periostum and an equilibrium between the virulence of the causal agent and the host resistance.

Specific attention should be given to the clinical and radiographic explorations in case of mandibular swelling in order not to miss a possible malignant bone disease.

The treatment goal of periostitis ossificans is to eradicate the source of infection. Whenever the clinical situation permits, endodontic therapy should be the main treatment choice. Antibiotherapy is not systemic.

In our reported cases, endodontic treatment was the approach of choice and it led to a favorable evolution with complete regression.

References

[1] M. T. Brazão-Silva and T. N. Pinheiro, "The so-called garrè's osteomyelitis of jaws and the pivotal utility of computed tomography scan," *Contemp Clin Dent*, vol. 8, no. 4, pp. 645-646, 2017.

[2] F. R. Karjodkar, *Textbook of Dental and Maxillofacial Radiology*, Panama, Jaypee Brothers Medical Pub, 2nd edition, 2009.

[3] B. W. Neville, D. D. Damm, C. M. Allen, and J. E. Bouquot, "Pulp and periapical diseases," in *Oral and Maxillofacial Pathology*, B. W. Neville, Ed., pp. 118-119, Saunders and Co, Pennsylvania, 1st edition, 1995.

[4] R. Suma, C. Vinay, M. C. Shashikanth et al., "Garre's sclerosing osteomyelitis," *Journal of the Indian Society of Pedodontics and Preventive Dentistry*, vol. 25, pp. 30–33, 2007.

[5] M. Neelima, "Osteomyelitis and osteo radionecrosis of the jaw bones," in *Textbook of Oral and Maxillofacial Surgery*, M. Neelima, Ed., pp. 608–611, Jaypee Brothers Medical Pub, Panama, 3rd edition, 2012.

[6] C. Garré, "UeberbesondreFormen und Folgezustande d. akuteninfekt," *Osteomyelitis Beitr z klin Chir*, vol. 10, p. 257, 1893.

[7] M. Erişen, Bayar OF, and G. Ak, "Garre osteomyelitis: a case report," *J Dent Fac Atatürk Univ*, vol. 9, pp. 49–53, 2014.

[8] M. Gonçalves, D. P. Oliveira, E. O. Oya, and A. Gonçalves, "Garre's osteomyelitis associated with a fistula: a case report," *The Journal of Clinical Pediatric Dentistry*, vol. 26, no. 3, pp. 311–313, 2002.

[9] S. K. Kannan, G. Sandhya, and R. Selvarani, "Periostitis ossificans (Garrè's osteomyelitis) radiographic study of two cases,"

International Journal of Paediatric Dentistry, vol. 16, no. 1, pp. 59–64, 2006.

[10] C. Oulis, E. Berdousis, G. Vadiakas, and G. Goumenos, "Garre's osteomyelitis of an unusual origin in a 8-year-old child. a case report," *International Journal of Paediatric Dentistry*, vol. 10, no. 3, pp. 240–244, 2000.

[11] S. Cohen and R. Burns, *Pathways of the Pulp*, St. Louis: Mosby, 1980.

[12] D. Liu, J. Zhang, T. Li et al., "Chronic osteomyelitis with proliferative periostitis of the mandibular body: report of a case and review of the literature," *Annals of the Royal College of Surgeons of England*, vol. 101, no. 5, pp. 328-332, 2019.

[13] Y. Suei, A. Taguchi, and K. Tanimoto, "Diagnosis and classification of mandibular osteomyelitis," *Oral Surgery, Oral Medicine, Oral Pathology, Oral Radiology, and Endodontics*, vol. 100, no. 2, pp. 207–214, 2005.

[14] A. Zaghbani, S. Ben Yousef, L. Oualha, W. Hasni, K. Souid, and C. Baccouche, "Jaw malignancies: signs that should alert the dentist," *Tunis Med*, vol. 89, no. 6, pp. 580–584, 2011.

[15] E. Belli, C. Matteini, and T. Andreano, "Sclerosing osteomyelitis of Garré periostitis ossificans," *The Journal of Craniofacial Surgery*, vol. 13, no. 6, pp. 765–768, 2002.

[16] D. Schulze, M. Blessmann, P. Pohlenz, K. W. Wagner, and M. Heiland, "Diagnostic criteria for the detection of mandibular osteomyelitis using cone-beam computed tomography," *Dento Maxillo Facial Radiology*, vol. 35, no. 4, pp. 232–235, 2006.

[17] H. Nakano, T. Miki, K. Aota, T. Sumi, K. Matsumoto, and Y. Yura, "Garré's osteomyelitis of the mandible caused by an infected wisdom tooth," *Oral Sci Int*, vol. 5, no. 2, pp. 150–154, 2008.

[18] S. C. White and M. J. Pharoah, *Oral Radiology: Principles and Interpretation*, St. Louis: MO Mosby, 2009.

[19] L. Barnes, J. W. Eveson, P. Reichart, and D. Idransky, *Pathology and Genetics of Head and Neck Tumours*, International Agency for Research on Cancer, Geneva, 2005.

[20] P. Pitak-Arnnop, S. Bellefqih, C. Bertolus et al., "Ewing's sarcoma of jaw bones in adult patients: 10-year experiences in a Paris university hospital," *Journal of Cranio-Maxillo-Facial Surgery*, vol. 36, no. 8, pp. 450–455, 2008.

[21] S. M. Stern and P. J. Ferguson, "Autoinflammatory bone diseases," *Rheumatic Disease Clinics*, vol. 39, no. 4, pp. 735–749, 2013.

[22] C. Berglund, K. Ekströmer, and J. Abtahi, "Primary chronic osteomyelitis of the jaws in children: an update on pathophysiology, radiological findings, treatment strategies, and prospective analysis of two cases," *Case Reports in Dentistry*, vol. 2015, Article ID 152717, 12 pages, 2015.

[23] R. Kalaiarasi, C. Vijayakumar, R. Archana, and R. Natarajan, "Pediatric primary tuberculous osteomyelitis of the mandible mimicking parotitis," *Cureus*, vol. 10, no. 1, article e2071, 2018.

[24] G. Natarajarathinam, A. V. Rao, S. Palanimuthu, and J. Kannaperuman, "Primary tuberculous osteomyelitis of the mandible: a rare case report," *Dental Research Journal*, vol. 10, no. 2, pp. 283–286, 2013.

[25] P. G. Benca, R. Mostofi, and P. C. Kuo, "Proliferative periostitis (Garré's osteomyelitis)," *Oral Surgery, Oral Medicine, and Oral Pathology*, vol. 63, no. 2, pp. 258–260, 1987.

[26] G. J. Felsberg, R. L. Gore, M. E. Schweitzer, and V. Jui, "Sclerosing osteomyelitis of Garrè (periostitis ossificans)," *Oral Surgery, Oral Medicine, and Oral Pathology*, vol. 70, no. 1, pp. 117–120, 1990.

[27] R. Martin-Granizo, D. Garcia-Gonzalez, J. Sastre, and F. J. Diaz, "Mandibular sclerosing osteomyelitis of Garré," *Otolaryngology–Head and Neck Surgery*, vol. 121, no. 6, pp. 828-829, 2016.

[28] P. A. Krakowiak, "Alveolar osteitis and osteomyelitis of the jaws," *Oral and Maxillofacial Surgery Clinics of North America*, vol. 23, no. 3, pp. 401–413, 2011.

[29] G. D. Batcheidor, J. S. Giansanti, E. D. Hibbard, and C. A. Waldron, "Garré's Osteomyelitis of the Jaws: A Review and Report of Two Cases," *Journal of the American Dental Association (1939)*, vol. 87, no. 4, pp. 892–897, 1973.

[30] H. M. Akgül, F. Çağlayan, S. Günen Yılmaz, and G. Derindağ, "Garre's osteomyelitis of the mandible caused by infected tooth," *Case Reports in Dentistry*, vol. 2018, Article ID 1409539, 4 pages, 2018.

[31] A. Jayasenthil, P. V. Aparna, and S. Balagopal, "Non-surgical endodontic management of Garre's osteomyelitis: a case report," *British Journal of Medicine and Medical Research*, vol. 9, no. 3, pp. 1–4, 2015.

[32] H. L. J. Jacobson, J. C. Baumgartner, J. G. Marshall, and W. J. Beeler, "Proliferative periostitis of Garré: report of a case," *Oral Surgery, Oral Medicine, Oral Pathology, Oral Radiology, and Endodontics*, vol. 94, no. 1, pp. 111–114, 2002.

[33] G. D. Mattison, A. R. Gould, D. I. George, and J. L. Neb, "Garre's osteomyelitis of the mandible: the role of endodontic therapy in patient management," *Journal of Endodontia*, vol. 7, no. 12, pp. 559–564, 1981.

[34] G. M. McWalter and S. J. Schaberg, "Garre's osteomyelitis of the mandible resolved by endodontic treatment," *Journal of the American Dental Association (1939)*, vol. 108, no. 2, pp. 193–195, 1984.

[35] S. Eliyas, P. F. Briggs, and R. W. Porter, "Antimicrobial irrigants in endodontic therapy: 1. Root canal disinfection," *Dental Update*, vol. 37, no. 6, pp. 390–397, 2010.

[36] J. F. Siqueira Jr. and I. N. Rôças, "Optimising single-visit disinfection with supplementary approaches: a quest for predictability," *Australian Endodontic Journal*, vol. 37, no. 3, pp. 92–98, 2011.

[37] J. Vera, J. F. Siqueira Jr., D. Ricucci et al., "One- versus two-visit endodontic treatment of teeth with apical periodontitis: a histobacteriologic study," *Journal of Endodontia*, vol. 38, no. 8, pp. 1040–1052, 2012.

[38] A. Bah, S. Camara, F. Vaysse, and I. Bailleul-Forestier, "Prise en charge de l'Ostéopériostite chronique dentaire chez l'enfant: A propos d'un cas," *Afr J Dent Implantol*, vol. 7, pp. 52–60, 2016.

[39] C. Schultz, P. M. Holterhus, A. Seidel et al., "Chronic recurrent multifocal osteomyelitis in children," *The Pediatric Infectious Disease Journal*, vol. 18, no. 11, pp. 1008–1013, 1999.

9

The Integration of a Dual-Wavelength Super Pulsed Diode Laser for Consistent Tissue Ablation in the Esthetic Zone: A Case Series

Nur Hafizah Kamar Affendi,[1] **Rohana Ahmad,**[1] **Farhad Vahidi,**[2] **Mohd Zulkifli Hassan,**[3] **and Siti Nadia Rahimi**[4]

[1]*Unit of Prosthodontics, Centre of Restorative Dentistry Studies, Faculty of Dentistry, Universiti Teknologi MARA, Sungai Buloh Campus, Jalan Hospital, 47000 Sungai Buloh, Selangor, Malaysia*
[2]*Department of Prosthodontics, New York University, College of Dentistry, 205 E. 64th St., Ste 403, New York, NY 10065, USA*
[3]*Universiti Kebangsaan Malaysia, Jalan Raja Muda Abdul Aziz, 50300 Kuala Lumpur, Federal Territory of Kuala Lumpur, Malaysia*
[4]*Faculty of Dentistry, Islamic Science University of Malaysia (USIM), Malaysia*

Correspondence should be addressed to Nur Hafizah Kamar Affendi; hafizah_kamar@uitm.edu.my

Academic Editor: Sukumaran Anil

Introduction. A diode laser is one of the universally compact accepted laser systems used fundamentally for soft tissue applications. Most diode laser devices have a single wavelength of either 810 nm for superior coagulation or 980 nm for tissue ablation. In these case series, the use of dual wavelengths (810 nm and 980 nm) in combination with super pulsing has provided a cleaner cut (no charring) with faster healing that eases the placement of the final restoration in the esthetic zone. *Case Description.* The present case series describe four cases in the esthetic zone that achieved hemostasis ablation without collateral damage to enhance gingival balance of definitive restoration. The gingivoplasty and gingivectomy modes are used to achieve efficient tissue ablation. Although there is no specific mode indicated in the FDA laser requirement for gingival depigmentation, the procedure could be safely performed with the dual-wavelength diode laser *Result.* All four patients revealed a good esthetic outcome and reported no pain postoperatively. Healing was uneventful, and definitive restoration was delivered within two to four weeks postoperatively. *Conclusion.* Within the limitation of these case series, the dual-wavelength super pulsed diode laser has the capacity to deliver peak powers resulting in efficient cutting and less tissue charring and also as an alternative tool for removal of gingival pigmentation. Prospective clinical research with larger sample size is needed for conclusive results.

1. Introduction

Lasers have been widely used in dentistry since the 1980s as an adjunct therapy for the removal of pathologic lesions and for esthetic procedures [1]. One of the universally compact accepted laser systems is the diode laser that is primarily used for soft tissue applications. The near-infrared (NIR) wavelength that radiates from this laser is absorbed by chromophobes (mainly hemoglobin and melanin), which produces hemostatic ablation of the targeted tissue [2, 3]. The NIR produces efficient cutting that seals well-vascularized tissue resulting in low morbidity and excellent healing as compared to traditional scalpel and electrocautery [4, 5]. Dry field surgery is permitted, and suturing is usually not necessary, resulting in an improved treatment outcome and patient comfort [6].

Nevertheless, the slow cutting effect as a result of the limitation associated with the watts and single wavelength used has been a major concern of dental practitioners. To overcome the cutting inefficiency, a "continuous wave" was used instead to provide constant energy, but this will inevitably produce collateral damage to the soft tissues [7]. This collateral damage includes tissue necrosis and delayed wound healing, which affect the tissue management in the esthetic zone. Therefore, a new generation of a diode laser with a super pulsed mode was developed to achieve efficient cutting with low heat output and decreased collateral damage [8]. The beam is modulated with high energy levels (up to 20000 Hz) with very short pulses in milliseconds for optimum clinical results [9–11]. Additionally, the incorporation of dual wavelengths of 810 and 980 nm in one unit has enhanced the coagulative and cutting efficiency which translates into cleaner cut, less charring, and better soft tissue management [11, 12]. Therefore, the purpose of these case series was to demonstrate excellent tissue management with super pulsed dual-wavelength diode lasers, which provide consistent ablation to create gingival harmony in the esthetic zone.

2. Methods

These case series were based on four patients who were referred to the prosthodontics department for hard and soft tissue aesthetic management of their maxillary anterior teeth. For soft tissue management, minimally invasive excision of gingival tissue was performed with a super pulsed dual-wavelength diode laser of 810 and 980 nm (Gemini Ultradent, USA), using the parameters listed in Table 1. The surgical procedure with the diode laser and its possible complications were explained to the patients, who then gave their consent. The operator, patient, and assistants wore safety glass to protect their eyes and avoided the use of mirrored surface instruments to prevent laser beam reflections. The fiber tip was initiated with a carbon paper provided in the package. The surgical area was first dried, and gingivectomy performed with a maximum peak of 2 W, in a super pulsed mode under local anaesthesia (xylocaine 2% with adrenaline, 1 : 200000). The tip was cleaned regularly with damped gauze (in normal saline) to remove any tissue debris. No periodontal dressing was used and no medication prescribed. Postoperative healing was uneventful, and no pain was reported. The final restorations were delivered within two to four weeks after surgery.

Table 1: The parameters used for the diode laser device.

Product	Gemini
Type of laser	Diode (class IV)
Emission mode	Super pulsed
Time on/time off	Variable
Delivery system	Optical fiber
Wavelength	810 nM or 980 nM ± 10 nM Dual wavelength ± 10 nM (50% 810 nM and 980 nM ± 10 nM)
Peak power	2.0 watts
Average power	0.1 watt to 2.0 watts
Aiming beam power	5 mW max
Aiming beam wavelength	650 ± 10 nM
Beam divergence	617 mRad
Pulse frequency	50 Hz
Pulse width	Variable
Duty cycle	Variable
Voice confirmation	Yes
Power requirement	100-240 VAC @50 to 60 Hz–13 V

2.1. Case 1. A healthy 20-year-old female was unhappy with the shape and color of her maxillary anterior tooth. She has a congenitally missing upper right central incisor that was replaced with the lateral incisor, moved orthodontically into the place and built up with composite resin to resemble a central incisor (Figure 1(a)). Although this procedure was relatively successful in closing the anterior gap, there was noticeable discrepancy in shape, color, and gingival architecture with those of the contralateral central incisor. In addition, the overhanging margin of the composite build-up has resulted in inflammation of the gingiva and the interdental papilla (Figure 1(b)). The composite resin was removed and the tooth prepared for a porcelain veneer. To ablate the excess gingival tissue, a preset gingivoplasty mode was used with pulse duration of 140 μs. The remnants of the inflamed tissue were removed and conditioned with wet sterile gauze (Figure 1(c)). The final impression for the veneer was made immediately after the procedure, and the patient was recalled after 3 days. Excellent healing has occurred, and the patient reported no pain. The lithium disilicate veneer was cemented two weeks later, and the patient expressed immense satisfaction with the outcome (Figure 1(d)).

2.2. Case 2. A young male patient complained of uneven smile and discoloration of his front teeth. Upon examination, it was noted that he has mild anterior crowding, spacing, and peg-shaped right lateral incisor restored with composite resin. The maxillary right central and lateral incisors were endodontically treated (Figure 2(a)). Various treatment options were discussed including tooth realignment with orthodontics. He declined orthodontic treatment and opted for partial and complete coverage restorations. The maxillary right central and lateral incisors and maxillary left central incisor were prepared for crowns and veneer, respectively. Gingivoplasty was then performed with a diode laser on the lateral incisor to gain tooth structure for a ferrule effect (Figures 2(b) and 2(c)). Impression was made immediately after gingivoplasty, and no periodontal dressing was necessary. Uneventful healing occurred after 5 days. The patient was ecstatic of the final outcome (Figure 2(d)).

2.3. Case 3. A female patient aged 54 years complained of unsightly appearance and requested prosthesis to replace her missing maxillary teeth. Clinical examination revealed several missing teeth and moderately worn down dentition resulting in shortened clinical crown and gingival contour disharmony (Figure 3(a)). Gingivectomy on the maxillary anterior teeth was planned to increase the crown height and improve the gingival contour before final tooth preparation and fabrication of a fixed prosthesis. A preset gingivectomy mode with a diode laser was chosen to correct the gingival zenith. Periodontal examination and bone sounding were first performed to ensure that the biologic width was preserved. The sulcular epithelium was removed under local

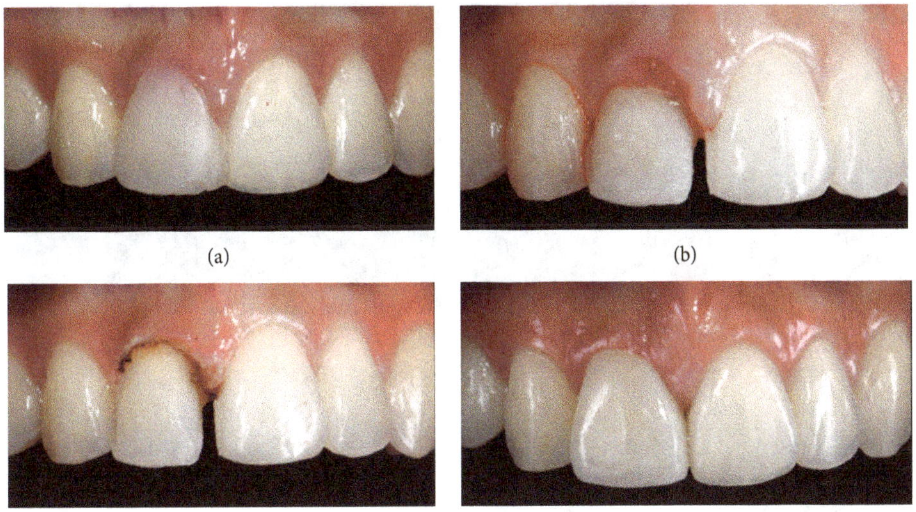

(a) (b) (c) (d)

FIGURE 1: (a) Right lateral incisor in the position of the central incisor and built up with composite resin. (b) Gingival inflammation underneath the overhanging composite restoration. (c) Gingivoplasty with a diode laser. (d) Cemented veneer with excellent postoperative gingival healing.

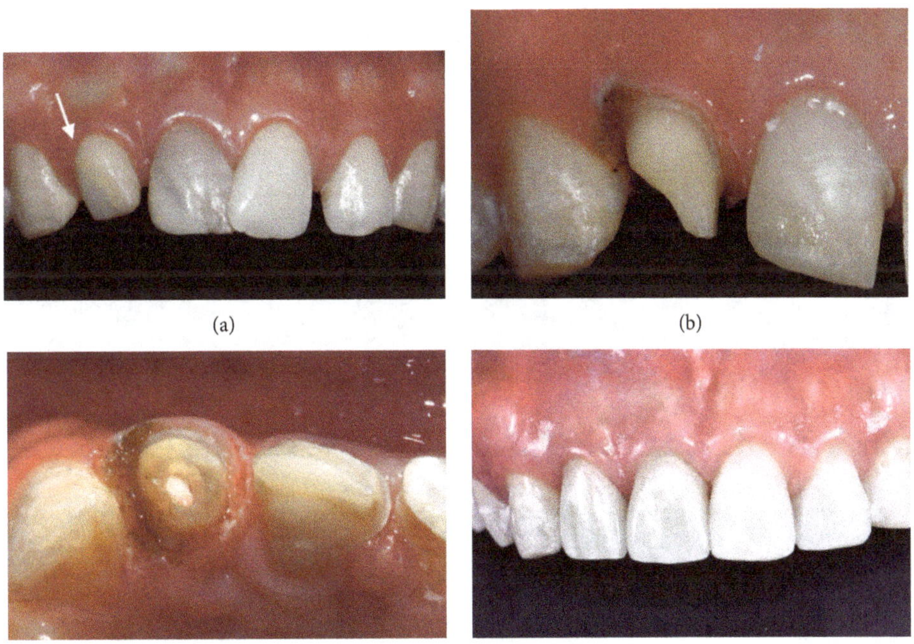

(a) (b) (c) (d)

FIGURE 2: (a) Overlapping of maxillary central incisors and a peg-shaped lateral incisor built up with composite resin (arrow), (b, c) gingivoplasty on a lateral incisor, and (d) restored maxillary incisors and healed gingiva.

anaesthesia by using the optic fiber tip at about 30-degree angle and passed along the marginal gingiva (Figure 3(b)). The postoperative event was uneventful, and healing of the gingival tissue was observed after two weeks (Figure 3(c)). The fixed prostheses were delivered a month after surgery, and the patient was satisfied with the final outcome (Figure 3(d)).

2.4. Case 4. A 49-year-old female patient complained of dark gingiva and corroded crown margins and requested replacement of the metal ceramic crowns (Figure 4(a)). The gingival pigmentation has a score of 3 according to the gingival pigmentation index, with diffuse brown/black pigmentation on the attached and marginal gingiva [13]. Gingivoplasty was planned to remove the pigmentation, and new all ceramic crowns were fabricated to replace the unesthetic crowns. The preset gingivoplasty mode was selected to remove the melanin pigments on the marginal and attached gingiva at the output power range of 1.0 to 2.0 watts under local anesthesia (Figure 4(b)). A depigmentation procedure was carried

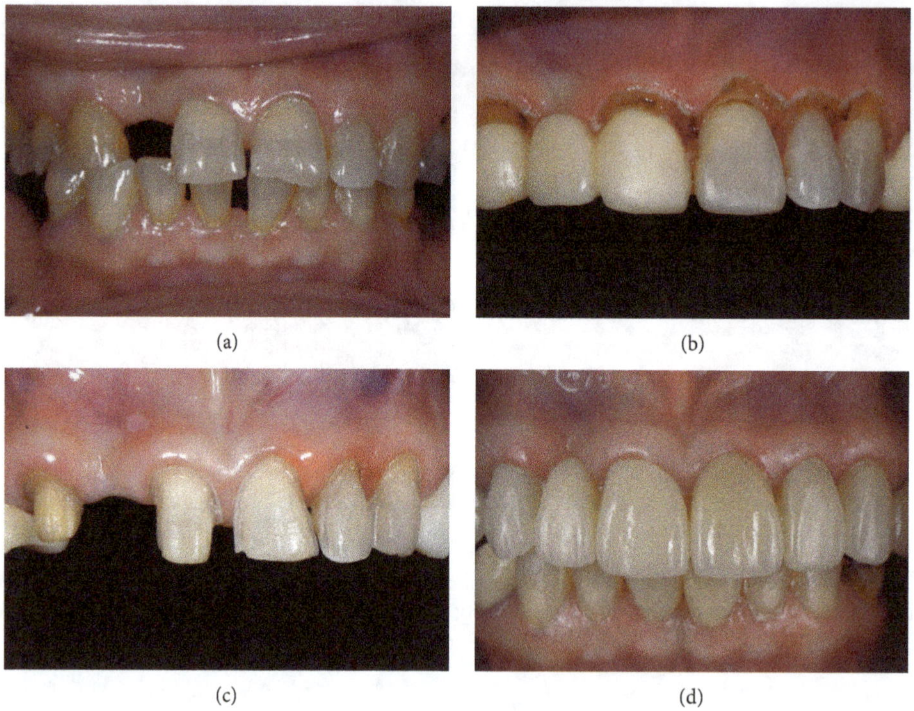

FIGURE 3: (a) Moderately worn down maxillary anterior teeth and missing a right lateral incisor. (b) Gingivectomy performed with the diode laser. (c) Final tooth preparation on healed gingiva. (d) Final prosthesis cemented showing good crown length and gingival harmony.

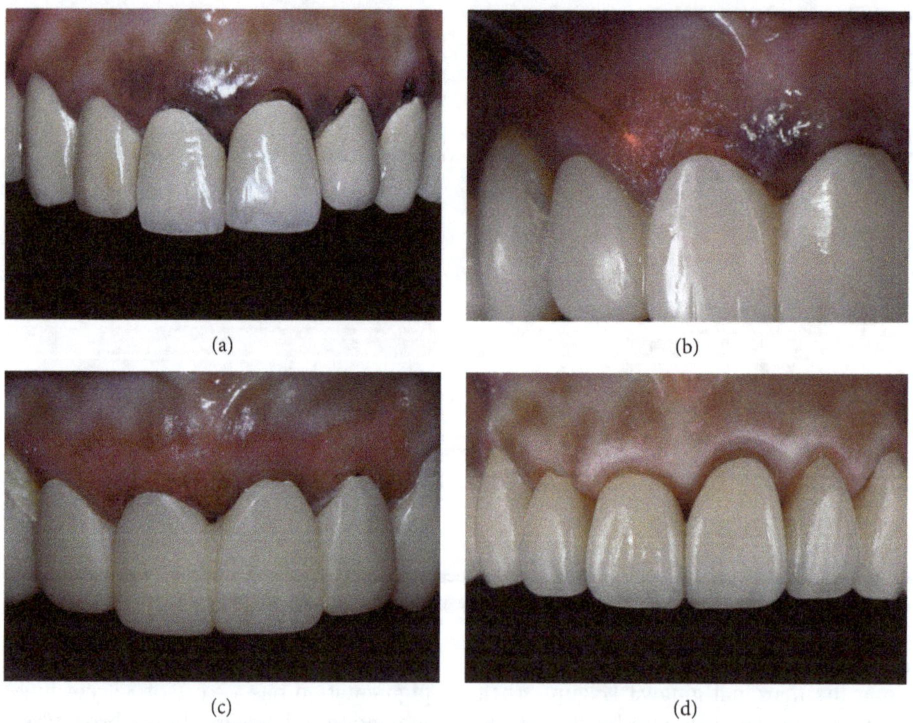

FIGURE 4: (a) Gingival pigmentation and discolored crown margins. (b) Gingivoplasty with a diode laser. (c) Immediate postoperative state of gingival peeling. (d) One-year recall showing minimal redeposition of melanin and minimal gingival recession.

out on the marginal and attached gingiva at the output power range of 1.0 to 2.0 watts (Figure 4(c)). The ablation was performed with a steady brushing stroke, and the tip was kept in motion all the time. Remnants of the ablated tissue were removed using sterile gauze dampened with saline solution. Postoperative healing was uneventful after 5 days, and the crowns were cemented in a supragingival manner a month later. She was recalled after a year, and very minimal melanin redeposition was seen on the attached gingiva and the mucogingival junction (Figure 4(d)).

3. Discussion

Gingival health is one of the essential components that create the harmony of smile in the esthetic area. To create balance in a clinical situation which displays surplus of the gingiva, a preprosthetic gingival procedure with a diode laser has shown to be precise, sterile, and suture-less and provides superior healing [14–17]. When compared to a retraction cord for the gingival displacement technique, the diode laser is more effective and simpler to use and causes less pain [18]. As shown in cases 1 and 2, hemostatic ablations from the diode laser permit a dry field and enable gingival troughing to be done for margin accessibility and ease of impression making within the same visit. In addition, the diode laser produces wider gingival sulci, less epithelial injury, and post-treatment gingival recession as compared with the use of a conventional presaturated retraction cord prior to impression making [19, 20]. However, it has been reported that the difference in the amount of recession associated with the use of either a diode laser or a retraction cord is not significant, with an average loss of gingival height of 0.26 mm for the cord technique and 0.27 mm for the diode laser [21]. The difference was probably due to the double-cord technique applied and the single wavelength used with a continuous pulse. Hence, larger samples with more variables including tissue thickness, keratinized tissue, wavelengths, and type of pulses used are needed for a more conclusive result.

A histological study on an animal model showed that the diode laser causes more tissue damage and delayed healing as compared to erbium, chromium-doped yttrium, scandium, gallium, and garnet (Er: Cr, YSGG) and scalpel [22]. Another in vivo study has shown that histologic specimens from the diode laser cause more degenerative changes to the epithelium and stromal cells as compared to a scalpel and electrocautery in the gingivectomy procedure [17]. However, the result should be interpreted cautiously as the lateral heat may impede histologic interpretation in small lesions (<3 mm diameter) [23]. When comparing patient perception, less discomfort and pain were recorded with the diode laser [12, 24, 25], but a few studies found a higher pain value in the laser group [26, 27]. These contradictory findings could be due to the different parameters used such as wave length, laser mode, and surgical technique. Nonetheless, as shown in case number 3, the dual-wavelength diode laser had provided efficient cutting and good bleeding control without the need for suture or dressing.

One of the remarkable advantages of the diode laser was the capability to remove a thin layer of a pigmented epithelium while preserving the connective layer and capillary vessel as shown in case 4 [28]. It was demonstrated to have a lower pain score, superior bleeding control, and less incidence of repigmentation [29, 30]. A clinical study that compared different wavelengths has found that melanin pigments effectively absorb the diode laser energy, enhance faster peeling, and cause no relapse as compared to an erbium laser. [31]. Although no specific mode for depigmentation is available in the system, it showed that this procedure could be performed safely with the dual-wavelength diode laser. Further prospective studies with a longer follow-up are necessary to confirm this "gingivoplasty" mode as one of the options to remove gingival pigmentation.

Diode laser devices have a single wavelength that ranges between 810 and 980 nm. The lower wavelength closer to 810 nm is reported to be better at coagulation, while the higher 980 nm wavelength diodes are better at tissue ablation. As documented in these case series, the combination of dual wavelengths (810 nm and 980 nm) into one unit has provided a clean cut (no charring) with uneventful healing that eases the placement of the final restoration within a month [12, 32]. While continuous and traditional pulse modes can be effective, a featured advantage of a super pulsed mode allows a more precise cut without a thermal side effect and minimal involvement of the adjacent tissue [7]. However, further studies are recommended to confirm the efficacy of the dual-wavelength approach with low laser power settings to achieve more conclusive results.

4. Conclusion

Within the limitation of these case series, the following conclusion could be drawn: the dual-wavelength super pulsed diode laser has the capacity to deliver peak powers resulting in fast cutting and minimal tissue charring and as an alternative tool for the removal of gingival pigmentation that was well tolerated by patients. Prospectively, it is suggested to have larger sample sizes with histological studies to explore the different impacts of wavelengths and pulse on the gingival tissue.

Acknowledgments

The authors would like to thank Ultradent Inc. (USA/Malaysia) for providing the diode lasers used in these case series.

References

[1] S. Parker, "Introduction, history of lasers and laser light production," *British Dental Journal*, vol. 202, no. 1, pp. 21–31, 2007.

[2] S. Parker, "Surgical lasers and hard dental tissue," *British Dental Journal*, vol. 202, no. 8, pp. 445–454, 2007.

[3] C. M. David and P. Gupta, "Lasers in dentistry: a review," *International Journal of Advanced Health Sciences*, vol. 2, no. 8, pp. 7–13, 2015.

[4] M. Dang and S. Ram, "Integrating laser dentistry into esthetic dentistry," *International Journal of Laser Dentistry*, vol. 2, no. 2, pp. 63–68, 2012.

[5] F. Sobouti, V. Rakhshan, N. Chiniforush, and M. Khatami, "Effects of laser-assisted cosmetic smile lift gingivectomy on postoperative bleeding and pain in fixed orthodontic patients: a controlled clinical trial," *Progress in Orthodontics*, vol. 15, no. 1, pp. 1–5, 2014.

[6] S. Pirnat, "Versatility of an 810 nm diode laser in dentistry: an overview," *Journal of Laser and Health Academy*, vol. 4, no. 2, pp. 1–9, 2007.

[7] A. A. Al-Khatib and A. S. Al-Azzawi, "Comparative study of diode laser 940 nm in performing frenectomy in both: continuous and pulsed modes: an in vivo study," *Journal of Dental Lasers*, vol. 9, no. 2, p. 50, 2015.

[8] R. Borchers, *Comparison of diode lasers in soft-tissue surgery using CW-and superpulsed mode: an in vivo study*, RWTH Aachen University: Master thesis for Master of Science in Laser in Dentistry, 2008.

[9] C. Maiorana and S. Salina, "Versatility of a superpulsed diode laser in oral surgery: a clinical report," *Journal of Oral Laser Applications*, vol. 6, no. 3, 2006.

[10] N. Derikvand, Z. Chinipardaz, S. Ghasemi, and N. Chiniforush, "The versatility of 980 nm diode laser in dentistry: a case series," *Journal of Lasers in Medical Sciences*, vol. 7, no. 3, pp. 205–208, 2016.

[11] A. Gutiérrez-Corrales, Y. Rizcala-Orlando, P. Montero-Miralles et al., "Comparison of diode laser–oral tissue interaction to different wavelengths. In vitro study of porcine periodontal pockets and oral mucosa," *Medicina Oral, Patología Oral y Cirugía Bucal*, vol. 25, no. 2, pp. e224–e232, 2020.

[12] H. Borjian, "Preprosthetic oral surgery by dual wavelength diode laser: a case report study," *EC Dental Science*, vol. 18, pp. 228–236, 2019.

[13] S. Kumar, G. S. Bhat, and K. M. Bhat, "Comparative evaluation of gingival depigmentation using tetrafluoroethane cryosurgery and gingival abrasion technique: two years follow up," *Journal of Clinical and Diagnostic Research*, vol. 7, no. 2, pp. 389–394, 2013.

[14] A. Meenawat, S. C. Verma, V. Govila, V. Srivastava, and K. Punn, "Histological and clinical evaluation of gingival healing following gingivectomy using different treatment modalities," *Journal of the International Clinical Dental Research Organization*, vol. 5, no. 1, p. 31, 2013.

[15] P. Kumar, V. Rattan, and S. Rai, "Comparative evaluation of healing after gingivectomy with electrocautery and laser," *Journal of Oral Biology and Craniofacial Research*, vol. 5, no. 2, pp. 69–74, 2015.

[16] G. Sagar, N. Rajesh, T. Kumar, K. K. M. Reddy, B. S. Shankar, and V. Sandeep, "Comparative evaluation of two surgical techniques using conventional scalpel method and diode laser for treatment outcome of depigmentation: 6 months follow-up study," *Journal of Dental Lasers*, vol. 10, no. 1, p. 2, 2016.

[17] A. Bhatsange, E. P. Meshram, A. Waghamare, L. Shiggaon, V. Mehetre, and A. Shende, "A clinical and histological comparison of mucosal incisions produced by scalpel, electrocautery, and diode laser: a pilot study," *Journal of Dental Lasers*, vol. 10, no. 2, p. 37, 2016.

[18] D. Melilli, R. Mauceri, A. Albanese, D. Matranga, and G. Pizzo, "Gingival displacement using diode laser or retraction cords: a comparative clinical study," *American Journal of Dentistry*, vol. 31, no. 3, pp. 131–134, 2018.

[19] A. Gupta, N. Jain, and P. G. Makhija, "Clinical applications of 980 nm diode laser for soft tissue procedures in prosthetic restorative dentistry (case report)," *Journal of Lasers in Medical Sciences*, vol. 3, no. 4, pp. 185–188, 2012.

[20] H.-L. Wang, "Comparison of gingival troughing by laser and retraction cord," *The International Journal of Periodontics & Restorative Dentistry*, vol. 38, pp. 527–532, 2018.

[21] M. Stuffken and F. Vahidi, "Preimpression troughing with the diode laser: a preliminary study," *The Journal of Prosthetic Dentistry*, vol. 115, no. 4, pp. 441–446, 2016.

[22] J.-Y. Jin, S.-H. Lee, and H.-J. Yoon, "A comparative study of wound healing following incision with a scalpel, diode laser or Er, Cr: YSGG laser in guinea pig oral mucosa: a histological and immunohistochemical analysis," *Acta Odontologica Scandinavica*, vol. 68, no. 4, pp. 232–238, 2010.

[23] F. Angiero, L. Parma, R. Crippa, and S. Benedicenti, "Diode laser (808 nm) applied to oral soft tissue lesions: a retrospective study to assess histopathological diagnosis and evaluate physical damage," *Lasers in Medical Science*, vol. 27, no. 2, pp. 383–388, 2012.

[24] H. M. Akram, O. H. Ali, N. K. Omran, and A. O. Ali, "Diode laser versus scalpel gingivectomy," *Biomedical and Pharmacology Journal*, vol. 10, no. 4, pp. 1799–1804, 2017.

[25] Ö. Elif, "Comparison of gingivectomy procedures for patient satisfaction: conventional and diode laser surgery," *Selcuk Dental Journal*, vol. 4, no. 1, pp. 6–9, 2017.

[26] B. Guler, S. C. Isler, A. Uraz, S. Bozkaya, and F. D. Cetiner, "The comparison of postoperative wound healing following different gingivectomy techniques: a randomized prospective clinical trial," *Annals of Medical Research*, vol. 26, no. 3, pp. 382–388, 2019.

[27] B. D. Jonnalagadda, S. N. Gottumukkala, C. Dwarakanath, and S. Koneru, "Effect of diode laser-assisted flap surgery on postoperative healing and clinical parameters: a randomized controlled clinical trial," *Contemporary Clinical Dentistry*, vol. 9, no. 2, pp. 205–212, 2018.

[28] M. Giannelli, L. Formigli, and D. Bani, "Comparative evaluation of photoablative efficacy of erbium: yttrium-aluminium-garnet and diode laser for the treatment of gingival hyperpigmentation. A randomized split-mouth clinical trial," *Journal of Periodontology*, vol. 85, no. 4, pp. 554–561, 2014.

[29] G. Suragimath, M. H. Lohana, and S. Varma, "A split mouth randomized clinical comparative study to evaluate the efficacy of gingival depigmentation procedure using conventional scalpel technique or diode laser," *Journal of Lasers in Medical Sciences*, vol. 7, no. 4, pp. 227–232, 2016.

[30] S. Chandna and S. D. Kedige, "Evaluation of pain on use of electrosurgery and diode lasers in the management of gingival hyperpigmentation: a comparative study," *Journal of Indian Society of Periodontology*, vol. 19, no. 1, pp. 49–55, 2015.

[31] M. Taher Agha and P. Polenik, "Laser treatment for melanin gingival pigmentations: a comparison study for 3 laser wavelengths 2780, 940, and 445 nm," *International Journal of Dentistry*, vol. 2020, 11 pages, 2020.

[32] R. A. Lowe and F. D. Fiadfe, *Tissue Management in Restorative Dentistry: The "Super Pulsed" Diode Laser*, Oral Health Group, 2018.

10

Periapical Microsurgery with an Endoscope and Microscope of Two Upper Central Incisors Already Subjected to Periapical Surgery 25 Years Ago

Pablo Glera-Suarez,[1] Blanca Serra-Pastor,[2] David Peñarrocha-Oltra,[1] Miguel Peñarrocha-Diago,[1,3] and Cosme Gay-Escoda[3,4]

[1]*Department of Stomatology, Faculty of Medicine and Dentistry, University of Valencia, Spain*
[2]*Prosthodontics Unit, Department of Stomatology, Faculty of Medicine and Dentistry, University of Valencia, Spain*
[3]*IDIBELL Institute, Barcelona, Spain*
[4]*Oral and Maxillofacial Surgery Department, Faculty of Medicine and Health Sciences (School of Dentistry), University of Barcelona, Spain*

Correspondence should be addressed to David Peñarrocha-Oltra; dpenarrocha@gmail.com

Academic Editor: Samir Nammour

Introduction. The present clinical case describes periapical microsurgery with an endoscope and microscope in a patient already treated 25 years ago due to persistent periapical disease of the two central upper incisors, restored with poorly adapted crowns. *Clinical Case.* The first periapical surgery had been performed with silver amalgam as a retrograde filler material, causing grayish staining of the buccal mucosa. Periapical surgery was performed raising a submarginal flap with ostectomy and apicoectomy, retrograde cavity preparation with ultrasound tips, and filling with mineral trioxide aggregate (MTA). After soft tissue healing and complete bone regeneration of the lesion, retreatment of the incisors with a fixed prosthesis was carried out, adopting the biologically oriented preparation technique (BOPT). *Conclusions.* The described periapical microsurgery approach with magnification and illumination of the surgical field was found to be effective, avoiding the need to extract the two central upper incisors.

1. Introduction

Important advances have been made in periapical surgery, including the introduction of surgical field illumination and magnification with a microscope or endoscope and the use of high-quality filler materials. The aim of retrograde filling is to secure good sealing of the cavity and the accessory canals and dentinal tubules—avoiding bacterial microleakage in order to ensure success of the surgical technique [1]. In the period between 1940 and 2000, silver amalgam was the most widely used retrograde filler material. However, since the year 2000, different alternative materials have been introduced, such as glass ionomers, zinc oxide-eugenol cements, and gold or mineral trioxide aggregate (MTA) [2]. The properties of these newer materials have been studied in order to determine which is the best option for use in periapical surgery. In this regard, MTA has been shown to be the most stable material over the long term, minimizing leakage, with lesser inflammation of the periapical tissues and with a higher treatment success rate than the rest of the materials [3–8]. The development of ultrasound tips for retrograde cavity preparation, together with the incorporation of microsurgery (field amplification with an endoscope and illumination and magnification with a microscope), has allowed periapical surgery to become a predictable solution for the management of persistent chronic periapical periodontitis, with a success rate of approximately 92% [2].

In the event of persistent chronic periapical periodontitis affecting an incisor already previously subjected to periapical surgery that has failed, a possible solution is to remove the tooth and place a dental implant—though this involves more aggressive surgery, with greater morbidity and higher costs for the patient.

Endodontic microsurgery with the use of new filler materials, ultrasound tips, and magnification techniques [9] has increased the treatment success rates. We thus decided to perform periapical microsurgery with an endoscope and microscope in a patient already treated 25 years ago with silver amalgam cavity filling due to persistent periapical disease of the two central upper incisors. Our approach avoided removal of the incisors, and retreatment of the incisors was completed with a fixed prosthesis, adopting the biologically oriented preparation technique (BOPT).

2. Case Presentation

A 54-year-old woman who had undergone periapical surgery 25 years ago to solve persistent chronic periapical periodontitis of the two central upper incisors reported with discomfort in the periapical zones of the mentioned teeth. The intraoral exploration revealed reddening and inflammation at the buccal level of 1.1 and 2.1 and of the interdental papilla, as well as grayish buccal and apical staining of the central incisors, caused by the presence of the silver amalgam filler material (Figure 1). The periapical radiographs revealed radiolucencies around the apexes of 1.1 and 2.1 (Figure 2). Cone beam computed tomography (CBCT) (Planmeca®, Helsinki, Finland) evidenced bone destruction at 1.1 (Figure 3) and 2.1, with the involvement also of the buccal cortical layer of 2.1 (Figure 4).

Periapical surgery of the affected teeth was carried out. Infiltration anesthesia was performed in the vestibular depth of both teeth using two carpules of 4% articaine with epinephrine 1 : 100,000 (Inibsa®, Lliça de Vall, Spain). Magnification was provided by an EXTARO 300 dental microscope (Zeiss®, Oberkochen, Germany). A number 15C scalpel was used to perform a horizontal submarginal incision (Figure 5) at 3-4 mm from the gingival margin, with vertical releasing incisions distal to 1.2 and 2.2 and the raising of a full-thickness mucoperiosteal flap (Figure 6).

An ostectomy was performed for full visualization of the lesion, using a 6-blade tungsten carbide drill mounted in a handpiece with abundant sterile saline irrigation. The periapical inflammatory tissue was removed for posterior histopathological study (Figure 7), and inspection of the roots of 1.1 (Figure 8) and 2.1 (Figure 9) was made using a rigid endoscope (Karl Storz®, Tuttlingen, Germany), with the application of methylene blue dye to the zone in order to discard possible root fractures. The silver amalgam was removed from the retrograde cavities using ultrasound tips (Piezomed®, W&H, Bürmoos, Austria) (Figure 10).

The endoscope was used to check that the retrograde cavities of 1.1 (Figure 11) and 2.1 (Figure 12) were well prepared and clean. Bleeding was controlled with dressing impregnated with epinephrine, and the retrograde cavities of both teeth were filled with MTA (ProRoot®, Dentsply, York, USA) (Figure 13). Once the filler material had set, the endoscope was used to confirm correct completion of the retrograde filling of 1.1 (Figure 14) and 2.1 (Figure 15). Regeneration of the bone defect was secured with beta-tricalcium phosphate particles (KeraOs-Keramat®, Santiago de Compostela, Spain) (Figure 16), and suturing was carried out with a non-reabsorbable 4/0 multifilament suture (Tevdek®, Teleflex®, Wayne, USA) (Figure 17).

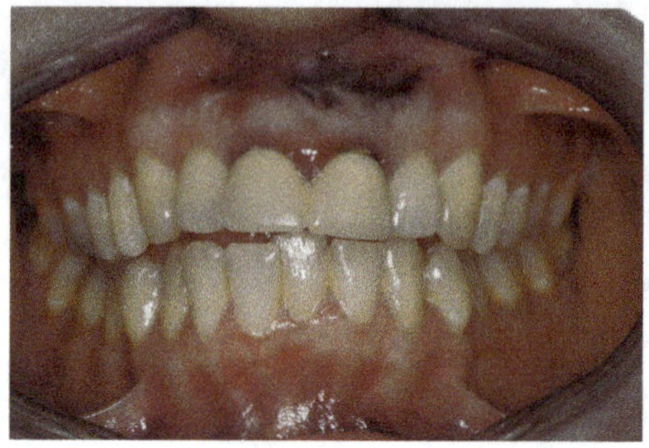

Figure 1: Preoperative clinical view. Note the reddening and inflammation at the buccal level of 1.1 and 2.1 and of the interdental papilla, as well as grayish buccal and apical staining of the central incisors, caused by the presence of the silver amalgam filler material.

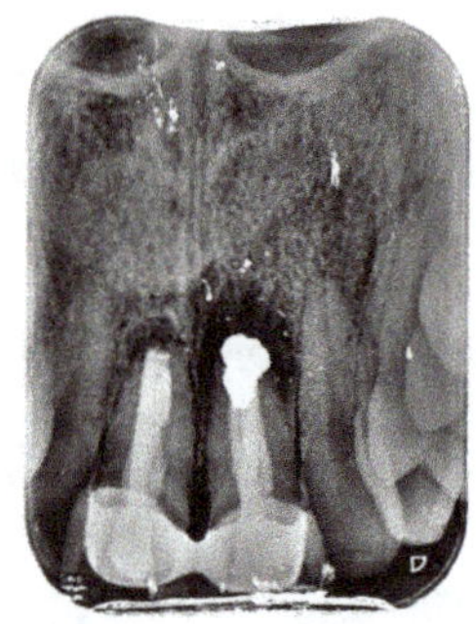

Figure 2: Preoperative periapical radiograph showing a radiolucent image around the root of 1.1 and a larger radiolucency around 2.1.

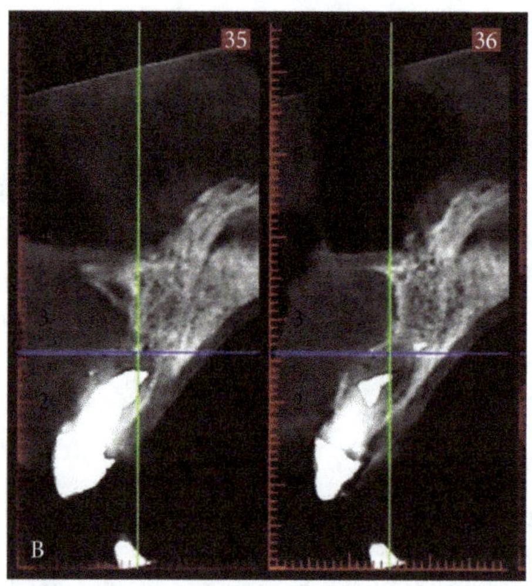

Figure 3: Preoperative sagittal CBCT view showing destruction of the buccal cortical layer of 2.1.

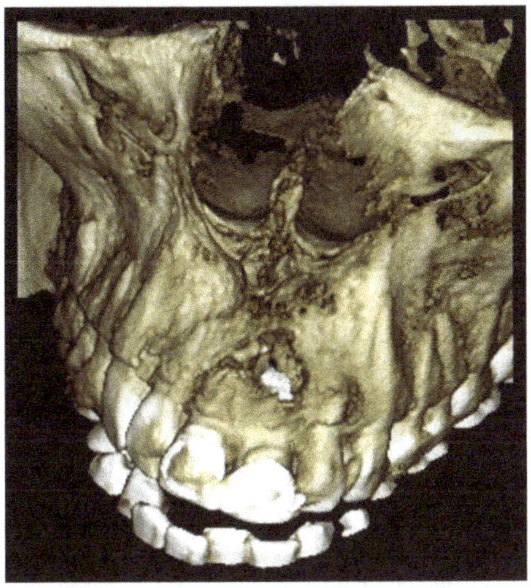

FIGURE 4: Preoperative three-dimensional radiographic reconstruction showing destruction of the buccal cortical layer of 2.1.

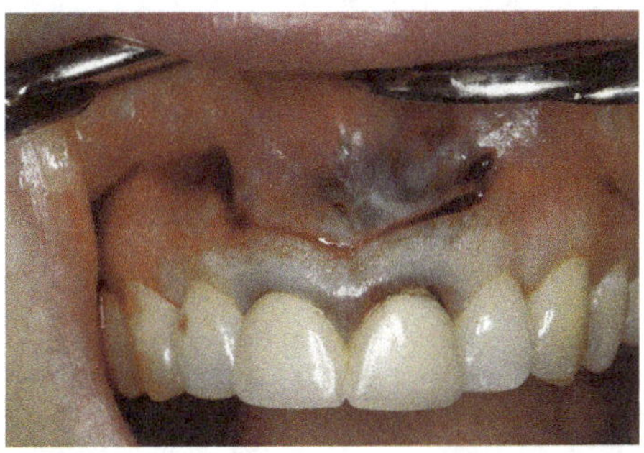

FIGURE 5: Submarginal incision.

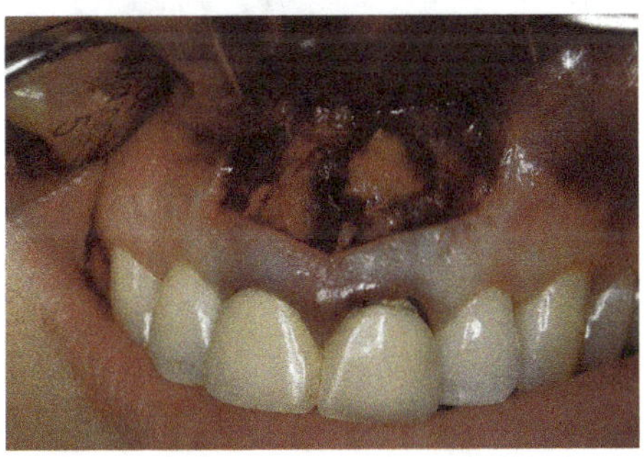

FIGURE 6: Raising of the full-thickness mucoperiosteal flap.

Amoxicillin 500 mg (Laboratorios Normon, Paterna, Spain) every 8 hours during 6 days was prescribed, along with ibuprofen 600 mg (Laboratorios Normon, Paterna, Spain) every 8 hours during three days and 0.12% chlorhexidine rinses (Perio Aid, Dentaid, Barcelona, Spain) every 8 hours during 7 days. The sutures were removed after one week (Figure 18). The histopathological study showed the presence of generally dense fibrocellular connective tissue fragments with chronic inflammatory foci.

Clinical evaluation one month after surgery showed no suture dehiscences (Figure 19), and the periapical radiographic study confirmed correct retrograde filling

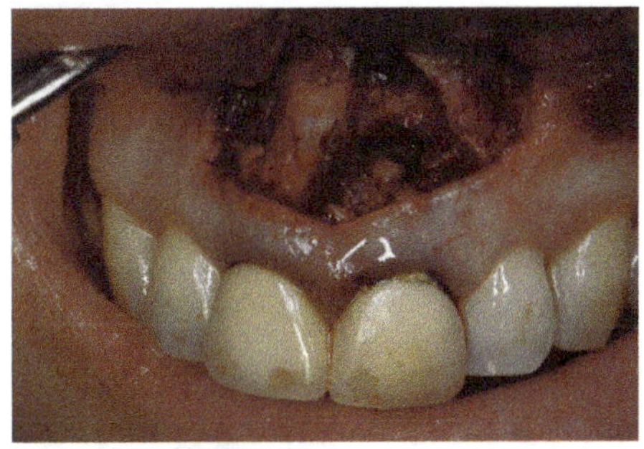

FIGURE 7: Ostectomy and curettage of the periapical lesions of 1.1 and 2.1.

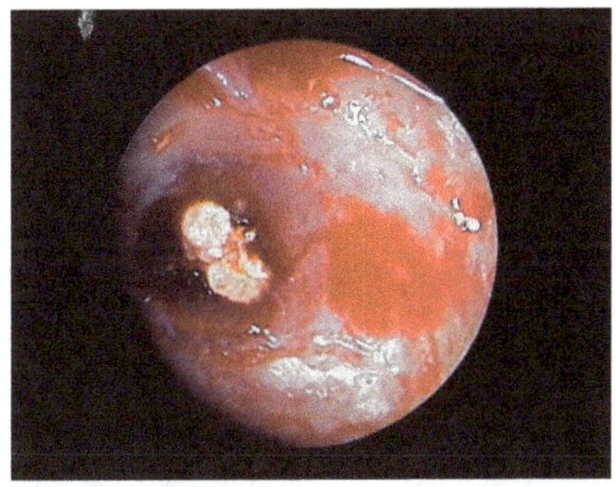

FIGURE 8: Endoscopic view of 1.1 before removal of the old filler material.

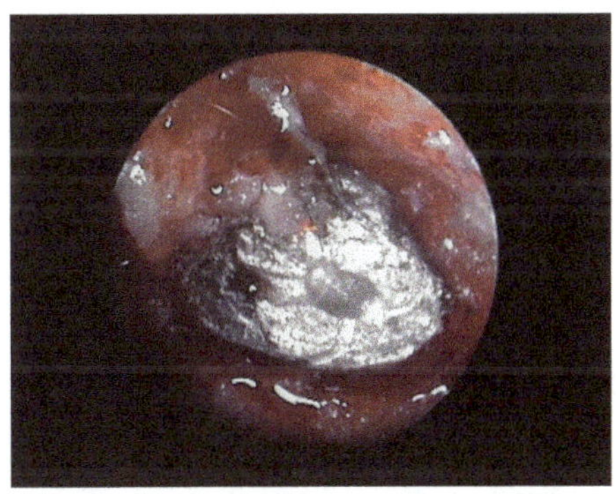

FIGURE 9: Endoscopic view of 2.1 before removal of the old filler material.

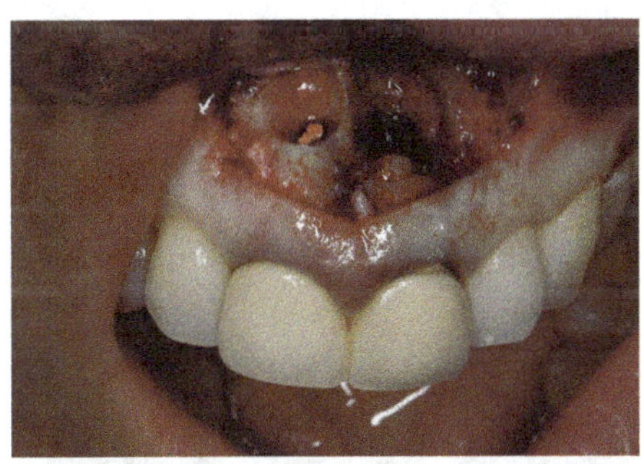

FIGURE 10: Clinical view of the removal of the old filler material of 1.1 and 2.1.

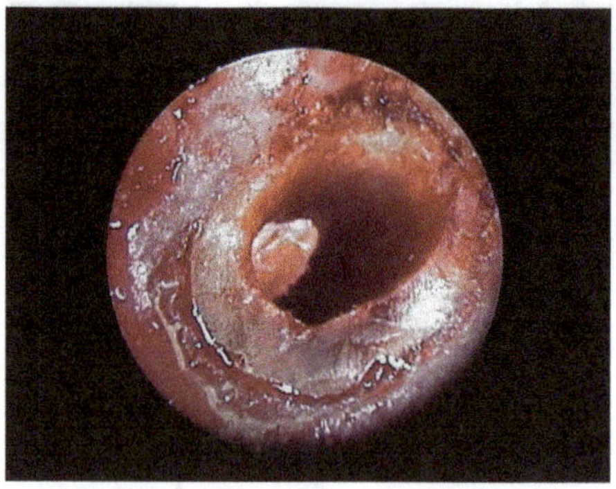

Figure 11: Endoscopic view of 1.1 after removal of the old filler material and checking of retrograde cavity integrity.

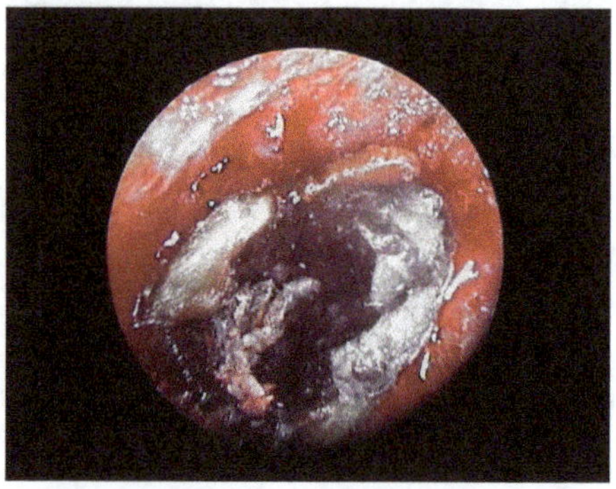

Figure 12: Endoscopic view of 2.1 after removal of the old filler material and checking of retrograde cavity integrity.

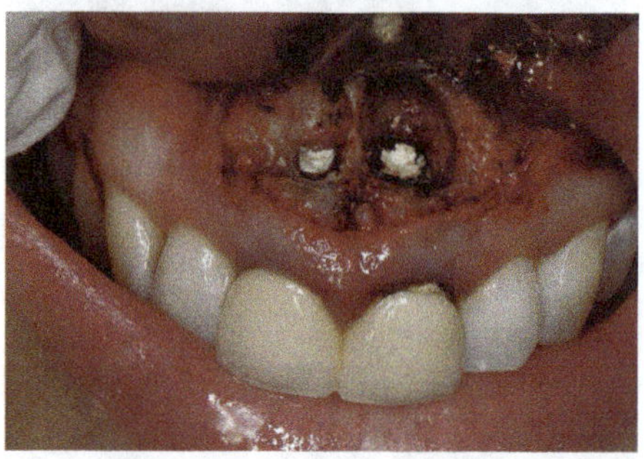

Figure 13: Clinical view of filling with MTA of the retrograde cavities of 1.1 and 2.1.

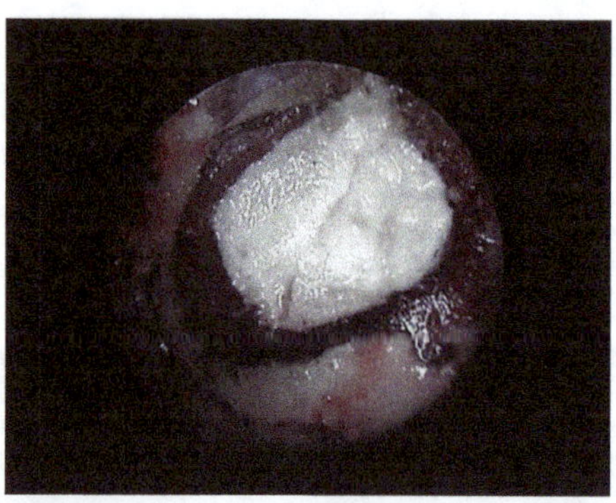

Figure 14: Endoscopic view of 1.1 after filling of the retrograde cavity with MTA.

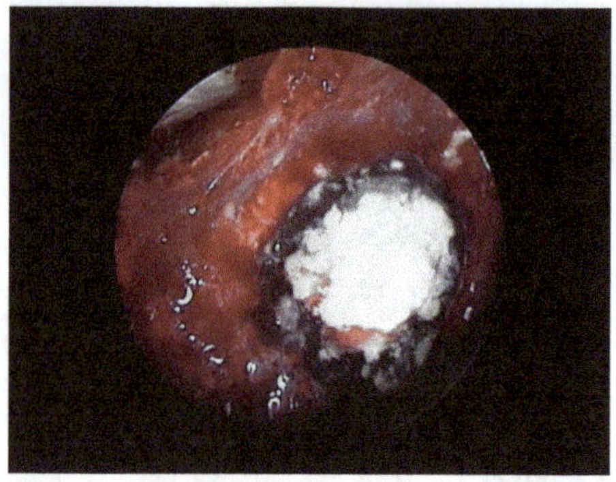

Figure 15: Endoscopic view of 2.1 after filling of the retrograde cavity with MTA.

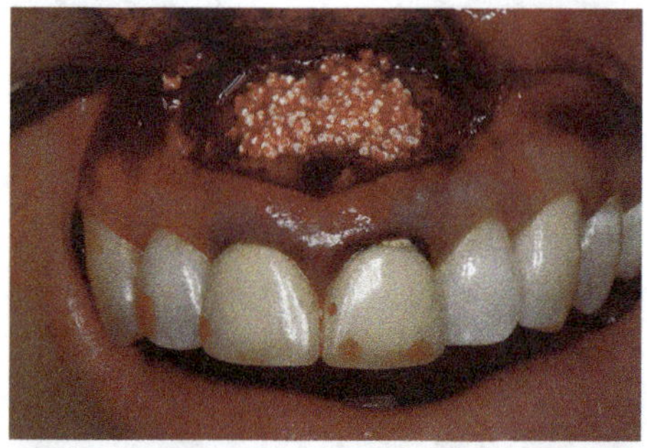

Figure 16: Regeneration of the defect with a synthetic bone graft.

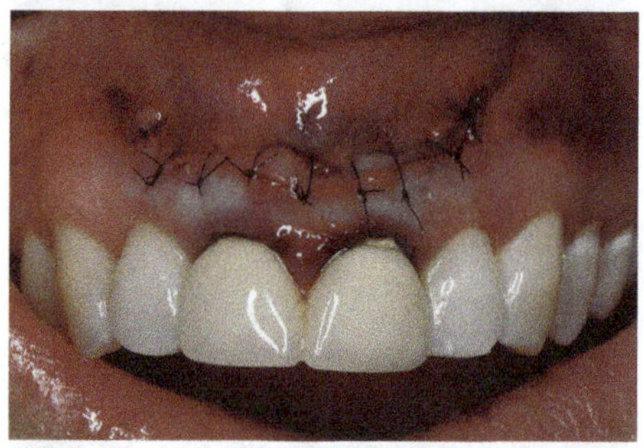

Figure 17: Flap suture with a non-reabsorbable 4/0 multifilament suture.

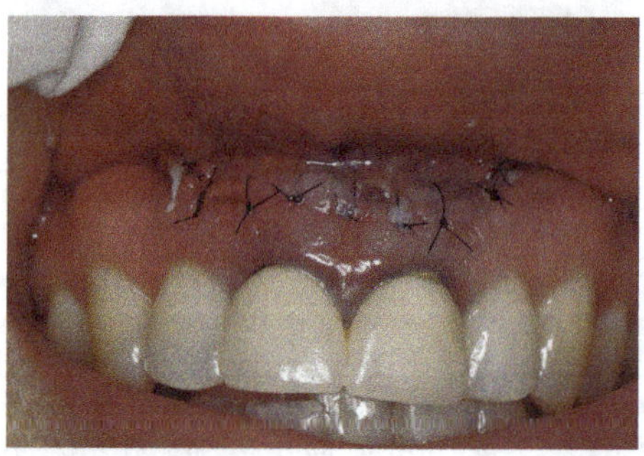

Figure 18: View after 7 days, before suture removal.

(Figure 20). After 6 months, clinical improvement of the soft tissues was evidenced (Figure 21), with adequate progression of bone healing of the defect on the periapical radiographs

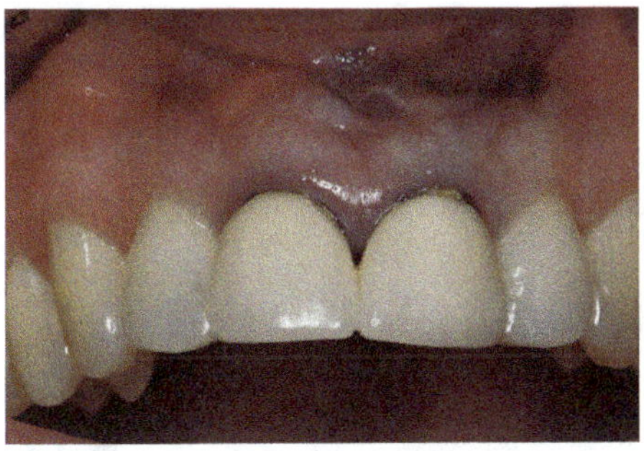

FIGURE 19: Clinical view one month after surgery: no suture dehiscence was noted.

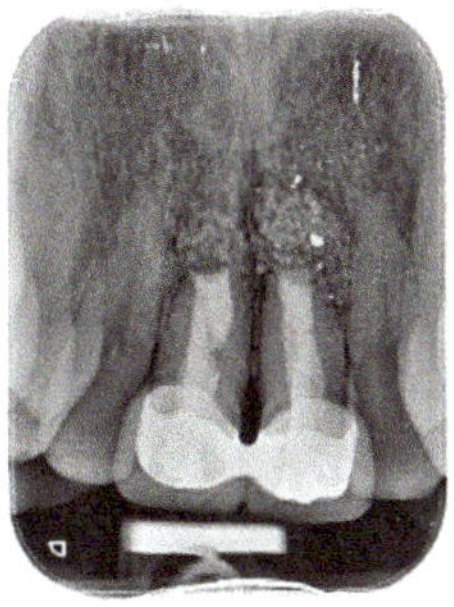

FIGURE 20: Periapical radiograph one month after surgery: correct retrograde cavity preparation is observed.

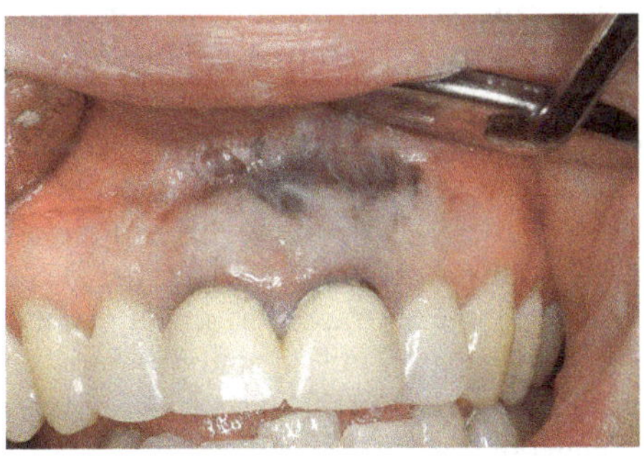

FIGURE 21: Clinical view 6 months after surgery, showing improvement of the soft tissues.

(Figure 22). After one year, correct soft tissue healing was confirmed (Figure 23), with complete bone regeneration in the radiographic study and no radiolucencies (Figure 24). The patient was informed of the advisability of replacing the crowns of 1.1 and 2.1 because of marginal misadjustment and the associated negative aesthetic impact. Three years later, the patient accepted 5the proposed treatment. The old crowns were replaced with new ones, and the biologically oriented preparation technique (BOPT) was used, eliminating the finishing line in both the frontal view (Figure 25) and occlusal view (Figure 26). Provisional crowns were placed during four weeks to stabilize the gingival tissue surrounding the teeth (Figure 27). The definitive crowns were made of monolithic zirconia with stratified feldspathic porcelain on

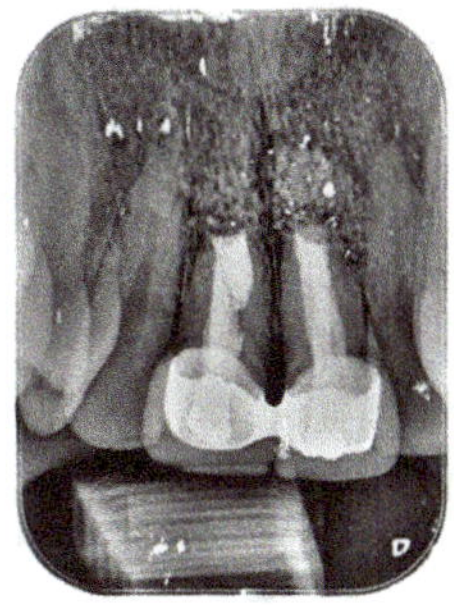

FIGURE 22: Periapical radiograph 6 months after surgery: correct progression of bone healing of the defect is observed.

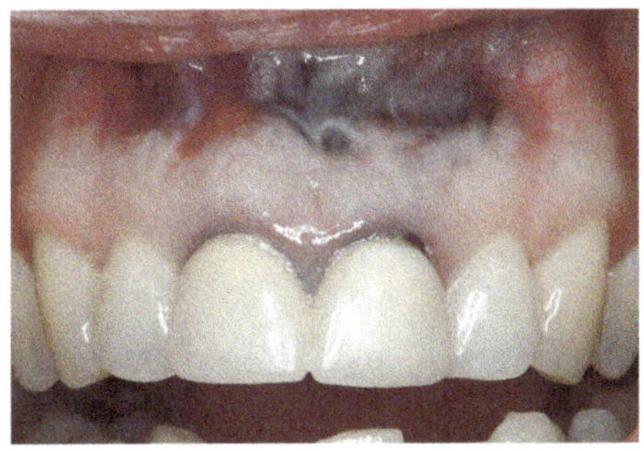

FIGURE 23: Clinical view one year after surgery: note the correct soft tissue healing.

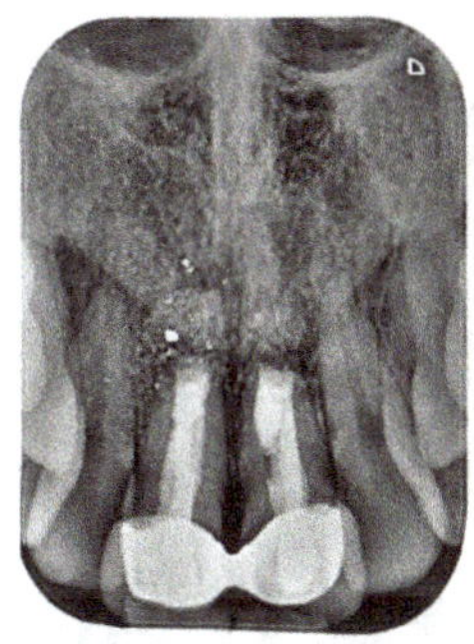

FIGURE 24: Periapical radiograph one year after surgery, showing complete bone regeneration of 1.1 and 2.1.

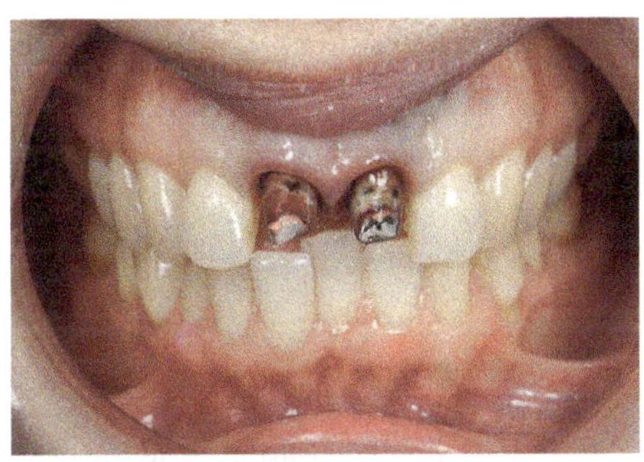

FIGURE 25: Frontal view of the stump of 1.1 and 2.1 based on the BOPT approach.

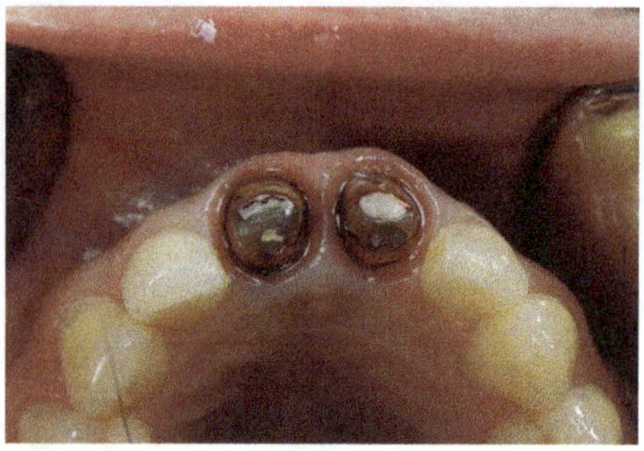

Figure 26: Occlusal view of the stump of 1.1 and 2.1 based on the BOPT approach.

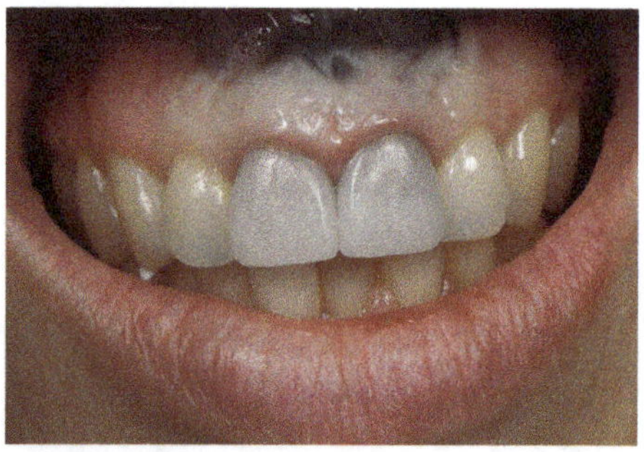

Figure 27: Fitting of the provisional crowns during four weeks to stabilize the surrounding gingival tissues.

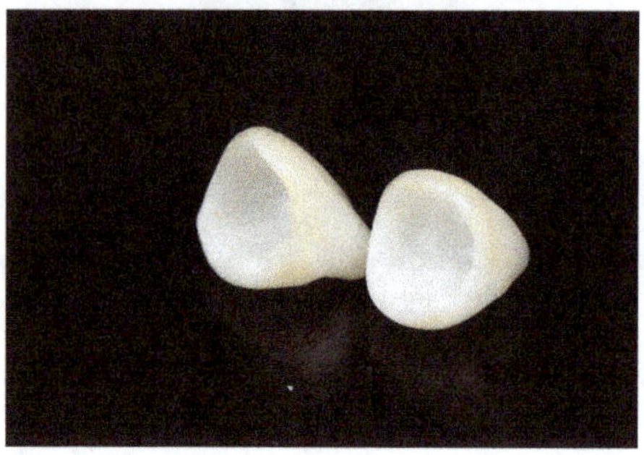

Figure 28: The definitive crowns made of monolithic zirconia with stratified feldspathic porcelain on the buccal aspect.

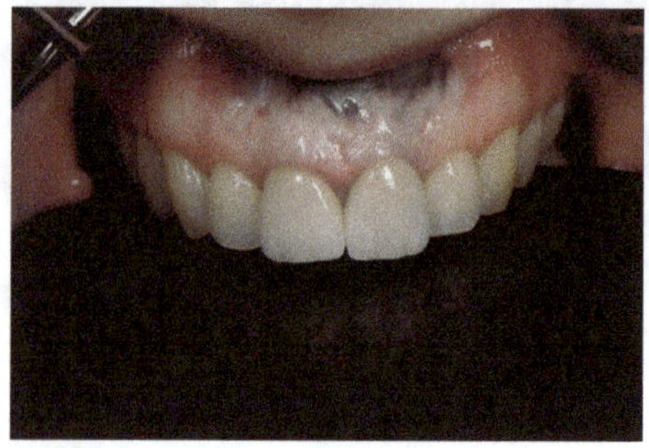

Figure 29: Clinical view after cementing the definitive crowns.

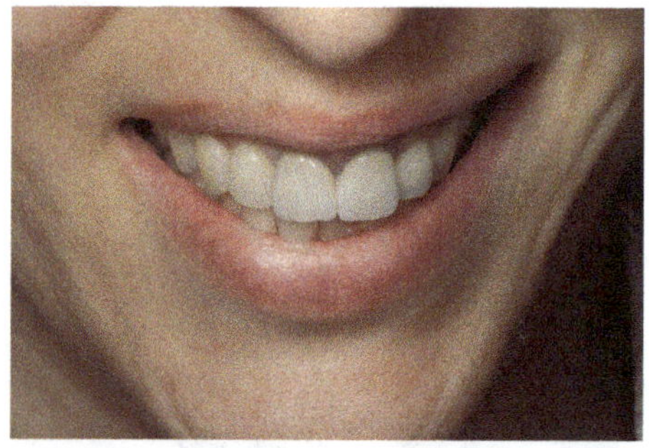

Figure 30: Extraoral view of smile after cementing the definitive crowns.

the buccal aspect (Figure 28), cemented with resin (RelyX Unicem, 3M®, Saint Paul, USA). Good periodontal health (Figure 29) and anterior aesthetic outcomes were achieved (Figure 30).

3. Discussion

In the present clinical case, periapical surgery was performed on two central upper incisors with persistent chronic periapical periodontitis that had already been subjected to periapical surgery 25 years ago, though without using the current magnification techniques. Over the years, conventional periapical surgery has evolved towards apical microsurgery, based on magnification and illumination of the surgical field with the endoscope and microscope [9–13]. The endoscope offers the surgeon excellent visibility [11], with an easier learning curve than the microscope, and both instruments afford a similar success rate [12]. The microscopic field is fixed, however, and the objective cannot be adjusted from different angles. Furthermore, in most cases, a mirror is needed for indirect visualization. In contrast, the endoscope offers easy adjustment, allowing visualization from different angles and providing direct images [13]. Endoscopy is therefore a versatile, rapid, and convenient magnification tool [12].

In addition to the introduction of ultrasound tips for retrograde cavity preparation [14], many materials have been used to secure correct cavity sealing, such as silver amalgam, zinc oxide-eugenol cements (IRM, Super-EBA), MTA, polycarboxylate cement (Durelon), or composites with dental adhesives (RetroPlast), among others.

At present, MTA is the most widely used material and with the strongest supporting evidence in the literature. A number of randomized clinical trials have compared MTA with other retrograde filler materials. Three such studies involving very low risk of bias [15–17] have reported success rates of 85-94.3% with the use of MTA. A meta-analysis published by Von Arx et al. [18] and a systematic review by Serrano-Giménez et al. [19] have defined MTA as the material of choice for retrograde cavity sealing in periapical surgery.

With regard to prosthetic rehabilitation, we chose the BOPT approach, involving elimination of the preexisting finishing line in the tooth stump, and rotary curettage of the gingival sulcus was performed using a diamond drill [20]—since a number of studies have evidenced improved periodontal tissue conditions of the teeth treated with this technique [21, 22].

4. Conclusions

In the reported patient with failed periapical surgical treatment of persistent chronic periapical periodontitis using the classical technique, the described periapical microsurgery approach with magnification and illumination of the surgical field was found to be effective, avoiding the need to extract the two central upper incisors.

References

[1] E. Martí-Bowen and M. Peñarrocha, "An update in periapical surgery," *Medicina Oral, Patología Oral y Cirugía Bucal*, vol. 11, pp. E503–E509, 2006.

[2] M. Peñarrocha-Diago, B. Ortega-Sánchez, B. García-Mira, E. Martí-Bowen, T. von Arx, and C. Gay-Escoda, "Evaluation of healing criteria for success after periapical surgery," *Medicina Oral, Patología Oral y Cirugía Bucal*, vol. 13, no. 2, pp. E143–E147, 2008.

[3] S. Sutimuntanakul, W. Worayoskowit, and C. H. Mangkornkarn, "Retrograde seal in ultrasonically prepared canals," *Journal of Endodontia*, vol. 26, no. 8, pp. 444–446, 2000.

[4] M. Torabinejad, T. R. Pitt Ford, D. J. McKendry, H. R. Abedi, D. A. Miller, and S. P. Kariyawasam, "Histologic assessment of mineral trioxide aggregate as a root-end filling in monkeys," *Journal of Endodontia*, vol. 23, no. 4, pp. 225–228, 1997.

[5] T. T. Nakata, K. S. Bae, and J. C. Baumgartner, "OR 40 perforation repair comparing mineral trioxide aggregate and amalgam," *Journal of Endodontia*, vol. 23, no. 4, pp. 259–262, 1997.

[6] T. von Arx, S. S. Jensen, S. Hänni, and S. Friedman, "Five-year longitudinal assessment of the prognosis of apical microsurgery," *Journal of Endodontia*, vol. 38, no. 5, pp. 570–579, 2012.

[7] T. von Arx, S. Hänni, and S. S. Jensen, "Clinical results with two different methods of root-end preparation and filling in apical surgery: mineral trioxide aggregate and adhesive resin composite," *Journal of Endodontia*, vol. 36, no. 7, pp. 1122–1129, 2010.

[8] Q. Zhu, K. E. Safavi, and L. S. W. Spangberg, "Cytotoxic evaluation of root-end filling materials in cultures of human osteoblast-like cells and periodontal ligament cells," *Journal of Endodontia*, vol. 25, no. 6, pp. 410–412, 1999.

[9] F. C. Setzer, M. R. Kohli, S. B. Shah, B. Karabucak, and S. Kim, "Outcome of endodontic surgery: a meta-analysis of the literature—part 2: comparison of endodontic microsurgical techniques with and without the use of higher magnification," *Journal of Endodontia*, vol. 38, no. 1, pp. 1–10, 2012.

[10] S. Taschieri, M. Del Fabbro, T. Testori, and R. Weinstein, "Endoscopic periradicular surgery: a prospective clinical study," *The British Journal of Oral & Maxillofacial Surgery*, vol. 45, no. 3, pp. 242–244, 2007.

[11] A. Pallarés-Serrano, P. Glera-Suarez, D. Soto-Peñaloza, D. Peñarrocha-Oltra, T. von Arx, and M. Peñarrocha-Diago, "The use of the endoscope in endodontic surgery: A systematic review," *Journal of Clinical and Experimental Dentistry*, vol. 12, no. 10, pp. e972–e978, 2020.

[12] S. Taschieri, M. Del Fabbro, T. Testori, and R. Weinstein, "Microscope versus endoscope in root-end management: a randomized controlled study," *International Journal of Oral and Maxillofacial Surgery*, vol. 37, no. 11, pp. 1022–1026, 2008.

[13] S. Taschieri and M. Del Fabbro, "Endoscopic endodontic microsurgery: 2-year evaluation of healing and functionality," *Brazilian Oral Research*, vol. 23, no. 1, pp. 23–30, 2009.

[14] T. von Arx and B. Kurt, "Root-end cavity preparation after apicoectomy using a new type of sonic and diamond-surfaced retrotip: a 1-year follow-up study," *Journal of Oral and Maxillofacial Surgery*, vol. 57, no. 6, pp. 656–661, 1999.

[15] R. Christiansen, L. L. Kirkevang, P. Hørsted-Bindslev, and A. Wenzel, "Randomized clinical trial of root-end resection followed by root-end filling with mineral trioxide aggregate or smoothing of the orthograde gutta-percha root filling–1-year follow-up," *International Endodontic Journal*, vol. 42, no. 2, pp. 105–114, 2009.

[16] J. A. H. Lindeboom, J. W. F. H. Frenken, F. H. M. Kroon, and H. P. van den Akker, "A comparative prospective randomized clinical study of MTA and IRM as root-end filling materials in single-rooted teeth in endodontic surgery," *Oral Surgery, Oral Medicine, Oral Pathology, Oral Radiology, and Endodontology*, vol. 100, no. 4, pp. 495–500, 2005.

[17] M. Song and E. Kim, "A prospective randomized controlled study of mineral trioxide aggregate and super ethoxy-benzoic acid as root-end filling materials in endodontic microsurgery," *Journal of Endodontia*, vol. 38, no. 7, pp. 875–879, 2012.

[18] T. Von Arx, M. Peñarrocha, and S. Jensen, "Prognostic factors in apical surgery with root-end filling: a meta-analysis," *Journal of Endodontia*, vol. 36, no. 6, pp. 957–973, 2010.

[19] M. Serrano-Gimenez, A. Sanchez-Torres, and C. Gay-Escoda, "Prognostic factors on periapical surgery: a systematic review," *Medicina Oral, Patología Oral y Cirugía Bucal*, vol. 20, no. 6, pp. e715–e722, 2015.

[20] I. Loi and A. Di Felice, "Biologically oriented preparation technique (BOPT): a new approach for prosthetic restoration of periodontically healthy teeth," *The European Journal of Esthetic Dentistry*, vol. 8, no. 1, pp. 10–23, 2013.

[21] R. Agustín-Panadero, B. Serra-Pastor, A. Fons-Font, and M. F. Solá-Ruíz, "Prospective clinical study of zirconia full-coverage restorations on teeth prepared with biologically oriented preparation technique on gingival health: results after two-year follow-up," *Operative Dentistry*, vol. 43, no. 5, pp. 482–487, 2018.

[22] B. Serra-Pastor, I. Loi, A. Fons-Font, M. F. Solá-Ruíz, and R. Agustín-Panadero, "Periodontal and prosthetic outcomes on teeth prepared with biologically oriented preparation technique: a 4-year follow-up prospective clinical study," *Journal of Prosthodontic Research*, vol. 63, no. 4, pp. 415–420, 2019.

11

Maxillary First Molars with Two Palatal Root Canals

Kun-Hwa Sung, Ho-Keel Hwang, and Hyoung-Hoon Jo

Department of Conservative Dentistry, School of Dentistry, Chosun University, Gwangju, Republic of Korea

Correspondence should be addressed to Hyoung-Hoon Jo; joyendo@hanmail.net

Academic Editor: Konstantinos Michalakis

Understanding the anatomical variations in the roots and root canal systems of a tooth is important for the success of root canal treatment. The palatal roots of the maxillary molars have fewer anatomical variations than the other roots, and fewer variations occur in the first molars than in the second molars. This case report describes two distinct cases of maxillary first molars with two palatal canals. For the root canal treatment of teeth with anatomical variations, it is essential to plan specific treatment strategies using cone-beam computed tomography and to execute them using a dental operating microscope. Knowledge of the anatomical variations in the palatal roots of maxillary first molars will help to increase the success rate of root canal treatments.

1. Introduction

Successful root canal treatment requires knowledge of the anatomy of the root and root canal [1]. However, anatomical variations can occur, which can complicate root canal treatment. Incomplete endodontic treatment is more likely to occur in teeth with such anatomical complexities, resulting in the failure of endodontic treatment [2].

More than 95% of the maxillary first molars have three roots—mesiobuccal, distobuccal, and palatal. The mesiobuccal root has the highest anatomical variability and has two or more canals in 56.8% of cases [1]. In contrast, the palatal root has the lowest variability, with a single canal in 99% and a single apical foramen in 98.8% of cases [1]. Stone and Stroner [3] reported very low proportions of maxillary molars with two palatal roots. However, Slowey [4] reported the root canal treatment of a maxillary molar with two palatal roots. In 1991, Christie et al. proposed a classification for maxillary molars with two palatal roots, depending on the shape and degree of root fusion [5]. According to this classification, type I maxillary molars have two widely divergent palatal roots, type II have four separate roots, which are short and parallel, while type III molars are constricted with the mesiobuccal, mesiopalatal, and distopalatal root dentin showing a web form. Following Christie's classification, Baratto-Filho et al. proposed an additional type IV, in which the mesiobuccal and palatal roots may be fused in the coronal two-thirds [6] Since then, rare cases of maxillary molars with palatal root abnormalities have been reported [7–16]; however, data on the various types of anatomical variations and their incidence are limited. These variations are more frequently reported in maxillary second molars than in maxillary first molars [8–11, 15, 17, 18]. This case report describes the nonsurgical root canal treatment of maxillary first molars with two palatal root canals in two patients.

2. Case Presentations

2.1. Case 1. A 53-year-old woman was referred to the Chosun University Dental Hospital with complaints of persistent pain in the left maxillary molar. Her medical history was noncontributory. The patient reported persistent pain in the left maxillary posterior area following a composite resin restoration. On clinical examination of the left maxillary first molar, spontaneous pain and tenderness on percussion were detected. The response of tooth 26 to cold and electric pulp testing (Parkell Electronics, Farmingdale, NY, USA) was negative. A periapical radiograph of the tooth showed divergent buccal roots and a palatal root that was not clearly distinguishable (Figure 1(a)). To clearly visualize the tooth anatomy, cone-beam computed tomography (CBCT) (CS9300; Carestream Health Inc., Rochester, NY, USA) was performed with a 10 × 5 field of view (FOV). The CBCT revealed that the mesiobuccal and distobuccal roots were fused from the cervical third to the apex, forming a C-shaped root (Figure 1(b)), and the root canal of the single palatal root was bifurcated at its middle third. Each branched root canal had an independent apical foramen (Figures 1(b) and 1(c)). The left maxillary first molar was diagnosed with symptomatic irreversible pulpitis and symptomatic apical periodontitis, and a nonsurgical root canal treatment was planned. An informed consent form was obtained after the treatment plan was established.

The tooth was anesthetised using 2% lidocaine containing 1 : 100,000 epinephrine and was isolated with a dental dam, and endodontic treatment was performed under a dental operating microscope (Global Surgical, St. Louis, MO, USA). A conventional access cavity was prepared using a no. 330 carbide bur and an Endo Access bur no. A0164 (Dentsply Maillefer, Ballaigues, Switzerland). On the pulpal floor, the orifices of the mesiobuccal, midbuccal, distobuccal, and palatal canal were observed (Figure 2(a)). Coronal flaring was performed using the ProTaper SX rotary file (Dentsply Maillefer, Ballaigues, Switzerland) to establish straight-line access. The glide path was established using a ProGlider file (Dentsply Maillefer, Ballaigues, Switzerland). The working lengths of the root canals were determined using ISO 10 K-files (Dentsply Maillefer, Ballaigues, Switzerland) and an electronic apex locator (Dentaport II; J. Morita, Tokyo, Japan). The three buccal root canals were shaped using ProTaper Next files (Dentsply Maillefer, Ballaigues, Switzerland) up to size ×2. Irrigation was performed using 3.5% sodium hypochlorite (NaOCl) solution between instrumentations. After access opening, only one orifice of the palatal canal was observed on the pulpal floor. Since bifurcation of the roots occurred in the middle third of the roots in the CBCT examination, the root canal was enlarged from the orifice to the bifurcation area using a long neck round bur (EndoTracer; Komet, Lemgo, Germany) with a specially designed long neck to prevent obstruction of the visual field on the dental microscope. After enlarging the root canal using a long neck round bur, two orifices were confirmed (Figure 2(b)). After scouting and working length determination, the two palatal root canals were prepared in the same way as the other root canals using ProTaper Next files. Finally, three and two root canals in the buccal and palatal roots, respectively, were subjected to root canal shaping. Excluding the palatal canals, the three buccal canals were filled with gutta-percha cones and a calcium-silicate-based sealer (EndoSeal MTA; Maruchi, Wonju, Korea) using a continuous wave compaction technique (Figure 2(c)). The two palatal canals beyond the bifurcation were filled with gutta-percha cones and calcium-silicate-based sealer using a one-cone technique. The root canal above the bifurcation area was back-filled with gutta-percha. The access cavity was restored using composite resin, and the tooth was permanently restored with a gold crown.

Twelve months later, the patient was recalled for follow-up and was asymptomatic. The 12-month follow-up radiograph showed a no evidence of pathology (Figure 2(d)).

2.2. Case 2. A 58-year-old man complaining of gingival swelling in the right maxillary molar area was referred to the Chosun University Dental Hospital. His medical history was noncontributory. On clinical examination, a sinus tract was found in the buccal gingival region of tooth 16. The response of tooth 16 to cold and electric pulp testing (Parkell Electronics, Farmingdale, NY, USA) was negative. Intraoral examination revealed a deep gingival pocket with a probing depth of 8 mm on the buccal aspect. Preoperative periapical radiography revealed a radiolucent periapical lesion and narrowed root canals. Two buccal roots and one palatal root were observed on the radiograph; however, the periodontal ligament space on the mesial side suggested the possibility of additional roots (Figure 3(a)). Shadows due to fractures of the crown in the mesiocervical area were observed on preoperative radiographs, and there were no additional caries. After a diagnosis of pulpal necrosis and chronic apical periodontitis was established, nonsurgical root canal treatment was planned. An informed consent was obtained after the treatment plan was established. Local anesthesia was induced using 2% lidocaine with 1 : 100,000 epinephrine, and endodontic treatment was performed under a dental operating microscope (Global Surgical, St. Louis, MO, USA). After dental dam isolation, an access cavity was prepared using a no. 330 carbide bur and Endo Access bur no. A0164 (Dentsply Maillefer, Ballaigues, Switzerland). As the preoperative radiograph suggested a possibility that two palatal roots existed, modification was required when preparing the access cavity. The access cavity was prepared in the conventional form on the buccal side, but when preparing the palatal side, it was made wider in the mesiodistal direction than the conventional preparation. The orifice of one palatal root canal was observed distopalatally on the pulpal floor, and an additional root canal orifice was observed at the mesiopalatal position. Four canal orifices, including the two palatal canal orifices, were identified on the pulpal floor, and endodontic treatment was performed. Glide paths were established using ProGlider files (Dentsply Maillefer, Ballaigues, Switzerland). The working lengths of all canals were determined using ISO 10 K-files (Dentsply Maillefer, Ballaigues, Switzerland) and an electronic apex locator (Root ZX; J. Morita, Tokyo, Japan). To understand the anatomy of the buccal and palatal root canals, intraoperative radiographs were obtained with K- and H-files in the buccal and palatal root canals, respectively (Figure 3(b)). All root canals were shaped using ProTaper Next files (Dentsply Maillefer, Ballaigues, Switzerland) up to size ×2 under copious irrigation with 3.5% NaOCl. Root canal filling was performed using the continuous wave compaction technique with gutta-percha cones and a calcium-silicate-based sealer (EndoSeal MTA; Maruchi, Wonju, Korea). Subsequently, the access cavity was sealed with composite resin, and the tooth was permanently restored with a gold crown. Postoperative periapical radiography revealed two long palatal and two short buccal canals (Figure 3(c)). Figure 3(d) shows the four canal orifices over the pulpal floor after obturation. At the 6-month follow-up, the patient was asymptomatic. Clinical examination showed that the probing depth of the buccal gingival sulcus recovered to within the normal range (<3 mm). The periapical radiograph shows

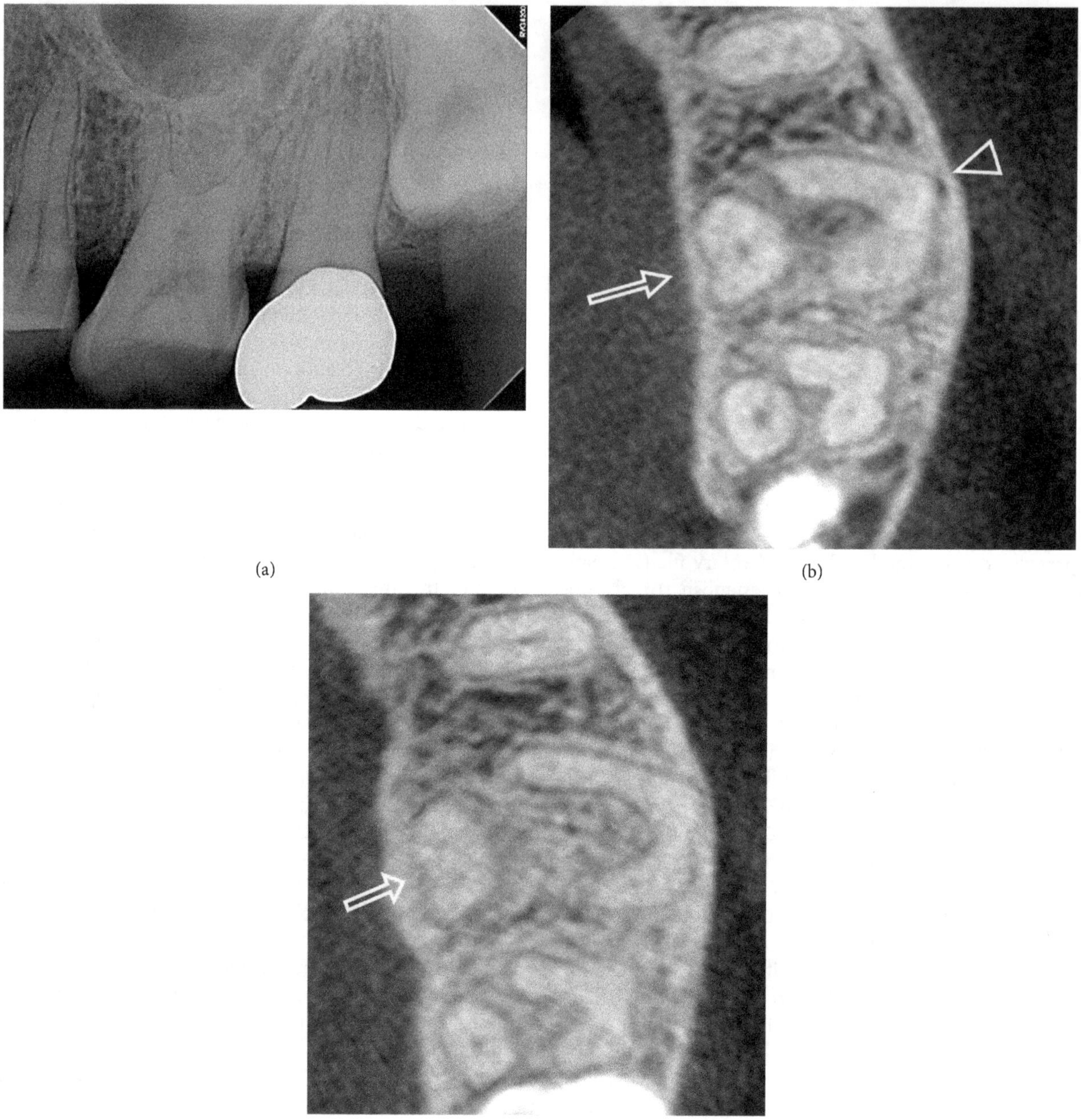

(a) (b) (c)

Figure 1: (a) Preoperative periapical radiograph. Note the divergence of the buccal roots and the unclear palatal root. (b) Axial CBCT image at the cervical third of the roots showing fusion of the buccal roots (triangle) and one palatal canal (arrow) in the palatal root. (c) Axial CBCT image at the middle third of the roots showing two canals in the palatal root (arrow).

partial resolution of the periradicular radiolucency (Figure 3(e)).

3. Discussion

Studies on the number and shape of the roots of the maxillary molars have shown higher anatomical variability in the maxillary second molars than in the first molars in various ethnic groups [19–22]. Previous studies on the anatomical variations in maxillary molars have focused mainly on the mesiobuccal root. In this regard, it has been reported that the maxillary first and second molars have two or more root canals in 40.3%–87.2% and 15.1%–57.94% of cases, respectively [23–29]. However, relatively few studies have been conducted on palatal root anatomy, which exhibits less variability. Stone and Stroner examined 500 extracted maxillary molars, excluding third molars, and reported that the palatal root had additional root canals in <2% of cases [3]. A CBCT study of the number of palatal root canals in 802 maxillary first molars and 660 upper second molars in Koreans showed that only 1.82% of the latter had two root canals [19]. In another study, Mohara et al. reported that in the maxillary first molars, the mesiobuccal and palatal roots had additional root canals in 64.22% and 0.31% of cases, respectively; in the

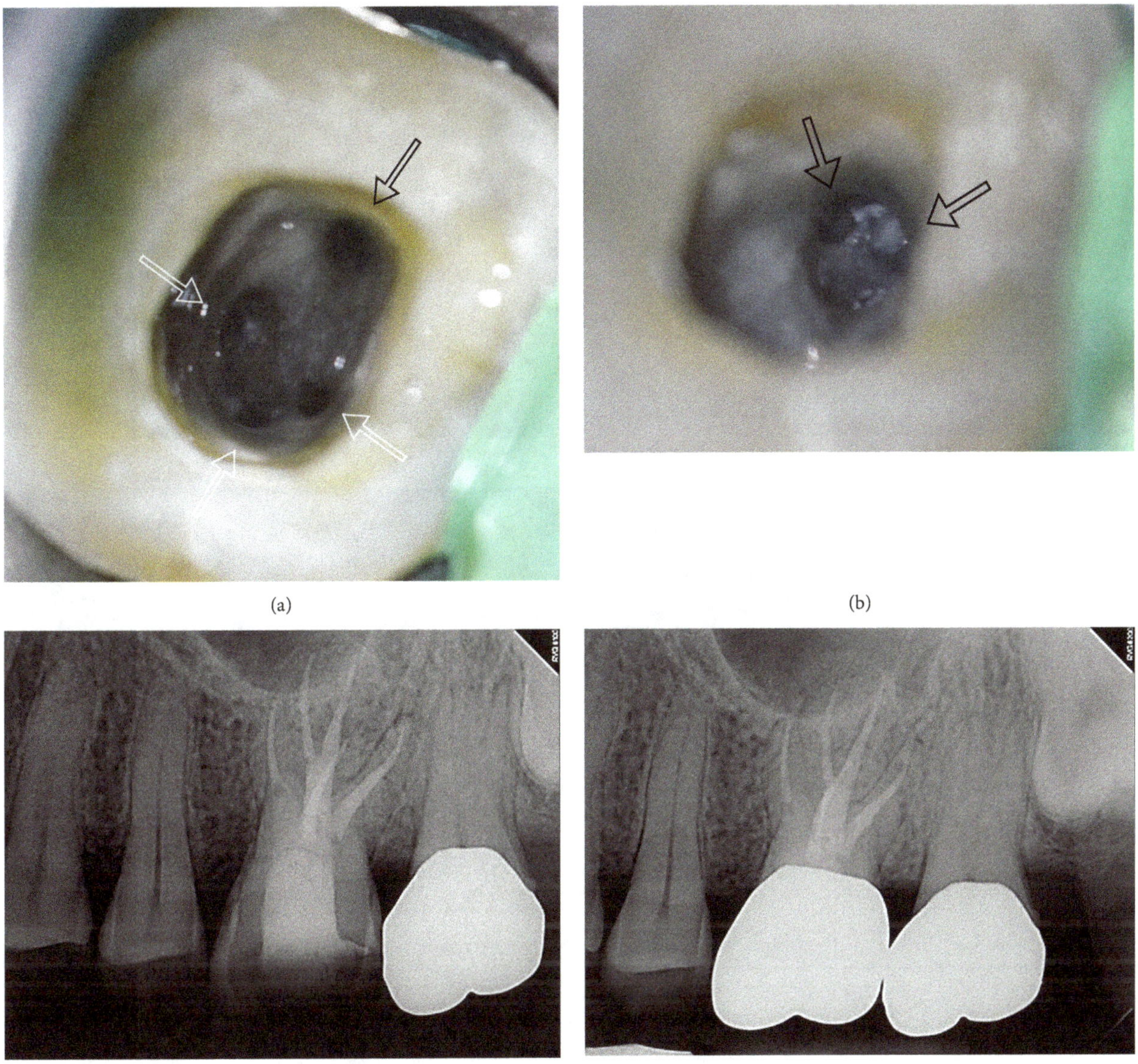

(a) (b) (c) (d)

FIGURE 2: (a) Microscopic image of the pulpal floor of tooth 26. At the level of the pulpal floor, one palatal canal orifice (black arrow) and three buccal canal orifices (white arrows) can be seen. (b) Microscopic image at the level of the bifurcation of the palatal canal. Two canal orifices (black arrows) can be seen. (c) Postoperative radiograph, showing two separate canals in the palatal root. (d) Radiograph at the 12-month follow-up visit.

second molars, additional root canals in the mesiobuccal and palatal roots were seen in 33.56% and 0.34% of cases, respectively [30].

The C-shaped root canal configuration is a unique anatomical variation that is caused by the fusion of the roots and characteristically occurs in mandibular molars. In the maxillary molars, C-shaped root canals due to the fusion of roots are rarely observed [31]. Studies of various ethnic groups have shown root fusions in 0.61%–7.1% and 9.91%–25.2% of the maxillary first and second molars, respectively [30, 32, 33]. The fusion of the distobuccal root to the palatal root occurs more frequently than that of the mesiobuccal root to the distobuccal root [1].

In the first patient, the distobuccal and mesiobuccal roots were fused, and canal bifurcation occurred inside the palatal root. This was an extremely rare case in which two types of anatomical abnormalities occurred simultaneously. In the second patient, tooth 16 had two separate palatal roots, each with one orifice, one canal, and one apical foramen. As seen in these two patients, various anatomical variations may occur in the palatal roots of maxillary first molars, and more cases may be reported with the increased use of CBCT and dental operating microscopes.

In the case of midroot bifurcation, as in the first case, it is important to allow the device to access the bifurcation area. For this, illumination using a dental operating microscope is essential, and a long neck round bur that does not interfere with the FOV is very useful. The EndoTracer bur (Komet, Lemgo, Germany) used in this case has a total length of 31 mm with a long neck portion, which helps to form an

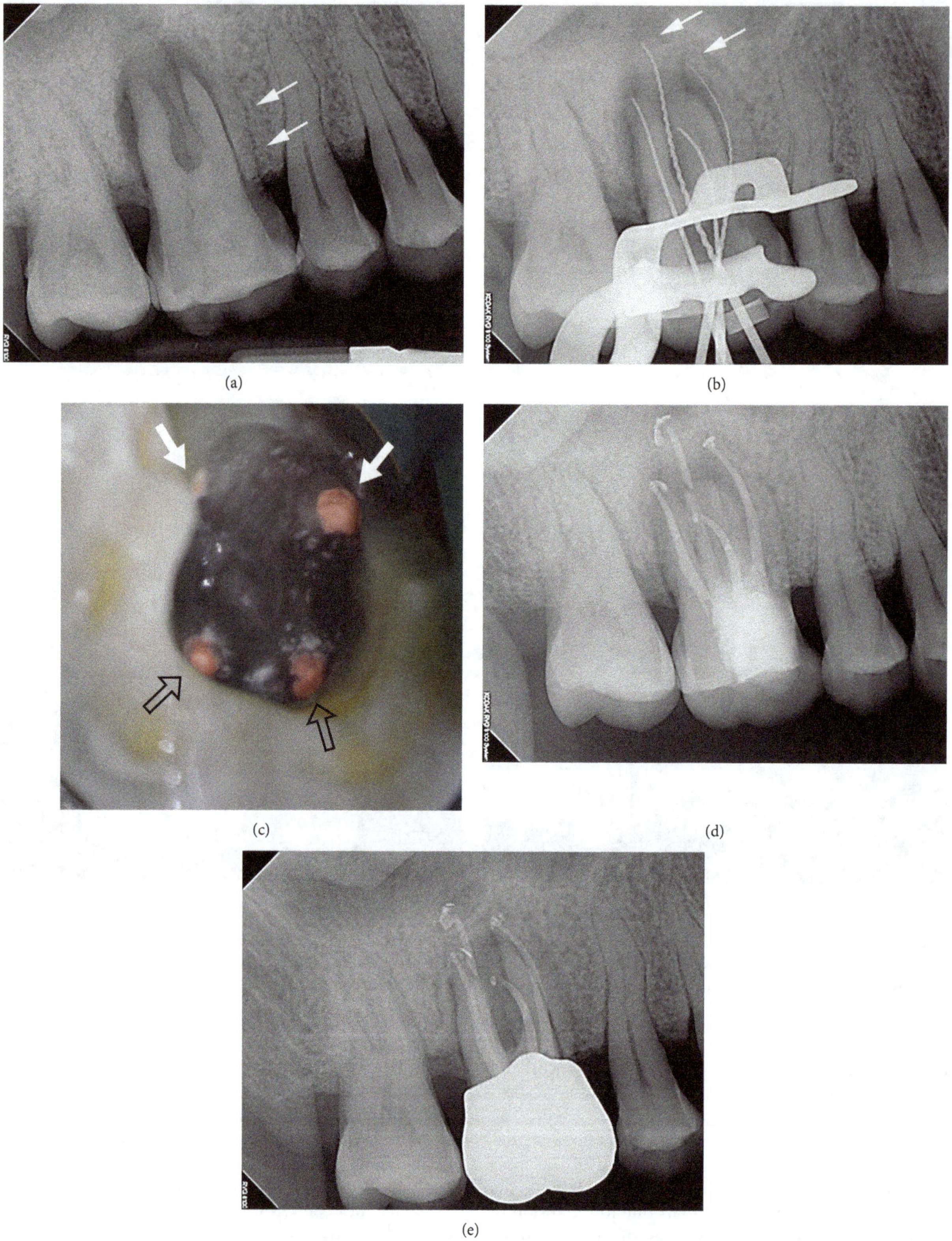

FIGURE 3: (a) Preoperative radiograph. Note the PDL space of the mesial side (white arrow) suggesting an additional root. (b) Intraoral radiograph shows two long palatal (white arrows) and two relatively short buccal root canals. Positioning of H-files on the palatal root canals and K-files in the buccal root canals to distinguish between the buccal and palatal sides. (c) Postoperative radiograph showing four separate canals. (d) Microscopic image of the pulpal floor of tooth 16 showing two buccal root canal orifices (black arrows) and two palatal root canal orifices (white arrows). (e) Radiograph at the recall visit at 6 months showing partial resolution of the periradicular radiolucency.

effective path without obstructing the FOV. For canal obturation beyond the bifurcation area, a one-cone technique using calcium silicate sealer and gutta-percha cone was performed, and backfill was performed from the bifurcation area to the pulpal floor.

In the second case, the possibility of the presence of an additional palatal root was suggested by the preoperative radiographs. When it is possible that two palatal roots exist, modification of the access cavity is required. In particular, if the orifice of the palatal root canal is not in the center relative to the tooth shape, but is located mesially or distally, the possibility of an additional root canal should be considered. In this case, the orifice of the first palatal root canal was located mesially, and the access cavity was expanded in the distal direction using a round bur. Checking the color of the pulpal floor through a dental operating microscope while preparing the access cavity may help to find the root canal orifice. Unlike the first case, in which bifurcation occurred in the midroot area, in the second case, two orifices were found on the pulpal floor, so a 31 mm long round bur was not used.

In this report, two important tools were used to manage anatomical variations. CBCT is a useful tool for identifying the internal anatomy of a tooth before treatment. In particular, it is useful to identify the number and curvature of the roots and the anatomical variation through 3D reconstruction [34, 35]. Clinicians can use CBCT for treatment planning before root canal treatment of maxillary molars with complex anatomy to understand the root structure. The second tool, the dental operating microscope, is essential for root canal treatment of teeth with complex anatomical structures. It provides better visualization of the operative field through effective illumination and higher magnification. Without it, detection of anatomical clues to find uncommon root canal bifurcation, such as that seen in the first patient, is difficult. The use of a dental operating microscope can help clinicians assess the treatment site and conduct complex treatment effectively.

Various anatomical variations can occur in the palatal root canal of the maxillary molar, and it is crucial that clinicians are aware of the possible aberrations or anomalies of the tooth. Through knowledge of the variations occurring in the palatal root and appropriate modifications, the clinician can increase the success rate of endodontic treatment. However, in some cases, the patient must be referred to an endodontist to receive specialized treatment.

4. Conclusion

In this case report, we presented the anomalies of the palatal roots and root canal system of the maxillary first molars. Clinicians should be aware of the possibility of anatomical variations, even though they rarely occur in the palatal root of the maxillary first molars.

In cases with two palatal root canals, CBCT can help establish a treatment plan, and a dental operating microscope can help with proper treatment. In addition, depending on the case, it is necessary to modify the shape of the access cavity according to the location of the orifice or to increase the accessibility by using a special long neck bur.

Finally, if a highly difficult endodontic treatment is expected, referral to an endodontist may be an option.

Authors' Contributions

All authors have contributed significantly to this study and have approved this manuscript.

Acknowledgments

This study was supported by a research fund from Chosun University Dental Hospital, 2020.

References

[1] B. M. Cleghorn, W. H. Christie, and C. C. Dong, "Root and root canal morphology of the human permanent maxillary first molar: a literature review," *Journal of Endodontics*, vol. 32, no. 9, pp. 813–821, 2006.

[2] M. Song, H. C. Kim, W. Lee, and E. Kim, "Analysis of the cause of failure in nonsurgical endodontic treatment by microscopic inspection during endodontic microsurgery," *Journal of Endodontics*, vol. 37, no. 11, pp. 1516–1519, 2011.

[3] L. H. Stone and W. F. Stroner, "Maxillary molars demonstrating more than one palatal root canal," *Oral Surgery, Oral Medicine, and Oral Pathology*, vol. 51, no. 6, pp. 649–652, 1981.

[4] R. R. Slowey, "Radiographic aids in the detection of extra root canals," *Oral Surgery, Oral Medicine, and Oral Pathology*, vol. 37, no. 5, pp. 762–772, 1974.

[5] W. H. Christie, M. D. Peikoff, and H. M. Fogel, "Maxillary molars with two palatal roots: a retrospective clinical study," *Journal of Endodontics*, vol. 17, no. 2, pp. 80–84, 1991.

[6] F. Baratto-Filho, L. F. Fariniuk, E. L. Ferreira, J. D. Pecora, A. M. Cruz-Filho, and M. D. Sousa-Neto, "Clinical and macroscopic study of maxillary molars with two palatal roots," *International Endodontic Journal*, vol. 35, no. 9, pp. 796–801, 2002.

[7] F. W. Benenati, "Segundo molar superior con dos conductos palatinos y un surco gingivo-palatino," *Journal of Endodontics*, vol. 11, no. 7, pp. 308–310, 1985.

[8] F. de Almeida-Gomes, C. Maniglia-Ferreira, and R. A. dos Santos, "Two palatal root canals in a maxillary second molar," *Australian Endodontic Journal*, vol. 33, no. 2, pp. 82-83, 2007.

[9] M. Eskandarinezhad and N. Ghasemi, "Nonsurgical endodontic retreatment of maxillary second molar with two palatal root canals: a case report," *Journal of Dental Research, Dental Clinics, Dental Prospects*, vol. 6, no. 2, pp. 75–78, 2012.

[10] M. Nabavizadeh, A. Abbaszadegan, H. Mirhadi, and Y. Ghahramani, "Root canal treatment of a maxillary second molar with two palatal canals: a case report," *Journal of Dentistry*, vol. 16, no. 4, pp. 371–373, 2015.

[11] M. B. Prashanth, P. Jain, and P. Patni, "Maxillary right second molar with two palatal root canals," *Journal of Conservative Dentistry*, vol. 13, no. 2, pp. 94–96, 2010.

[12] S. Shojaeian, J. Ghoddusi, and S. Hajian, "A case report of maxillary second molar with two palatal root canals and a furcal enamel pearl," *Iranian Endodontic Journal*, vol. 8, no. 1, pp. 37–39, 2013.

[13] T. T. Zhang, W. Qiu, and C. X. Ming, "Maxillary second molar with two palatal root canals: a case report," *Hua Xi Kou Qiang Yi Xue Za Zhi*, vol. 28, no. 6, pp. 678-679, 2010.

[14] P. M. Di Fiore, "A four-rooted quadrangular maxillary molar," *Journal of Endodontics*, vol. 25, no. 10, pp. 695–697, 1999.

[15] V. Gopikrishna, J. Reuben, and D. Kandaswamy, "Endodontic management of a maxillary first molar with two palatal roots and a single fused buccal root diagnosed with spiral computed tomography - a case report," *Oral Surgery, Oral Medicine, Oral Pathology, Oral Radiology, and Endodontics*, vol. 105, no. 4, pp. e74–e78, 2008.

[16] S. Holderrieth and C. R. Gernhardt, "Maxillary molars with morphologic variations of the palatal root canals: a report of four cases," *Journal of Endodontics*, vol. 35, no. 7, pp. 1060–1065, 2009.

[17] M. A. Versiani, J. D. Pecora, and M. D. de Sousa-Neto, "Root and root canal morphology of four-rooted maxillary second molars: a micro-computed tomography study," *Journal of Endodontics*, vol. 38, no. 7, pp. 977–982, 2012.

[18] V. Aggarwal, M. Singla, A. Logani, and N. Shah, "Endodontic management of a maxillary first molar with two palatal canals with the aid of spiral computed tomography: a case report," *Journal of Endodontics*, vol. 35, no. 1, pp. 137–139, 2009.

[19] Y. Kim, S. J. Lee, and J. Woo, "Morphology of maxillary first and second molars analyzed by cone-beam computed tomography in a Korean population: variations in the number of roots and canals and the incidence of fusion," *Journal of Endodontics*, vol. 38, no. 8, pp. 1063–1068, 2012.

[20] P. Neelakantan, C. Subbarao, R. Ahuja, C. V. Subbarao, and J. L. Gutmann, "Cone-beam computed tomography study of root and canal morphology of maxillary first and second molars in an Indian population," *Journal of Endodontics*, vol. 36, no. 10, pp. 1622–1627, 2010.

[21] K. Olczak and H. Pawlicka, "The morphology of maxillary first and second molars analyzed by cone-beam computed tomography in a Polish population," *BMC Medical Imaging*, vol. 17, no. 1, p. 68, 2017.

[22] Q. H. Zheng, Y. Wang, X. D. Zhou, Q. Wang, G. N. Zheng, and D. M. Huang, "A cone-beam computed tomography study of maxillary first permanent molar root and canal morphology in a Chinese population," *Journal of Endodontics*, vol. 36, no. 9, pp. 1480–1484, 2010.

[23] A. M. Ghobashy, M. M. Nagy, and A. A. Bayoumi, "Evaluation of root and canal morphology of maxillary permanent molars in an Egyptian population by cone-beam computed tomography," *Journal of Endodontics*, vol. 43, no. 7, pp. 1089–1092, 2017.

[24] N. Khosravifard, Z. D. Kajan, and H. Hasanpoor, "Cone beam computed tomographic survey of the mesiobuccal root canal anatomy in the maxillary first and second molar teeth of an Iranian population," *European Journal of Dentistry*, vol. 12, no. 3, pp. 422–427, 2018.

[25] J. N. R. Martins, D. Marques, A. Mata, and J. Caramês, "Root and root canal morphology of the permanent dentition in a Caucasian population: a cone-beam computed tomography study," *International Endodontic Journal*, vol. 50, no. 11, pp. 1013–1026, 2017.

[26] M. Pérez-Heredia, C. M. Ferrer-Luque, M. Bravo, P. Castelo-Baz, M. Ruíz-Piñón, and P. Baca, "Cone-beam computed tomographic study of root anatomy and canal configuration of molars in a Spanish population," *Journal of Endodontics*, vol. 43, no. 9, pp. 1511–1516, 2017.

[27] G. Plotino, L. Tocci, N. M. Grande et al., "Symmetry of root and root canal morphology of maxillary and mandibular molars in a White population: a cone-beam computed tomography study in vivo," *Journal of Endodontics*, vol. 39, no. 12, pp. 1545–1548, 2013.

[28] R. Ratanajirasut, A. Panichuttra, and S. Panmekiate, "A cone-beam computed tomographic study of root and canal morphology of maxillary first and second permanent molars in a Thai population," *Journal of Endodontics*, vol. 44, no. 1, pp. 56–61, 2018.

[29] R. Zhang, H. Yang, X. Yu, H. Wang, T. Hu, and P. M. Dummer, "Use of CBCT to identify the morphology of maxillary permanent molar teeth in a Chinese subpopulation," *International Endodontic Journal*, vol. 44, no. 2, pp. 162–169, 2011.

[30] N. T. Mohara, M. S. Coelho, N. V. de Queiroz et al., "Root anatomy and canal configuration of maxillary molars in a Brazilian subpopulation: a 125-μm cone-beam computed tomographic study," *European Journal of Dentistry*, vol. 13, no. 1, pp. 82–87, 2019.

[31] R. J. De Moor, "C-shaped root canal configuration in maxillary first molars," *International Endodontic Journal*, vol. 35, no. 2, pp. 200–208, 2002.

[32] H. H. Jo, J. B. Min, and H. K. Hwang, "Analysis of C-shaped root canal configuration in maxillary molars in a Korean population using cone-beam computed tomography," *Restorative Dentistry & Endodontics*, vol. 41, no. 1, pp. 55–62, 2016.

[33] J. N. Martins, A. Mata, D. Marques, C. Anderson, and J. Carames, "Prevalence and characteristics of the maxillary C-shaped molar," *Journal of Endodontics*, vol. 42, no. 3, pp. 383–389, 2016.

[34] T. C. Blattner, N. George, C. C. Lee, V. Kumar, and C. D. Yelton, "Efficacy of cone-beam computed tomography as a modality to accurately identify the presence of second mesiobuccal canals in maxillary first and second molars: a pilot study," *Journal of Endodontics*, vol. 36, no. 5, pp. 867–870, 2010.

[35] P. Neelakantan, C. Subbarao, and C. V. Subbarao, "Comparative evaluation of modified canal staining and clearing technique, cone-beam computed tomography, peripheral quantitative computed tomography, spiral computed tomography, and plain and contrast medium-enhanced digital radiography in studying root canal morphology," *Journal of Endodontics*, vol. 36, no. 9, pp. 1547–1551, 2010.

12

Erosion Infiltration in the Management of Molar-Incisor Hypomineralization (MIH) Defects

Rym Mabrouk[1], Souha Yahia[2], Afef Oueslati[1] and Nadia Frih[3]

[1]*Endodontics and Restorative Dentistry, Department of Dental Medicine, Hospital of Charles Nicolle, Tunis, Tunisia*
[2]*Endodontics and Restorative Dentistry, Service of Dental Medicine, Military Principal Hospital of Instruction, Tunis, Tunisia*
[3]*Forensic Dentistry and Head of Service, Department of Dental Medicine, Hospital of Charles Nicolle, Tunis, Tunisia*

Correspondence should be addressed to Rym Mabrouk; rim.mabrouk.rm@gmail.com

Academic Editor: Yuk Kwan Chen

White spot lesions caused by enamel demineralization are frequently encountered in dental practice. Their management has always been an important issue in modern dentistry. However, the real dilemma was treating aesthetic demands with noninvasive or minimally invasive techniques preserving the natural tissues. The introduction of resin infiltration technique seems to provide an intermediary treatment modality between prevention and restorative therapy. This case report is aimed at reporting the management of MIH opacities in anterior teeth with resin infiltration technique.

1. Introduction

White spot lesions (WSLs), defined as "white opacity," occur as a result of subsurface enamel demineralization that is located on smooth surfaces of teeth [1]. The resulting reduction of the mineral phase compared to healthy enamel leads to intrinsic optical modifications causing white marks. The etiologies are multiple involving preeruptive damages: fluorosis, traumatic hypomineralization, molar-incisor hypomineralization (MIH), or posteruptive lesions: white spots due to carious disease. Among the different clinical presentations of white defects, MIH is the least well-known [2, 3]. Molar-incisor hypomineralization (MIH) is defined as a developmental condition characterized by hypomineralization defects of the enamel on the first permanent molars associated with the permanent incisors. In the literature, the defects have been connected to environmental changes, breast feeding (milk dioxin), respiratory diseases, oxygen shortage of the ameloblasts, and high-fever diseases [4]. The defining clinical features of MIH are demarcated opacities with clear, distinct borders with the adjacent enamel. The opacities range from white to yellow/brown in appearance, and in lesions with a severe mineral deficit, rapid progression to posteruptive enamel breakdown can occur [5].

Incisal enamel defects are frequently quite extensive and most common on the buccal surfaces of the teeth, giving rise to more esthetic concerns [6]. Several techniques have been proposed to improve the appearance of MIH spot lesions. The common treatment strategy comprises restorative procedures, improvement of remineralization using CCP-ACP-containing or fluoride-containing products, microabrasion, and bleaching technique laminate veneer restoration. Recently, a resin infiltration technique was introduced with the development of highly flowable resin material [7].

This paper is aimed at describing and illustrating the aesthetic management of white opacities caused by MIH using a resin infiltration technique.

2. Case Presentation

A 29-year-old woman was referred to the Department of Dental Medicine of Hospital of Charles Nicolle, Tunis, with the chief complaint of restoring her smile before her wedding soon. The anamnesis did not specify any systemic illnesses of the patient. Intraoral examination revealed white spots in the upper bilateral central and lateral incisors. The spots were easily noticeable in the frontal view of the anterior teeth: big chalky white spots on tooth number 21 and 11 and two less pronounced spots on tooth 12 and 22. The spots were well limited, with distinct borders from the adjacent enamel (Figures 1(a) and 1(b)). The periodontal status of the patient was healthy and free from visible plaque, and the radiographic examination revealed no abnormalities of the supporting tissues. After the clinical and radiographic examination, the occurrence of hypomineralization of the upper first molars characterizing MIH confirmed the diagnosis. The erosion infiltration technique, a minimally invasive approach of management of enamel white spots, was proposed and discussed with the consent of the patient. The patient was informed of the infiltration technique's unpredictability, and those possible outcomes ranged from complete disappearance of the lesion to a partial aesthetic improvement. Under her agreement, a decision was made to perform the resin infiltration technique with Icon® (DMG, Hamburg, Germany) on the teeth. Teeth were cleaned with a prophylactic paste at the beginning of the procedure. A rubber dam was applied, and the lesion was locally isolated using a light-cured resin barrier (OpalDam™ Green Ultradent®) to ensure a more focalized treatment throughout the different steps of the process (Figure 1(c)). The resin infiltration technique was performed according to the manufacturer's instructions on the upper central and lateral incisors. The enamel surface layer was eroded by the application of 15% hydrochloric acid gel (Icon-Etch, DMG, Hamburg, Germany) for two minutes (Figure 1(d)). To achieve a homogeneous etching pattern, the manufacturer's recommendation to stir the gel from time to time, during application, using the smooth surface tips included in the respective product kit was followed. The etching procedure serves to remove superficial discolorations and the higher mineralized surface layer and expose the lesion body. Then, the acid gel was evacuated with a surgical aspirator. Teeth were rinsed for 30 seconds using a water spray, and the enamel surfaces were dried. At this time, the lesions were assessed for color modification; no visual color change was obtained. So, the etchant was applied again and reactivated for additional two minutes, until some color alteration could be observed at the wet eroded surface.

Next, the surfaces were air-dried, and ethanol (99%; Icon-Dry, DMG) was applied for 30 seconds to maximize the water removal inside the lesions (Figure 1(e)). To boost water removal, this step should be repeated at least once. The lesions were air-dried again, and the whitish appearance of enamel lesions was more pronounced (Figures 1(f) and 1(g)).

The resin infiltrant (Icon®) was then applied on the lesion surface, and it was allowed to penetrate for three minutes (Figure 1(h)). Excess resin was removed using a blow of air, and light-curing was performed for 40 seconds. The primary result was controlled, and the Icon infiltrant was applied again and allowed to set for one min and then light-cured for 40 s. Finally, the rubber dam was removed. The surfaces were polished using fine-grained abrasive flexible discs, silicone polishers, and finishing strips, depending on the treated area. An immediate esthetic improvement, with total color masking, was observed after treatment (Figure 1(i)).

3. Discussion

Enamel developmental defects are caused by various etiological factors, such as amelogenesis imperfecta, fluorosis, trauma hypomineralization, and molar-incisor hypomineralization (MIH). MIH is a qualitative defect of the enamel, characterized by the hypomineralization of one to four permanent first molars, frequently associated with affected incisors. It is also called as hypomineralized permanent first molars (PFMs), idiopathic enamel hypomineralization, nonfluoride hypomineralization, and dysmineralized PFMs [8, 9]. MIH prevalence varied from 3.6% to 37.5% among studies [10]. MIH can sometimes present with opacities in the upper and lower incisors. The characteristic feature of MIH is the clear demarcation between the affected and sound enamels [9]. The incisor defects are usually without loss of enamel substance and are generally less serious than those seen in molars due to the absence of chewing forces [11]. The risk of defects to the upper incisors appears to increase with an increasing number of affected FPMs. Enamel opacities associated with MIH can be problematic for the patients with much esthetic concern. Several techniques have been proposed to improve the appearance of these spots [6]. The described case showed an immediate improvement following the application of the low-viscosity resin, which could be an aesthetic alternative to masking the white opacities caused by molar-incisor hypomineralization [12].

Resin enamel infiltration is described as a microinvasive technology that fills, reinforces, and stabilizes demineralized enamel without drilling or sacrificing healthy tooth structure. This mini-invasive technique can be used to treat smooth surface and proximal carious lesions up to the first third of dentin (D-1) [13]. The procedure for resin infiltration is fairly simple. As the mineralized surface layer of the affected enamel impedes resin from penetrating into the lesion, this layer should be removed using hydrochloric acid gel (15%) which has been demonstrated to be superior to 37% phosphoric acid gel in removing the surface layer of natural enamel lesions when applied for 120 seconds. Its penetration depth etching is more than twice (58 μm) that of phosphoric acid, enabling penetration into the deepest part of the lesion and eliminating the decalcified areas. The lesion was then desiccated with 99% ethanol (Icon-Dry) to facilitate the drying process. Icon® works on the principle of infiltration and requires a very dry field. Apart from keeping the environment moisture-free, additional steps must be taken to dry the lesion. This is accomplished by treating the lesion area with alcohol, which evaporates the water within the porosities that could inhibit the process of infiltration [11, 13, 14].

The last step involved the infiltration of the resin and its light-curing for three minutes. The principle of resin infiltration is to perfuse the porous enamel with resin by capillary action, thereby arresting lesion progression by occluding the microporosities that provide diffusion pathways for the acids and dissolved materials. A positive side effect of resin infiltration is that enamel lesions lose their whitish appearance when these microporosities are filled with the resin. The principle of masking enamel lesions by resin infiltration is based on changes in light scattering within the lesions.

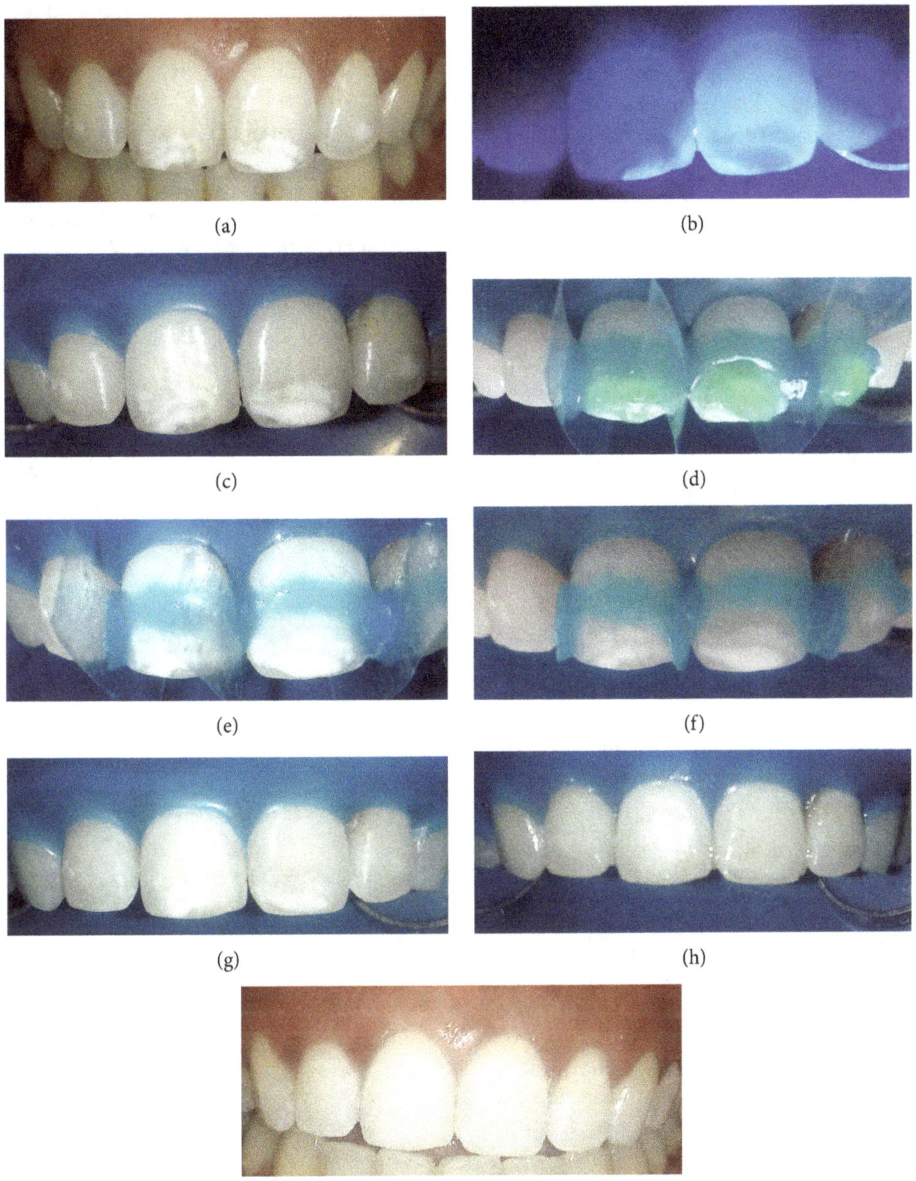

(a) (b) (c) (d) (e) (f) (g) (h) (i)

FIGURE 1: (a) White spot lesion related to molar-incisor hypomineralization. (b) Evaluation of the depth of the lesion under transillumination. (c) Isolation with a rubber dam. (d) Application of the acid gel (120 s) and washing with water spray. (e) Application of an ethanol drier. (f) The appearance of enamel surfaces after ethanol application. (g) Second application of an ethanol drier. (h) Application of a low-viscosity resin infiltration and polymerization. (i) Immediately final result.

Once infiltrated, white spot lesions take on the appearance of the surrounding healthy enamel [11, 15, 16]. In this case report, the resin infiltration technique was applied to the maxillary central and lateral incisors giving an aesthetically satisfactory result, in accordance with the finding of previous studies [8].

Biologically, the resin infiltration technique is a therapeutic of choice to aesthetically manage MIH white enamel spots. In addition to masking enamel opacities, resin infiltration increases the enamel surface hardness improving the mechanical properties of such lesions [17, 18]. Even though the resin infiltration technique is a noninvasive aesthetic treatment, preserving tooth structure, it still has some limitations such as inefficient isolation, incomplete resin polymerization, and the depth of the lesion that may affect the success of the treatment [16, 18]. Furthermore, organic materials, such as biofilm remnants, carbohydrates, lipids, and proteins, attached to the inner enamel surfaces, could possibly occlude the (underlying) pores in lesions, leading to an incomplete resin penetration of the porous structures and limiting the procedure results.

4. Conclusion

White spots caused by molar-incisor hypomineralization could be eradicated using a minimally invasive technique which shifts to enamel removal procedures. The patient's motivation would probably play a major role in the success of this approach. This technique is considered to be a micro-invasive procedure and might bridge the gap between noninvasive and minimally invasive treatments.

References

[1] D. Sundararaj, S. Venkatachalapathy, A. Tandon, and A. Pereira, "Critical evaluation of incidence and prevalence of white spot lesions during fixed orthodontic appliance treatment: a meta-analysis," *Journal of International Society of Preventive and Community Dentistry*, vol. 5, no. 6, pp. 433–439, 2015.

[2] M. Denis, A. Atlan, E. Vennat, G. Tirlet, and J. P. Attal, "White defects on enamel: diagnosis and anatomopathology: two essential factors for proper treatment (part 1)," *International Orthodontics*, vol. 11, no. 2, pp. 139–165, 2013.

[3] J. P. Attal, A. Atlan, M. Denis, E. Vennat, and G. Tirlet, "White spots on enamel: treatment protocol by superficial or deep infiltration (part 2)," *International Orthodontics*, vol. 12, no. 1, pp. 1–31, 2014.

[4] K. L. Weerheijm, B. Jälevik, and S. Alaluusua, "Molar-incisor hypomineralisation," *Caries Research*, vol. 35, no. 5, pp. 390-391, 2001.

[5] A. Ghanim, R. Mariño, and D. J. Manton, "Validity and reproducibility testing of the molar incisor hypomineralisation (MIH) index," *International Journal of Paediatric Dentistry*, vol. 29, no. 1, pp. 6–13, 2019.

[6] S. A. Fayle, "Molar incisor hypomineralisation: restorative management," *European Journal of Paediatric Dentistry*, vol. 4, no. 3, pp. 121–126, 2003.

[7] S. Jeong-Hye, H. Bock, K. Hyeon-Cheol, and P. Jeong-Kil, "Management of white spots: resin infiltration technique and microabrasion," *Journal of Korean Academy of Conservative Dentistry*, vol. 36, no. 1, pp. 66–71, 2011.

[8] H. S. Bahadır, G. Karadağ, and Y. Bayraktar, "Minimally invasive approach for improving anterior dental aesthetics: case report with 1-year follow-up," *Case Reports in Dentistry*, vol. 2018, Article ID 4601795, 5 pages, 2018.

[9] S. Padavala and G. Sukumaran, "Molar incisor hypomineralization and its prevalence," *Contemporary Clinical Dentistry*, vol. 9, Supplement 2, pp. S246–S250, 2018.

[10] P. Wogelius, D. Haubek, and S. Poulsen, "Prevalence and distribution of demarcated opacities in permanent 1st molars and incisors in 6 to 8-year-old Danish children," *Acta Odontologica Scandinavica*, vol. 66, no. 1, pp. 58–64, 2009.

[11] R. Bhandari, S. Thakur, P. Singhal, D. Chauhan, C. Jayam, and T. Jain, "Concealment effect of resin infiltration on incisor of grade I molar incisor hypomineralization patients: an *in vivo* study," *Journal of Conservative Dentistry*, vol. 21, no. 4, pp. 450–454, 2018.

[12] K. Srivastava, T. Tikku, R. Khanna, and K. Sachan, "Risk factors and management of white spot lesions in orthodontics," *Journal of Orthodontic Science*, vol. 2, no. 2, pp. 43–49, 2013.

[13] A. R. Cocco, R. G. Lund, E. N. Torre, and J. Martos, "Treatment of fluorosis spots using a resin infiltration technique: 14-month follow-up," *Operative Dentistry*, vol. 41-4, pp. 357–362, 2016.

[14] Z. Azizi, "Management of white spot lesions using resin infiltration technique: a review," *Open Journal of Dentistry and Oral Medicine*, vol. 3, no. 1, pp. 1 6, 2015.

[15] H. Meyer-Lueckel, S. Paris, and A. M. Kielbassa, "Surface layer erosion of natural caries lesions with phosphoric and hydrochloric acid gels in preparation for resin infiltration," *Caries Research*, vol. 41, pp. 223–230, 2007.

[16] V. Manoharan, S. A. Kumar, S. B. Arumugam, V. Anand, S. Krishnamoorthy, and J. J. Methippara, "Is resin infiltration a micro invasive approach to white lesions of calcified tooth structures?: a systemic review," *International Journal of Clinical Pediatric Dentistry*, vol. 12, no. 1, pp. 53–58, 2019.

[17] O. Marouane, N. Douki, and F. Chtioui, "A combined approach for the aesthetic management of stained enamel opacities: external bleaching followed by resin infiltration," *Case Reports in Dentistry*, vol. 2018, Article ID 1605842, 4 pages, 2018.

[18] S. A. Horuztepe, "Effect of resin infiltration on the color and microhardness of bleached white-spot lesions in bovine enamel (an in vitro study)," *Journal of Esthetic and Restorative Dentistry*, vol. 29, no. 5, pp. 378–385, 2017.

13

Dental Prosthetic Treatments in Cleidocranial Dysplasia: Case Report and Literature Review

Yosra Mabrouk[1] **Sinda Ammar,**[1] **Amel Labidi,**[1] **Lamia Mansour,**[1] **and Sonia Ghoul**[2]

[1]*Removable Prosthetics Department, ABCDF Laboratory (LR12ES10), Faculty of Dental Medicine, University of Monastir, Tunisia*
[2]*ABCDF Laboratory (LR12ES10), Faculty of Dental Medicine, University of Monastir, Tunisia*

Correspondence should be addressed to Yosra Mabrouk; mabroukyosra@gmail.com

Academic Editor: Giuseppe Alessandro Scardina

Cleidocranial dysplasia (CCD) is a rare inherited skeletal syndrome. There is no consensus regarding the dental treatment strategy. *Objectives.* To report a rare case of cleidocranial dysplasia and to summarize the current clinical and dental features and prosthetic treatment of similar CCD patients reported in the literature. *Results.* A 17-year-old girl was diagnosed with CCD. She had a short stature with the ability to bring the shoulders under the chest. All remaining teeth were deciduous except the four first molars were permanent. The maxilla was hypoplastic with a relative prognathism of the mandible. The cone-beam computed tomography examination showed a distorted and incomplete root formation of the permanent teeth. She was treated with both, complete and partial, removable overdentures. PubMed was used for the literature research using the following keys words "Cleidocranial Dysplasia"[Mesh], "Prosthodontics"[Mesh], "Dental Care"[Mesh], "cleidocranial dysostosis," and "dental treatment." The retention of deciduous teeth was described in the majority of cases. All the patients had supernumerary teeth. The most used treatments were dental prosthetics and orthodontics. The fixed prosthetic implant was the most used type of prosthetic treatment. Among the 15 cases who specified the type of prosthetic treatment, seven patients received removable dentures. Prosthetics was indicated especially for aged patients. *Conclusion.* Removable prostheses are a good solution that rapidly restores esthetics and functions. The use of implants for these patients needs to be validated by a long-term follow-up.

1. Introduction

Cleidocranial dysplasia (CCD) is a rare disease that occurs in 1 per million individuals worldwide [1]. It is a disorder involving an abnormal development of bones and teeth. This dysplasia affects the entire skeleton [2] and leads to several abnormalities threatening the patient's life. Diagnosis is always based on the clinical and radiological features and could be confirmed by a genetic analysis.

The bone-related manifestations include clavicular aplasia or hypoplasia and cone-shaped thorax with short ribs. The cephalic region presents a delayed closure of sutures and fontanels with the presence of wormian bones, frontal bossing, hypertelorism, and an enlarged nose base with a depressed bridge [3].

The tooth-related manifestations are considered as major characteristics of CCD which are almost the cause of complaint. The common dental features are the retention of deciduous dentition, the presence of many supernumerary teeth, and the noneruption of permanent dentition. Other disruptions could be described such as the underdevelopment of maxilla, upward and forward mandibular rotation, and skeletal class III malocclusion tendency. Although the presence of such problems, the child patient may have no pain, no swelling problems, and no difficulties for oral functions as long as deciduous teeth are still in the mouth. Child patients do not consult at an early age. Dental disability begins later with the progressive damage of deciduous dentition. Oral deterioration becomes rapidly progressive in few years giving the patient an edentulous and aged facial appearance [4]. At that time, the majority of patients consult with a complex clinical picture.

Several therapeutic approaches have been reported in the literature including the surgical procedure combined or not with orthodontics or implant placement and the prosthodontic procedure including a removable or fixed denture.

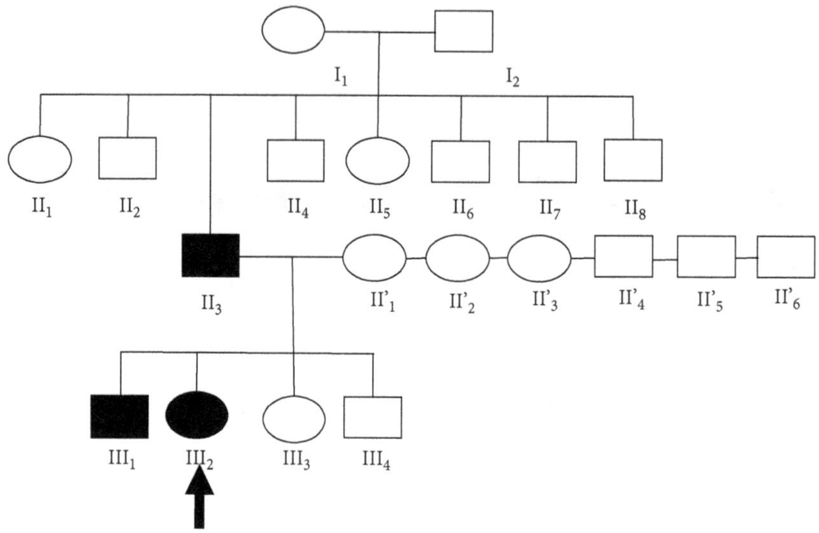

FIGURE 1: Pedigree of the studied family.

Concerning the invasive procedures, the surgical-orthodontic approach involves the extraction of unerupted supernumerary teeth, the exposure of permanent included teeth, their orthodontic traction, and their subsequent alignment [5]. The auto-transplantation of permanent teeth is another surgical alternative [5]. Concerning the implant surgical procedure, it is generally associated with the removal of deciduous and unerupted supernumerary teeth interfering with the implant placement [5]. Once osseointegration is obtained, a fixed or a removable prosthesis will be fabricated. This approach was reported since 1997 by Lombardas and Toothaker [6].

The noninvasive procedures include either fixed or removable tooth-supported prostheses. Concerning prosthetic rehabilitation with fixed prostheses, some authors propose the use of spontaneously erupted permanent teeth as abutments. However, CCD patients generally have a limited number of erupted permanent teeth. Therefore, fixed prostheses solely could not be used. Several authors [7–9] proposed the rehabilitation of this stomatognathic disorder with the removable prostheses by leaving permanent and supernumerary teeth in their positions as long as pathological changes did not occur and the use or not of deciduous teeth as abutments. This alternative is not only suitable for elderly patients, for whom orthodontic or surgical procedures could not be indicated, but also for child patients allowing them to integrate into society at an early age. In his literature review, D'Alessandro noted that the most reported cases treated with removable prostheses are children [5].

Although there is a great therapeutic choice, there is no consensus about the treatment strategy. According to Chang et al. [10], every author [11–13] almost proposes a treatment strategy that is based solely on his professional field. This ambiguity of treatment is associated with the presence of several factors in the therapeutic decision. These factors are almost related to the patients and not to the clinical findings such as their age at the time of consultation, their demands, and their treatment acceptance.

Theoretically, the surgical exposure of permanent teeth and their orthodontic traction seems to be a good option, but practically, it is a difficult and complicated treatment. In fact, after surgical extraction of supernumerary teeth and removal of the bone covering permanent teeth under general anesthesia, the prognosis of treatment remains unclear, and there is a risk for treatment failure [4]. In the past, the main treatment for these patients was prosthetic replacement [14]. That remains an interesting option that is always demanded by the patient as esthetics and function are restored rapidly and normal integration in the society is facilitated.

The need for a better understanding of this syndrome and the treatment options is necessary to better manage CCD patients. In this context, a systematic review was proposed to sum up the clinical and dental features which are almost described in CCD patients. The literature data about the treatment strategies were collected with an emphasis on prostheses. A CCD patient treated with removable prostheses was also reported.

2. Case Presentation

A 17-year-old girl presents at the removable prosthetics department. Her chief complaint was the unsightly retained deciduous teeth.

2.1. Clinical Evaluation. On examination, the patient had a short stature with lameness at walk. A cone-shaped thorax was noticed with an ability to bring the shoulders under the chest. The patient's father and brother also carry the same genetic defect. The transmission mode was recessive (Figure 1).

The facial examination revealed an enlarged nose base, cheeks sagging, an unsupported upper lip, and a decreased occlusal vertical dimension (OVD). The intraoral examination showed generalized chronic periodontitis with tartar deposits in the lower anterior region. All the remaining teeth,

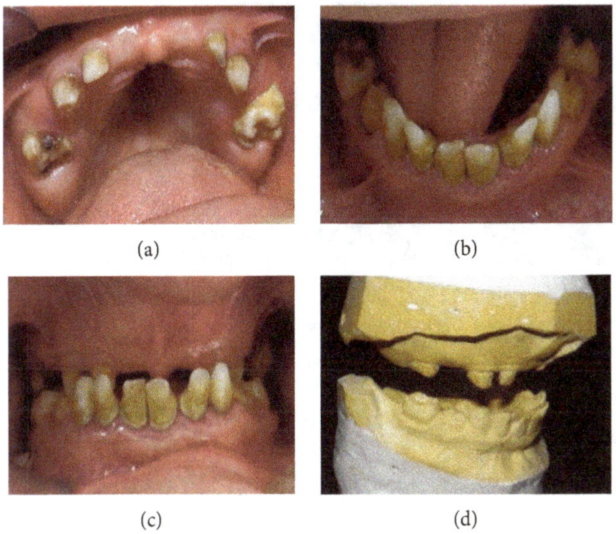

FIGURE 2: Clinical evaluation. (a) Occlusal view of maxillary arch. (b) Occlusal view of mandibular arch. (c) Intraoral photograph showing an anterior and posterior cross bite. (d) Bite registration in the correct occlusal vertical dimension.

in both the maxillary and mandibular arch, were deciduous except the four first molars were permanent. Mobility of the lower temporary incisors and canines was noticed. The upper anterior teeth were absent. The left maxillary molar was decayed (Figures 2(a) and 2(b)). The maxilla was hypoplastic with a relative prognathism of the mandible. An anterior and lateral crossbite was diagnosed (Figure 2(c)).

Casts were made and articulated at the patient's correct OVD. Registration was recorded with an interocclusal bite (Moycowax®, Aluwax®). An interocclusal rest space of 6 mm was evaluated (Figure 2(d)).

2.2. Radiographic Evaluation. The orthopantomogram revealed the presence of many unerupted supernumeraries and permanent teeth that had not achieved their root formation, especially in the maxillary premolar regions. The second upper left molar had a suprabony situation. Only its crown was formed. The lower permanent incisors achieved their root formation. They present a right eruption pathway (Figure 3(a)). A cone-beam computed tomography examination was performed. It showed a distorted and incomplete root formation of the permanent teeth. The two definitive upper central incisors present a juxta-bone situation with a right eruption pathway. However, only its crowns were formed. The lower permanent incisors had submucosal situation (Figure 3(c) and 3(d)). The frontal radiograph showed the presence of multiple wormian bones, a widened sagittal suture, and an underdevelopment of the maxilla and paranasal sinuses (Figure 3(b)). The left clavicle was hypoplastic with a deformation of the vertebral column in the thorax X-ray (Figure 3(e)).

2.3. Ultrastructural Evaluation. Upon a scanning electron microscopic examination, the extruded deciduous teeth showed normal structures either for the enamel, dentine, or pulp (Figures 4(a) and 4(b)).

2.4. Dental Treatment. After obtaining the patient's consent, the lower incisors and canines were extracted (Figure 5(a)). The patient had an incomplete root development of her permanent unerupted teeth with a generalized chronic periodontitis that did not allow orthodontic intervention. The treatment was oriented to the prosthodontic option. The patient had one permanent tooth in each hemiarch. Moreover, there was an important interocclusal rest space. These conditions could not allow the exploitation of the remaining permanent teeth as abutments for fixed prostheses. The use of implants was also eliminated because the patient refused a surgical extraction of the supernumerary teeth in the implant site. In addition, there was a risk of bone fragility given the high number of supernumerary and unerupted teeth to be extracted.

The decision was to make a complete removable overdenture at the maxilla and a partial removable denture at the mandible. The deciduous teeth were used as abutments for a complete prosthesis.

Individual trays were fabricated using diagnostic casts. Master impressions were recorded in polysulfide material (Surflex®). Occlusal registration was performed at the correct reestablished OVD. The mounted prosthetic teeth were checked and approved by the patient. The two removable prostheses were polymerized, fitted, and adjusted in the patient's mouth. Retention and stability of prostheses were excellent. The patient was very pleased and satisfied with her new appearance (Figure 3(b) and 3(c)).

The patient consulted every 2 months for a check-up. She has been followed for 4 years. The deciduous canines with mobility were extracted, and the prostheses were relined. Although the primary lower incisors and canines were avulsed, the corresponding permanent teeth did not erupt.

3. Literature Review

3.1. Statement of the Problem. Cleidocranial dysplasia is a rare inherited skeletal syndrome. It affects especially the clavicular bone and teeth. Several treatment options are used including orthodontics, surgery, and prosthodontics, but there is no consensus regarding the treatment strategy. The prosthodontic alternative remains a simple, cheap, and rapid solution.

3.2. Search Strategy. The explored database was Medline using the PubMed interface. The search strategy was conducted using the terms "Cleidocranial Dysplasia"[Mesh], "Prosthodontics"[Mesh], "Dental Care"[Mesh], "cleidocranial dysostosis," and "dental treatment." The review focused on combinations of these terms to collect the maximum of articles related to the subject. Four Boolean formula were made: ("Cleidocranial Dysplasia"[Mesh]) AND "Prosthodontics"[Mesh]), ("cleidocranial dysostosis" AND "Prosthodontics"[Mesh]), ("Cleidocranial Dysplasia"[Mesh]) AND "Dental Care"[Mesh]), and ("Cleidocranial Dysplasia"[-Mesh]) AND "dental treatment"). The final search update was in June 2016.

The exclusion criteria included the date of publication (<1996), and only the articles written in French or English

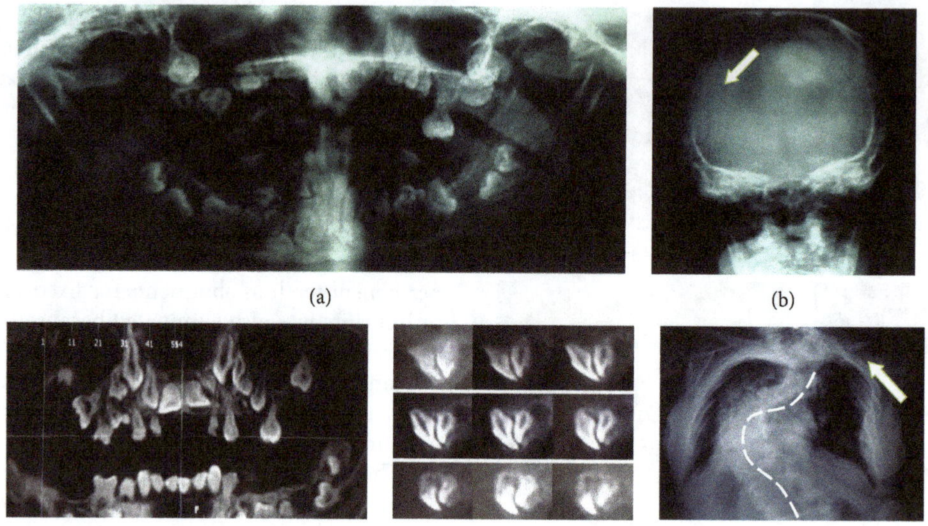

Figure 3: Radiographic evaluation. (a) Panoramic view of the jaws showing multiple unerupted supernumerary teeth. (b) Frontal radiograph showing a delayed closure of sagittal suture and the presence of Wormian bones. (c) Cone-beam radiograph of maxillary and mandibular arches showing a dilacerated root and inverted erupting pathway. (d) Sagittal cone-beam computed tomography section showing an incomplete formation of the left unerupted permanent incisor root. (e) Thorax radiograph showing hypoplasia of the left clavicle.

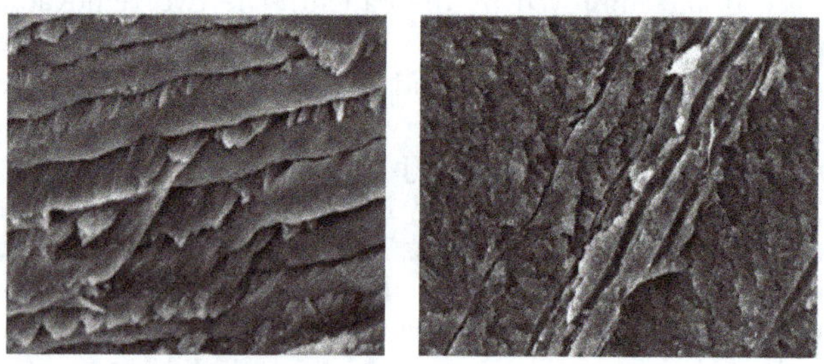

Figure 4: Ultrastructural evaluation. (a) A scanning electron microscopy (zoom ×2000) view showing the prismatic aspect of the enamel of the patient's temporary tooth. (b) A scanning electron microscopy (zoom ×2000) view showing some dentinal tubules in longitudinal section.

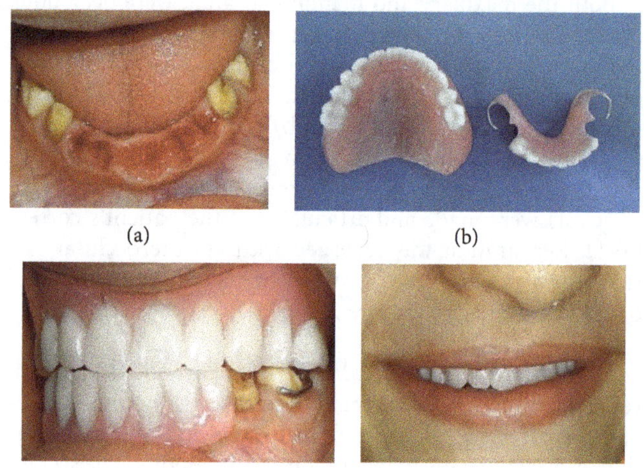

Figure 5: Dental treatment. (a) Extraction of the mandibular incisors and canines. (b) Interim maxillary and mandibular prostheses. (c) Prostheses adjusted in the mouth. (d) Final clinical view.

were retained. All types of articles were included except reviews. The data described by the authors in these papers were collected and analyzed by five reviewers independently using a preestablished checklist for data extraction (clinical photographs or radiographs were not used to include additional findings). In case of disagreement, a consensus was obtained by discussion among the reviewers.

3.3. Results

3.3.1. Article Selection. Sixty-four articles were obtained after the search. Considering the exclusion criteria and duplicates, 13 articles were retained. Three papers were excluded after reading (Figure 6). One article was not available.

3.3.2. Clinical Characteristics and Dental Features of the Patients That Were Included in This Systematic Review (Tables 1 and 2). Nine papers were included in the systematic review. Among these papers, eight concerned 10 case reports and 1 retrospective study described 15 patients. A total of 25 patients were included in the study, the youngest was 8 years old, and the oldest was 46. Twelve of them were male, and 13 were female. Twenty-one were in mixed dentition while four of them were in permanent dentition. Clavicular aplasia was noticed in 19 cases and hypoplasia in two cases while clavicular abnormalities were not specified in 4 cases. Delayed fontanel ossification was described in 15 patients. Inheritance was described in one case as autosomal dominant.

The dental features described in these patients covered retention of deciduous teeth (8 patients), unerupted permanent teeth (10 patients), dental shape abnormalities (3 patients), and skeletal class III (2 patients). All the patients showed supernumerary teeth while dental structure abnormalities were not specified in any case.

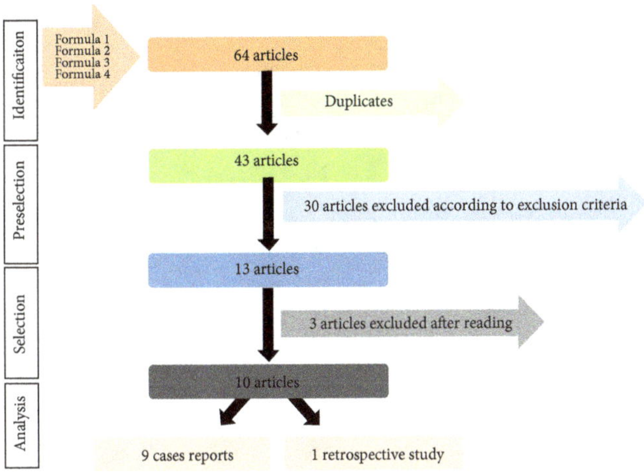

FIGURE 6: Articles selection.

3.3.3. Dental Therapies of the Patients That Were Included in This Systematic Review (Table 3). Seven treatment options were described in this review. The most used ones were the prosthetic (all patients) and orthodontic alternatives (22 patients). Periodontal surgery (16 patients) and conservative odontology (17 patients) were also frequently used. Extraction of supernumerary teeth was associated with treatment in 9 cases. The patients' follow-up was mentioned in three cases varying from 1 to five years.

3.3.4. Prosthetic Treatment (Table 4). The type of prosthetic treatment was not specified for the 15 patients of the retrospective study. Among the 10 other patients, 5 received implant fixed prosthetics (only one case described the treatment follow-up), 4 patients had removable partial prostheses, 3 patients were treated with complete prostheses, one patient fixed prosthesis, and one had patient implant-supported removable complete prostheses. No overdenture was described.

Twenty-two patients among the 25 received a combination of orthodontic and prosthodontic treatment. Concerning the chronology of these combined treatments, for the 15 patients included in the retrospective study, the author did not mention whether he started with the orthodontic or prosthodontic treatment. However, orthodontic treatment prior to prosthodontic treatment was described in 5 cases. Among these cases, orthodontic treatment was stopped or failed in 3 patients. In 2 cases, orthodontic treatment was achieved followed by prosthetic implants. All the patients who received an orthodontic treatment were lastly treated with prostheses. Three patients received only prostheses, the first case was treated with removable complete prostheses and implant-supported removable complete prostheses, the second with removable partial prostheses in the two dental arches, and the third with a fixed prosthetic implant.

4. Discussion

CCD patients present many challenges in diagnostics as well as in the treatment.

For diagnostics, the difficulty lies in the variability of the clinical and radiological manifestations of this syndrome. As it is described in the illustrated case, the common features are short stature, narrow chest with hypermobility of the shoulders, and dental disorders involving retention of the deciduous teeth, delayed eruption of permanent teeth, and the presence of many supernumerary teeth. Diagnosis could be confirmed by a genetic analysis. In fact, this condition is usually caused by a mutation of the RUNX2 gene located at chromosome 6p21. The difficulty also lies in the presence of other diseases having similar features such as crane-Heise syndrome, mandibuloacral dysplasia, pycnodysostosis, and Yanis-Varon syndrome [15]. Histopathological features are not frequently reported, but the findings are controversial in the literature. In fact, in the present case, there were no perturbations in the tooth structure. However, Vij et al. [16], in his histological analysis, found distorted dentinal tubules, prominent interglobular dentine, and acellular cementum with the absence of cellular cementum in the apical region. Yet, Lukinmaa et al. found a regular dentine structure in his observation [17].

The rarity of CCD syndrome makes the guidelines for its treatment scanty in the literature. So it is important to present any treated cases [18]. In this review, the majority of the published papers are case reports. In these lasts, the treatment philosophy was not the same and seemed to be based on the authors' experiences.

Planning treatment is difficult. A whole set of questions must be answered concerning the supernumerary teeth, removing them surgically or intervening only if pathological changes occur; concerning the remaining deciduous teeth, leaving them until they exfoliate naturally or removing them with the purpose of facilitating eruption of the permanent teeth into the arch; and concerning the age of intervention [2].

The literature analysis highlights the variety of therapeutic choices. They can involve orthodontics, surgery, or prosthodontics.

The surgical exposure of permanent teeth associated with orthodontic traction at an early age is an interesting solution. In fact, the patient's natural dentition will be spared and a good function and esthetics will be achieved. According to Kargul [19], the surgical exposure of unerupted teeth can lead to cementum formation and eruption of a dentition with normal root formation at an early age. The obvious disadvantage of this approach is the extensive duration of treatment, requiring multiple surgical procedures which could be expensive for the patient and challenging for the practitioner [20]. Several dental problems could not be resolved with this treatment option such as irregular dentition due to shape abnormalities. Besides, calcification and the loss of some teeth due to the presence of caries after orthodontic treatment are mentioned in the literature. Added to that, orthodontic treatment can be interrupted or failed. In fact, in the present review, among the 22 patients who had received orthodontic treatment, there were 3 cases for whom the treatment was stopped by the patients or failed, and several cases were described without follow-up.

Table 1: Clinical characteristics of the patients included in the systematic review.

No.	Authors	Study design	Age (years)	Sex	Dentition	Clavicular abnormalities	Delayed fontanels ossification	Inheritance
1 [10]	Chang et al.	RS	(9-46)	8 M, 7 F	Mx	15/15 aplasia	14/15 patients	Ns
2 [25]	Petropoulos et al.	CR (1)	45	F	P	Aplasia	Ns	Ns
3 [26]	Berg et al.	CR (1)	13	M	Mx	Ns	Ns	Ns
		(2)	13	F	Mx	Aplasia	Ns	Ns
4 [13]	Olszewska	CR (1)	40	M	P	Ns	Ns	Ns
5 [20]	Daskalogiannakis et al.	CR (1)	39	F	P	Ns	Ns	Ns
		(2)	8	M	Mx	Ns	Ns	Ns
6 [27]	Angle and Rebellato	CR (1)	10	F	Mx	Aplasia	Ns	Ns
7 [21]	Petropoulos et al.	CR (1)	42	F	P	Hypoplasia	Ns	Ns
8 [3]	Butterworth	CR (1)	9	M	Mx	Aplasia	Ns	Ns
9 [19]	Kargul et al.	CR (1)	12	F	Mx	Hypoplasia	Yes	Autosomal dominant

RS: retrospective study; CR: case report; F: female; M: male; P: permanent dentition; Mx: mixed dentition; Ns: not specified; FB: frontal bossing; FD: frontal depression.

Table 2: Dental features of the patients included in the systematic review.

No.	Retention of deciduous teeth	Unerupted permanent teeth	Shape abnormalities	Structure abnormalities	Skeletal class	Supernumerary teeth
1 [10]	Ns	Ns	Ns	Ns	Ns	12 yes
2 [25]	No	Yes	Yes[1]	Ns	Ns [2]	Yes
3 [26]	Yes	Yes	Ns	Ns	Ns	Yes
	Yes	Yes	Ns	Ns	Ns	Yes
4 [13]	Yes	Yes	Ns	Ns	Cl III	Yes
5 [20]	No	Yes	Ns	Ns	Ns	Yes
	Yes	Yes	Ns	Ns	Ns	Yes
6 [27]	Yes	Yes	Yes	Ns	Cl III	Yes
7 [21]	Yes	Yes	Ns	Ns	Ns	Yes
8 [3]	Yes	Yes	Yes	Ns	Ns	Yes
9 [19]	Yes	Yes	Ns	Ns	Ns	Yes

[1]Malformation and short conical roots. [2]Dental class I and anterior cross bite. Ns: not specified; Cl III: skeletal class III malocclusion.

Table 3: Dental therapies of the patients included in the systematic review.

No.	Orthodontic treatment	Prosthetic treatment	Orthognathic surgery	Periodontal surgery	Conductive osteotomy	Conservative odontology	Extraction of supernumerary teeth	Patients' follow-up (year)
1 [10]	+	+	-	+	+	+	-	Ns
2 [25]	+*[1]	+[2]	Ns	Ns	-	-	+	5
3 [26]	+[3]	+[3,2]	+	-	-	-	+	Ns
	+[3]	+[3]	-	-	-	-	+	
4 [13]	+*[1]	+[2]	-	-	+	-	+	Ns
5 [20]	(1)-	+	-	-	-	-	+	4
	(2)+[1]	+[2]	+	-	+	-	-	Ns
6 [27]	+[1]	+[2]	-	+	+	+	+	Ns
7 [21]	-	+	-	-	+	-	+	Ns
8 [3]	+*[1]	+[2]	-	-	+	+	+	1
9 [19]	-	+	-	-	-	-	+	Ns

[1]First-line treatment. [2]Second-line treatment. [3]Simultaneous treatment. *Failure or interruption of the treatment. Ns: not specified.

Table 4: Prosthetic treatment.

No.	Implant prosthetics	Complete prosthesis	Removable partial prosthesis	Fixed prosthesis	Over denture	Implant-supported removable complete prosthesis	Implant-supported removable partial prosthesis	Hybrid prosthesis
1 [10]	Ns	Ns	Ns	Ns	Ns	Ns	Ns	Ns
2 [25]	+	+[1]	-	-	-	-	-	-
3 [26]	(1) + (2)-	- -	+ +	- -	- -	- -	- -	- -
4 [13]	Ns	Ns	Ns	Ns	Ns	Ns	Ns	Ns
5 [20]	(1)- (2)+	+ -	- -	- -	- -	+ -	- -	- -
6 [27]	+	-	-	-	-	-	-	-
7 [21]	+	+	-	-	-	-	-	-
8 [3]	-	-	+	+	-	-	-	-
9 [19]	-	-	+	-	-	-	-	-

[1]Transitional complete prostheses after implant surgery. Ns: not specified.

The prosthodontic treatment was the most used alternative as all the patients included in this review were treated with prostheses. Chang et al. [10] thought that without prosthodontic treatment, occlusion and esthetics do not improve. In fact, in this review, the 2 cases that had a successful orthodontic treatment received a prosthodontic treatment. The majority of patients who were treated with only prostheses were aged more than 15 years. This treatment was indicated for aged patients for whom the displacement of teeth with orthodontics was difficult. Among the 10 patients, five had received implants. This alternative seemed to be an interesting option that provides a good result in a short time. The use of implants for CCD patients is controversial in the literature. In fact, according to Butterworth [3], the use of endosteal implants is generally contraindicated due to the presence of multiple unerupted teeth which reduce the amount of available bone. Petropoulos et al. [21] described a case of a CCD patient using 16 osseointegrated implants. After extraction of all the teeth, an alveoloplasty was carried out. The harvested bone was then put into the osseous defects. The entire treatment lasted 11 months. However, a long-term follow-up was needed to confirm the validity of this treatment and the quality of osseointegration of these implants regarding bone defects. In fact, the incriminated gene is not only expressed in the teeth but also in the bone. While bone abnormalities are described microscopically, little is known about the biological features of this tissue, particularly during osseointegration.

The placement of the implant through impacted teeth to avoid invasive surgery should be considered. While this option was described in the literature [22, 23], it was never described for CCD patients. More studies are needed before this unconventional procedure might be considered as a possible clinical option.

Removable prostheses and overdentures were used in five patients. They can be considered as a rapid solution that restores esthetics and functions. Deciduous teeth can be used as abutments for these dentures. But several questions can be raised whether they are able to withstand the forces applied to them when the prosthesis is in function or they will resorb prematurely [3]. The extraction of these teeth does not necessarily induce the eruption of permanent teeth [24]. So, these teeth could be preserved if removable prostheses were indicated. The prosthesis should be relined whenever some of these teeth are lost. For the presented case, the patient refused a long and surgical treatment. Removable prostheses were provided, and the patient was very pleased with the result.

5. Conclusion

The dental treatment of CCD patients is complex. Practitioners should be aware of the different therapeutic options to indicate the appropriate one according to the patients' age, their demands, and their compliance with the treatment. At an early age, a long treatment such as surgical-orthodontic approach can be proposed. But at late age, a rapid solution is almost used such as the prosthetic treatment. The removable denture offers a good result, but retention depends on the number of teeth remaining in the arch. Implants are frequently used. However, there is a need for clinical long-term studies to confirm the validity of the treatment.

Authors' Contributions

All authors have contributed equally to this work and are in agreement with the content of this paper.

References

[1] P. Singhal, A. Singhal, C. Jayam, and A. Bandlapalli, "Cleidocranial dysplasia syndrome (CCD) with an unusual finding in a young patient," *BMJ case reports*, vol. 2015, no. nov17 2, p. bcr2015210514, 2015.

[2] L. Lo Muzio, S. Tetè, F. Mastrangelo et al., "A novel mutation of gene CBFA1/RUNX2 in cleidocranial dysplasia," *Annals of*

Clinical and Laboratory Science, vol. 37, no. 2, pp. 115–120, 2007.

[3] C. Butterworth, "Cleidocranial dysplasia: modern concepts of treatment and a report of an orthodontic resistant case requiring a restorative solution," *Dental Update*, vol. 26, no. 10, pp. 458–462, 1999.

[4] A. Becker, J. Lustmann, and A. Shteyer, "Cleidocranial dysplasia: Part 1-General principles of the orthodontic and surgical treatment modality," *American journal of orthodontics and dentofacial orthopedics*, vol. 111, no. 1, pp. 28–33, 1997.

[5] G. D'Alessandro, T. Tagariello, and G. Piana, "Craniofacial changes and treatment of the stomatognathic system in subjects with cleidocranial dysplasia," *European journal of paediatric dentistry*, vol. 11, no. 1, pp. 39–43, 2010.

[6] P. Lombardas and R. W. Toothaker, "Bone grafting and osseointegrated implants in the treatment of cleidocranial dysplasia," *Compendium of continuing education in dentistry*, vol. 18, pp. 509–512, 1997.

[7] M. J. Fardy, "Cleidocranial dysostosis: some problems in the dental management of occlusion," *Dental Update*, vol. 11, no. 6, pp. 363–368, 1984.

[8] E. Kelly and R. Y. Nakamoto, "Cleidocranial dysostosis–a prosthodontic problem," *The Journal of Prosthetic Dentistry*, vol. 31, no. 5, pp. 518–526, 1974.

[9] G. S. Weintraub and I. L. Yalisove, "Prosthodontic therapy for cleidocranial dysostosis: report of case," *Journal of the American Dental Association (1939)*, vol. 96, no. 2, pp. 301–305, 1978.

[10] H. Chang, J. Wei, Y. Wang et al., "Restorative treatment strategies for patients with cleidocranial dysplasia," *Acta Odontologica Scandinavica*, vol. 73, no. 6, pp. 447–453, 2014.

[11] G. Farronato, C. Maspero, D. Farronato, and S. Gioventu, "Orthodontic treatment in a patient with cleidocranial dysostosis," *The Angle Orthodontist*, vol. 79, no. 1, pp. 178–185, 2009.

[12] Z. Suba, G. Balaton, S. Gyulai-Ga??l, P. Balaton, J.??. Barab??s, and I.??. Tarj??n, "Cleidocranial dysplasia: diagnostic criteria and combined treatment," *The Journal of Craniofacial Surgery*, vol. 16, no. 6, pp. 1122–1126, 2005.

[13] A. Olszewska, "Dental treatment strategies in a 40-year-old patient with cleidocranial dysplasia," *Journal of Applied Genetics*, vol. 47, no. 2, pp. 199–201, 2006.

[14] B. L. Jensen and S. Kreiborg, "Dental treatment strategies in cleidocranial dysplasia," *British Dental Journal*, vol. 172, no. 6, pp. 243–247, 1992.

[15] R. Mendoza-Londono and B. Lee, "Cleidocranial Dysplasia," in *GeneReviews(R), Seattle WA: University of Washington, Seattle*, R. A. Pagon, M. P. Adam, H. H. Ardinger, S. E. Wallace, A. Amemiya, and L. J. H. Bean, Eds., GeneReviews is a registered trademark of the University of Washington, Seattle, 1993.

[16] R. Vij, P. Batra, and H. Vij, "Cleidocranial dysplasia: complete clinical, radiological and histological profiles," *BMJ case reports*, vol. 2013, article bcr2013009015, 2013.

[17] P. L. Lukinmaa, B. L. Jensen, I. Thesleff, J. O. Andreasen, and S. Kreiborg, "Histological observations of teeth and peridental tissues in cleidocranial dysplasia imply increased activity of odontogenic epithelium and abnormal bone remodeling," *Journal of Craniofacial Genetics and Developmental Biology*, vol. 15, no. 4, pp. 212–221, 1995.

[18] A. Richardson and F. F. Deussen, "Facial and dental anomalies in cleidocranial dysplasia: a study of 17 cases," *International Journal of Paediatric Dentistry*, vol. 4, no. 4, pp. 225–231, 1994.

[19] S. I. Kargul B1, L. Yilmaz, and A. Dumlu, "Cleidocranial dysostosis: report of a case," *The Journal of Clinical Pediatric Dentistry*, vol. 22, pp. 83–86, 1997.

[20] J. Daskalogiannakis, L. Piedade, T. C. Lindholm, G. K. B. Sándor, and R. P. Carmichael, "Cleidocranial dysplasia: 2 generations of management," *Journal of the Canadian Dental Association*, vol. 72, pp. 337–342, 2006.

[21] V. C. Petropoulos, T. J. Balshi, S. F. Balshi, and G. J. Wolfinger, "Treatment of a patient with cleidocranial dysplasia using osseointegrated implants: a patient report," *The International Journal of Oral & Maxillofacial Implants*, vol. 19, pp. 282–287, 2004.

[22] M. Davarpahah and S. Szmukler-Moncler, "Unconventional implant placement. 2: placement of implants through impacted teeth. Three case reports," *The International Journal of Periodontics & Restorative Dentistry*, vol. 29, no. 4, pp. 405–413, 2009.

[23] A. Labidi, S. Bekri, L. Mansour, and S. Ghoul-Mazgar, "Implants placement in contact with dental tissue: a potential paradigm shift? Systematic literature review," *European Journal of Dentistry*, vol. 13, no. 4, pp. 642–648, 2019.

[24] S. W. C. HM and B. M. Levy, *A textbook of oral pathology*, 625-626, 1985.

[25] V. C. Petropoulos, T. J. Balshi, G. J. Wolfinger, and S. F. Balshi, "Treatment of a patient with cleidocranial dysplasia using a single-stage implant protocol," *Journal of Prosthodontics*, vol. 20, pp. S26–S31, 2011.

[26] R. W. Berg, K. S. Kurtz, I. Watanabe, and A. Lambrakos, "Interim prosthetic phase of multidisciplinary management of cleidocranial dysplasia:"the Bronx approach"," *Journal of Prosthodontics*, vol. 20, pp. S20–S25, 2011.

[27] A. D. Angle and J. Rebellato, "Dental team management for a patient with cleidocranial dysostosis," *American journal of orthodontics and dentofacial orthopedics*, vol. 128, no. 1, pp. 110–117, 2005.

14

Type 1–3 Canal Configuration in the Buccal Root of a Maxillary Second Molar

Hui Li,[1] Qiang Wang,[1] Mingwen Fan,[1] and Qingan Xu[1,2]

[1]*Department of Operative Dentistry and Endodontics, Wuhan First Stomatological Hospital, No. 675 Jianshe Avenue, Jianghan District, Wuhan 430000, China*
[2]*Department of Stomatology, School of Medicine, Jianghan University, No. 8 SanJiao Lake Road, Economic and Technological Development District, Wuhan 430000, China*

Correspondence should be addressed to Qingan Xu; xu.qa@wuhankq.com

Academic Editor: Maria Beatriz Duarte Gavião

Objectives. A major challenge in root canal treatment is the complex and variable root canal system. There are several methods of classification of root canal systems. Herein, we report a case of a maxillary second molar, the root canal system of which could not be classified according to any of the previous methods. *Case Report.* Cone-beam computed tomography (CBCT), used to visualize the root canal system of a maxillary left second molar with fused roots, revealed a type 1–3 root canal system in the buccal root and a type 1–1 root canal system in the palatal root. A dental operating microscope was used throughout the treatment, and the root canals were successfully obturated. *Conclusion.* To the best of our knowledge, this is the first report on the classification of buccal roots of maxillary second molars. *Clinical Significance.* A dental operating microscope and CBCT play a vital role in mapping the root canal system to ensure that no canal is missed.

1. Introduction

A major challenge in root canal therapy is the existence of complex and variable root canal systems. To fully understand the internal morphological changes in different teeth, several studies have been conducted, and root canal systems have been classified into different categories [1, 2]. This provides the dentist with information about the root canal system. When encountering root canal systems beyond the classification, the dental operating microscope (DOM) is an effective device to help dentists identify specific anatomic features of the root canal [3]. The minimum distance that the human eye can distinguish is 0.1 mm, and more details can be visualized using a DOM. Moreover, use of a DOM ensures that the ultrasonic tip accurately removes the calcification that blocks the root canal orifice, reduces unnecessary grinding of healthy dentin, and improves the fracture resistance of the teeth [4]. In addition, cone-beam computed tomography (CBCT) can predict root canal location in teeth with unusual root canal anatomy [5]. Vertucci described three types of root canal systems in maxillary second molars. The variation mainly occurs in the mesiobuccal root, which is divided into type I, type II, and type IV [1]. Regarding the maxillary second molar, some studies have reported three canals in the mesiobuccal root [6], while other studies have reported two canals in the palatal root [7–10]. Herein, we present a case of a maxillary left second molar with a trifurcated buccal root canal. The DOM and CBCT showed two canals at the orifice level; however, the buccal canal trifurcated at the middle third of the root. To the best of our knowledge, there is no relevant report on the classification of buccal roots of the maxillary second molar.

2. Case Presentation

A 44-year-old woman presented to the Department of Operative Dentistry and Endodontics with pain, both spontaneous and to extreme temperatures, on the left side of the face, two days prior to her visit. Clinical examination revealed dental restoration in teeth #15, which had been placed one year prior at a different hospital. Tooth #15 had severe pain on percussion, and a severe lingering painful

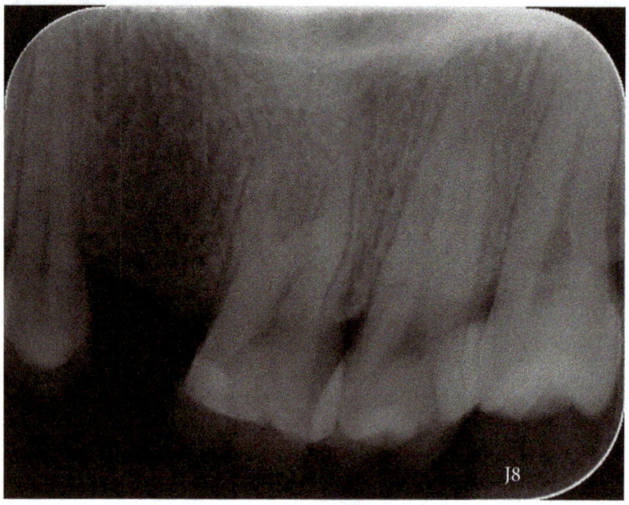

FIGURE 1: Preoperative radiograph.

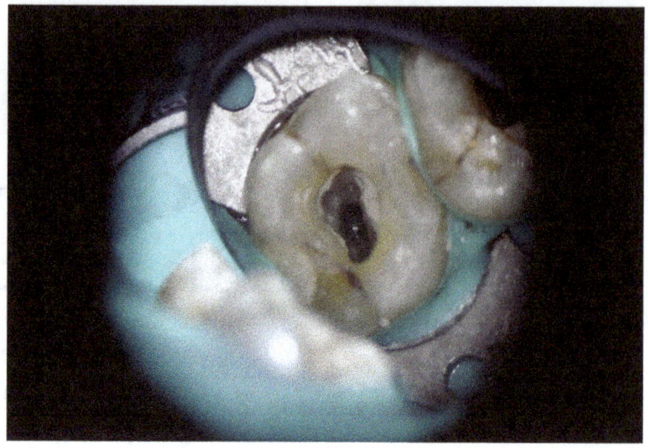

FIGURE 2: Three canals in the buccal root.

response to cold water, whereas tooth #14 was only tender to percussion. The periodontal conditions of teeth #14 and #15 were normal. Tooth #15 was diagnosed with irreversible pulpitis. The patient was informed about the conditions of her teeth and was advised to undergo root canal treatment (RCT) on tooth #15. The patient provided informed consent for RCT. The preoperative radiograph (Figure 1) showed dental restoration approximating the pulp chamber in tooth #15.

After administration of local anesthesia, an access cavity was prepared in tooth #15 and paraformaldehyde was placed into the pulp chamber to inactivate the dental pulp. Seven days later, the temporary seal was removed, and the root canals were visualized under a DOM (Zumax, Suzhou, China). A #10 K file (Dentsply Sirona, York, PA) was used to explore the root canals under 5× magnification using the DOM. The resistance to exploration was significantly lesser in the buccal root canal than in the palatal root canal. Next, the magnification was set to 20×, and a C-shaped root canal was observed in the buccal root with some dentin blocking the direct access. An ultrasonic working tip (ET20, Satelec, France) was used to remove part of the dentin; four root canals were found, three of which were in the buccal root and had a common orifice, and one was in the palatal root (Figure 2). The patient was recommended to undergo CBCT (NewTom, Italy) because of the morphological variation in tooth #15 to avoid missing other canals. CBCT showed that the root canal was trifurcated at the middle third of the fused buccal root, and the palatal root contained a single independent root canal (Figure 3). An electronic apex locator (Propex II, Dentsply, USA) was used to measure the length of the root canal, and pathfiles #13, #16, and #19 (Dentsply Sirona, York, PA) were used sequentially to dredge the root canals. The canals were prepared using #20 and #25 Protaper-next nickel–titanium rotary instruments (Dentsply Sirona, York, PA). Ethylenediaminetetraacetic acid (EDTA; Glyde, Dentsply, USA) was used for each root canal preparation. Frequent irrigation was performed using 2.5% NaOCl with P5 Newtron ultrasonic agitation (Satelec, France). The canals were rinsed, dried, and filled with calcium hydroxide paste. The access opening was sealed with a zinc oxide and eugenol dressing.

Seven days later, the canals were emptied and copiously flushed with 2.5% NaOCl. Ultrasonic irrigation of the root canals was performed, followed by drying with paper points. Master gutta-percha cones were selected for all canals (Figure 4a), and the canals were obturated using iRoot SP (Innovative BioCreamix, Vancouver, Canada), using the single-cone technique. Two weeks later, a computer-aided design/manufacturing ceramic crown was fabricated on tooth #15. A final radiograph (Figure 4b) was taken to confirm the completeness and extension of the root filling.

3. Discussion

Despite the high success rate achieved in RCT, morphological variations in the root canal are an unresolved mystery. Variations in root canal anatomy are closely associated with failure of RCT because of the difficulty in locating, cleaning, and filling the aberrant canals [1, 2, 6–12]. Owing to the many dissimilarities in selection, the results of previous studies cannot be compared directly. In an *in vitro* study, 42.25% of 187 extracted maxillary second molars had fused roots. Among teeth with fused roots, those with three-root fusion had a high frequency of merged canals [10]. Another study using CBCT to evaluate the incidence of root fusion and root-canal fusion in 4120 molars *in vivo* found that a complex root canal system is often present in fused roots. In this study, the incidence of root fusion and root-canal fusion in the maxillary second molar was 25.2% and 8.6%, respectively [13]. Another *in vivo* study using CBCT showed a 23.9% incidence of fused roots in maxillary second molars, with root-canal fusion within fused roots observed in 10.6% of cases [11]. In our patient, CBCT showed a three-root fusion in tooth #15. Ordinola-Zapata et al. reported that maxillary second molars with fused roots have a high incidence of merged and C-shaped canals [12].

In our case, tooth #15 showed a distinctive variation. Two separate root canals originated from the pulpal floor: one buccal and one palatal canal. Under the DOM, a

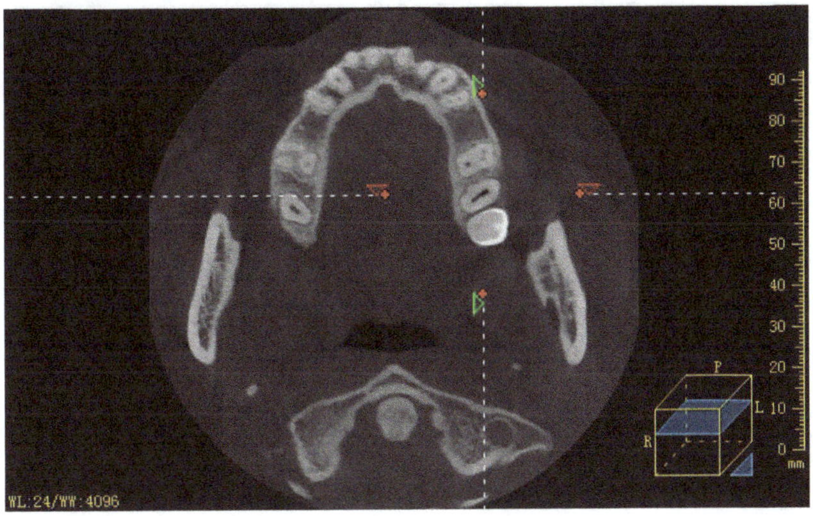

(a)

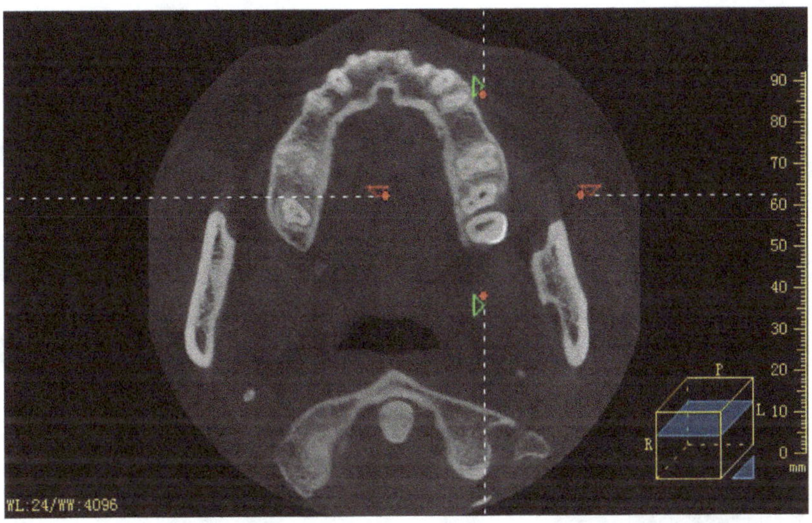

(b)

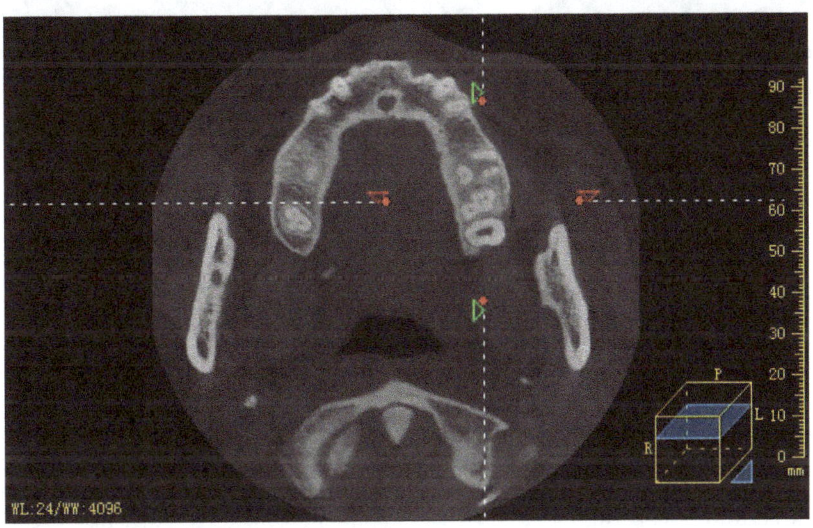

(c)

FIGURE 3: Continued.

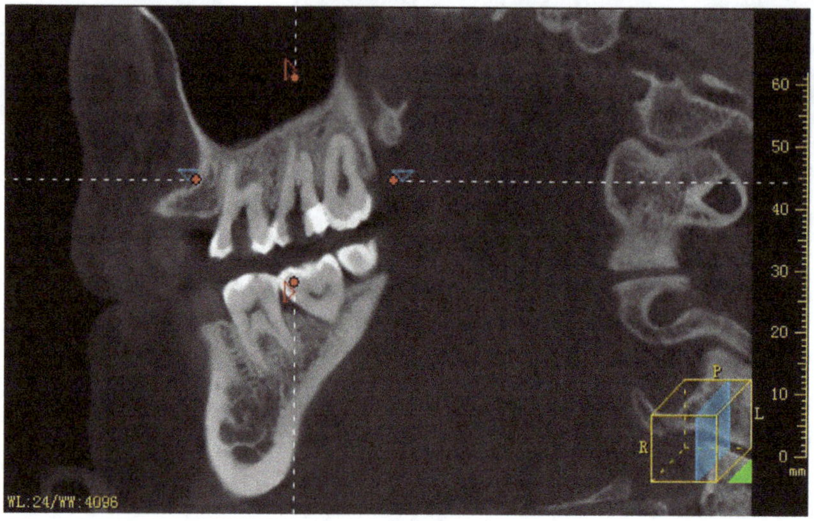

(d)

FIGURE 3: Cone-beam computed tomography images. Horizontal sections at (a) orifice level, (b) midroot level, (c) apical level, and (d) sagittal view reveal a type 1–3 canal.

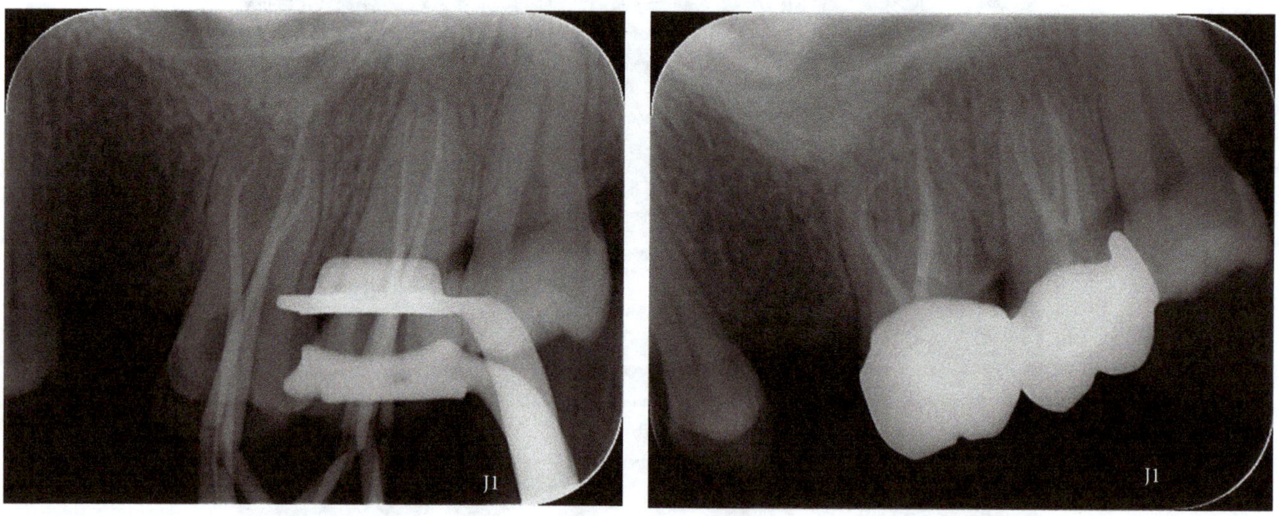

(a) (b)

FIGURE 4: (a) Radiograph to confirm the working length, (b) postoperative radiograph.

C-shapedconfiguration was visualized till the middle third of the buccal root, which trifurcated in the mesial, buccal, and distal directions and formed three independent root canals with independent apical foramina. In this case, the treatment was difficult because we had to locate and clean the three buccal canals and put three gutta-percha cones through the same orifice at the same time. Fortunately, DOMs are being increasingly used for endodontic treatment, and are especially useful in such cases. CBCT can accurately image the maxillofacial hard tissue and confirm the internal anatomy of the teeth that need RCT [14–16].

At present, irrespective of the instruments used, some areas of the root canal cannot be cleaned. Therefore, chemical disinfection of root canals is the key to successful treatment [17]. In our case, EDTA was used to remove the smear layer and NaOCl and ultrasonic irrigation were used to reduce bacterial load and dissolve organic tissues, thereby improving the success rate.

4. Conclusion

Finding and treating additional root canals can improve the success rate of RCT. Therefore, clinicians should be aware of the typical root canal configuration. On encountering an aberration, clinicians should ask questions and use the DOM and CBCT in a timely manner to deal with various complex situations. Particularly, during RCT of the maxillary second molar, if a fused root canal is suspected on radiographs, it is recommended that the entire treatment be performed under a DOM. CBCT should be performed to confirm the root shape and number of root canals to avoid missing root canals. We believe that the prognosis of RCT can be improved with standardized treatment combined with the use of advanced equipment.

References

[1] F. J. Vertucci, "Root canal anatomy of the human permanent teeth," *Oral Surgery, Oral Medicine, Oral Pathology and Oral Radiology*, vol. 58, pp. 589–599, 1984.

[2] R. N. Weller and G. R. Hartwell, "The impact of improved access and searching techniques on detection of the mesiolingual canal in maxillary molars," *Journal of Endodontics*, vol. 15, pp. 82–83, 1989.

[3] N. Khalighinejad, A. Aminoshariae, J. C. Kulild, K. A. Williams, J. Wang, and A. Mickel, "The effect of the dental operating microscope on the outcome of nonsurgical root canal treatment: a retrospective case-control study," *Journal of Endodontics*, vol. 43, pp. 728–732, 2017.

[4] A. Iandolo, G. Landolo, M. Malvano, G. Pantaleo, and M. Simeone, "Modern technologies in endodontics," *Giornale Italiano di Endodonzia*, vol. 30, pp. 2–9, 2016.

[5] P. S. D'Addazio, A. C. Carvalho, C. N. Campos, K. L. Devito, and M. Özcan, "Cone beam computed tomography in endodontics," *International Endodontic Journal*, vol. 49, pp. 311–312, 2016.

[6] N. Eskoz and F. S. Weine, "Canal configuration of the mesiobuccal root of the maxillary second molar," *Journal of Endodontics*, vol. 21, pp. 38–42, 1995.

[7] Y. Gu, W. Wang, and L. Ni, "Four-rooted permanent maxillary first and second molars in a northwestern Chinese population," *Archives of Oral Biology*, vol. 60, pp. 811–817, 2015.

[8] O. I. Ulusoy and G. Görgül, "Endodontic treatment of a maxillary second molar with 2 palatal roots: a case report," *Oral Surgery Oral Medicine Oral Pathology Oral Radiology Endodontology*, vol. 104, pp. e95–e97, 2007.

[9] B. Pasternak Júnior, C. S. Teixeira, R. G. Silva, L. P. Vansan, and M. D. S. Neto, "Treatment of a second maxillary molar with six canals," *Australian Endodontic Journal*, vol. 33, pp. 42–45, 2007.

[10] Q. Zhang, H. Chen, B. Fan, W. Fan, and J. L. Gutmann, "Root and root canal morphology in maxillary second molar with fused root from a native Chinese population," *Journal of Endodontics*, vol. 40, pp. 871–875, 2014.

[11] X. M. Tian, X. W. Yang, L. Qian, B. Wei, and Y. Gong, "Analysis of the root and canal morphologies in maxillary first and second molars in a Chinese population using cone-beam computed tomography," *Journal of Endodontics*, vol. 42, pp. 696–701, 2016.

[12] R. Ordinola-Zapata, J. N. R. Martins, C. M. Bramante, M. H. Villas-Boas, M. H. Duarte, and M. A. Versiani, "Morphological evaluation of maxillary second molars with fused roots: a micro-CT study," *International Endodontic Journal*, vol. 50, pp. 1192–1200, 2017.

[13] J. N. Martins, A. Mata, D. Marques, and J. Caramês, "Prevalence of root fusions and main root canal merging in human upper and lower molars: a cone-beam computed tomography in vivo study," *Journal of Endodontics*, vol. 42, pp. 900–908, 2016.

[14] C. K. Song, H. S. Chang, and K. S. Min, "Endodontic management of supernumerary tooth fused with maxillary first molar by using cone-beam computed tomography," *Journal of Endodontics*, vol. 36, pp. 1901–1904, 2010.

[15] J. Guo, A. Vahidnia, P. Sedghizadeh, and R. Enciso, "Evaluation of root and canal morphology of maxillary permanent first molars in a North American population by cone-beam computed tomography," *Journal of Endodontics*, vol. 40, pp. 635–639, 2014.

[16] Q. H. Zheng, Y. Wang, X. D. Zhou, Q. Wang, G.-N. Zheng, and D.-M. Huang, "A cone-beam computed tomography study of maxillary first permanent molar root and canal morphology in a Chinese population," *Journal of Endodontics*, vol. 36, pp. 1480–1484, 2010.

[17] A. Iandolo, M. Simeone, S. Orefice, and S. Rengo, "3D cleaning, a perfected technique: thermal profile assessment of heated NaOCl. Detersione 3D, una tecnica perfezionata: valutazione dei profili termici dell'NaOCl riscaldato," *Giornale Italiano di Endodonzia*, vol. 31, pp. 58–61, 2017.

15

Hemodialysis-Related Amyloidosis in the Tongue

Satoshi Nakamura,[1] Miki Yamada,[1] Yosuke Iijima,[1] Keisuke Sawada,[2] Shunsuke Hino,[1] Takahiro Kaneko,[1] and Norio Horie[1]

[1]*Department of Oral and Maxillofacial Surgery, Saitama Medical Center, Saitama Medical University, Saitama, Japan*
[2]*Department of Pathology, Saitama Medical Center, Saitama Medical University, Saitama, Japan*

Correspondence should be addressed to Shunsuke Hino; shunhino@saitama-med.ac.jp

Academic Editor: Paulo J. Palma

Dialysis-related amyloidosis (DRA) represents a group of relatively rare disorders characterized by the systemic extracellular deposition of insoluble fibrils of amyloid protein in long-term dialysis patients. We describe herein a case of relatively early DRA on the tongue of a long-term dialysis patient. A 67-year-old man with a 39-year history of dialysis was referred for diagnosis of a tongue mass. On examination, a collection of whitish-yellow papules was identified on the ventral surface of the tongue tip. The pathological diagnosis was DRA. Clinicians should be aware that long-term dialysis can cause oral amyloidosis of the tongue.

1. Introduction

In end-stage renal disease, as the final stage of chronic kidney disease, the kidneys no longer function and are thus unable to appropriately remove waste products or fluid from the blood. Chronic dialysis is the only option for patients with end-stage renal disease who are ineligible for renal transplantation [1, 2]. Amyloidosis represents a group of relatively rare disorders characterized by the extracellular deposition of insoluble fibrils of amyloid protein [3]. As a complication of long-term hemodialysis (HD), "dialysis-related amyloidosis" (DRA) represents the accumulation of amyloid fibrils from plasma concentrations of β2-microglobulin (β2m). DRA manifests first in the osteoarticular form and in some cases may appear peripherally on the skin and mucous membranes (tongue). Typical symptoms of DRA are carpal tunnel syndrome, bone cysts, scapula-humeral periarthritis, joint arthropathy, and destructive spondyloarthropathy [4]. DRA is rarely seen in the oral region but when present is found primarily on the tongue. Amyloid accumulation that becomes extensive may present as macroglossia [3].

Histopathologically, amyloid appears as amorphous eosinophilic extracellular deposits in hematoxylin and eosin staining. With Congo red stain, amyloid stains red under light microscopy and displays apple-green birefringence under polarized light. Other stains such as direct fast scarlet (DFS) can also confirm the presence of amyloid deposits [5].

Here, we report a case of relatively early-stage tongue amyloidosis in a long-term HD patient with systemic DRA.

2. Case Report

The patient was a 67-year-old man who had been on HD for 39 years due to chronic renal failure. About 3 months earlier, he had noticed discomfort in the tongue and was referred by a dialysis doctor for examination. His medical history other than chronic renal failure (at 27 years old) included right nephrectomy for renal cell carcinoma (at 47 years old), left nephrectomy for renal cell carcinoma (at 50 years old), parathyroidectomy (at 51 years old), surgery for lumbar spinal stenosis (at 56 years old), surgery for destructive spondyloarthropathy (at 59 years old), right-side colon resection for ileus due to intestinal tuberculosis (at 63 years old), surgical decompression of carpal tunnel syndrome (at 66 years old), and ileal biopsy suggestive of amyloidosis (at 67 years old). Histopathological examination of the specimen from ileal biopsy showed amorphous eosinophilic deposits on the vessel wall (Figures 1(a) and 1(b)). Immumohistochemically,

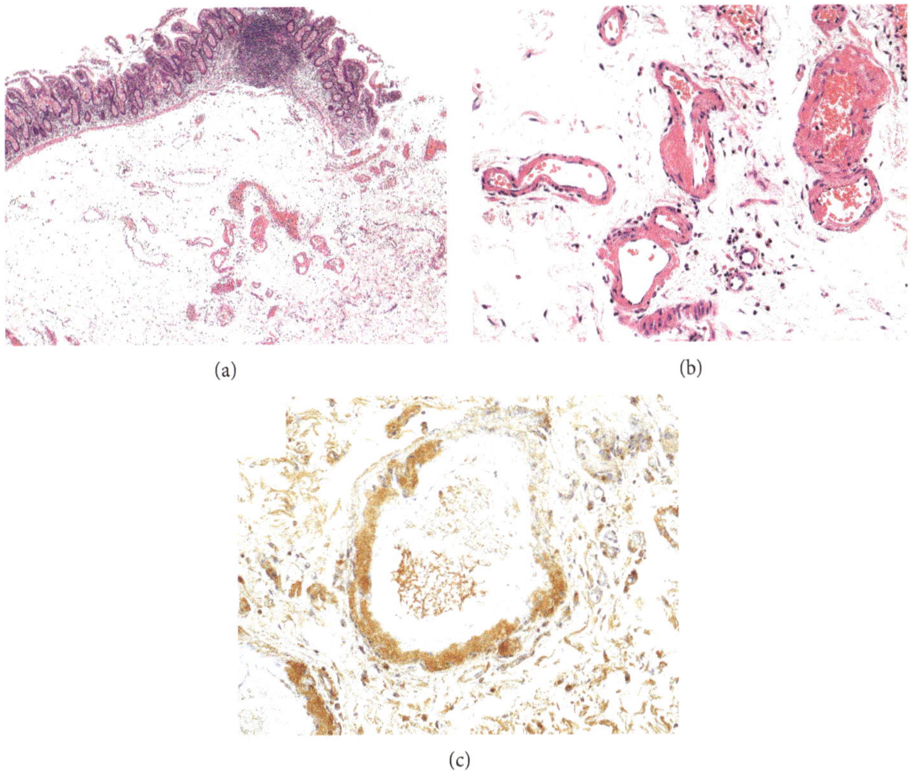

FIGURE 1: (a) A low-power view of the ileal biopsy specimen (hematoxylin and eosin stain; original magnification ×40). (b) Amorphous eosinophilic deposits are apparent on the vessel wall (hematoxylin-eosin stain, original magnification ×200). (c) Immunohistochemically, deposits show positive staining for β2-microglobulin (original magnification ×200).

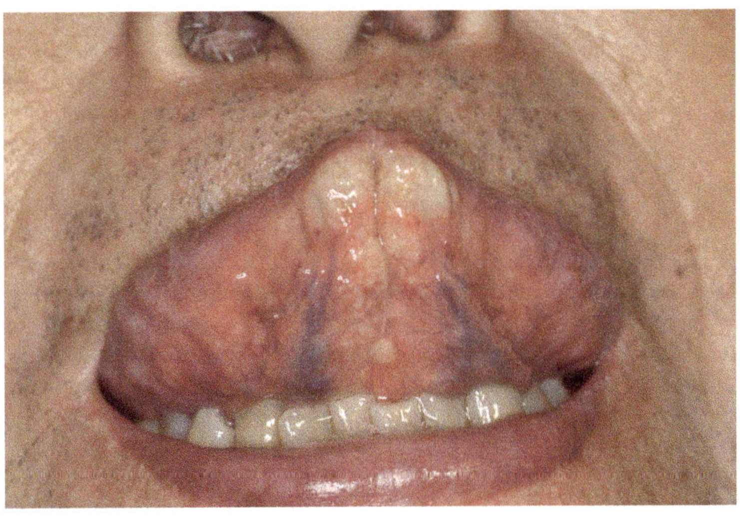

FIGURE 2: A collection of whitish-yellow papules is evident on the ventral surface of the tongue tip.

deposits were positive for β2m (Figure 1(c)). Current medications included alfacalcidol, ursodeoxycholic acid, sevelamer hydrochloride, and lanthanum carbonate hydrate, and the serum β2m level was 20.7 mg/L. In addition, the renal cell carcinomas and surgical decompression of carpal tunnel syndrome were not treated at the referring hospital and detailed data were not available. On oral examination, a collection of painless, relatively hard, rugged whitish-yellow papules was found on the ventral surface of the tongue tip (Figure 2). No movement disorder of the tongue was apparent. The patient showed no difficulty in eating or dysphagia. No abnormal findings were found in other sites of the oral cavity or regional lymph nodes. Biopsy was performed under local anesthesia. Histopathologically, the specimen showed amorphous eosinophilic extracellular deposits in the subepithelial region (Figure 3(a)). Extracellular deposits showed positive results from DFS staining, and also from potassium permanganate- ($KMnO_4$-) DFS staining and β2m staining

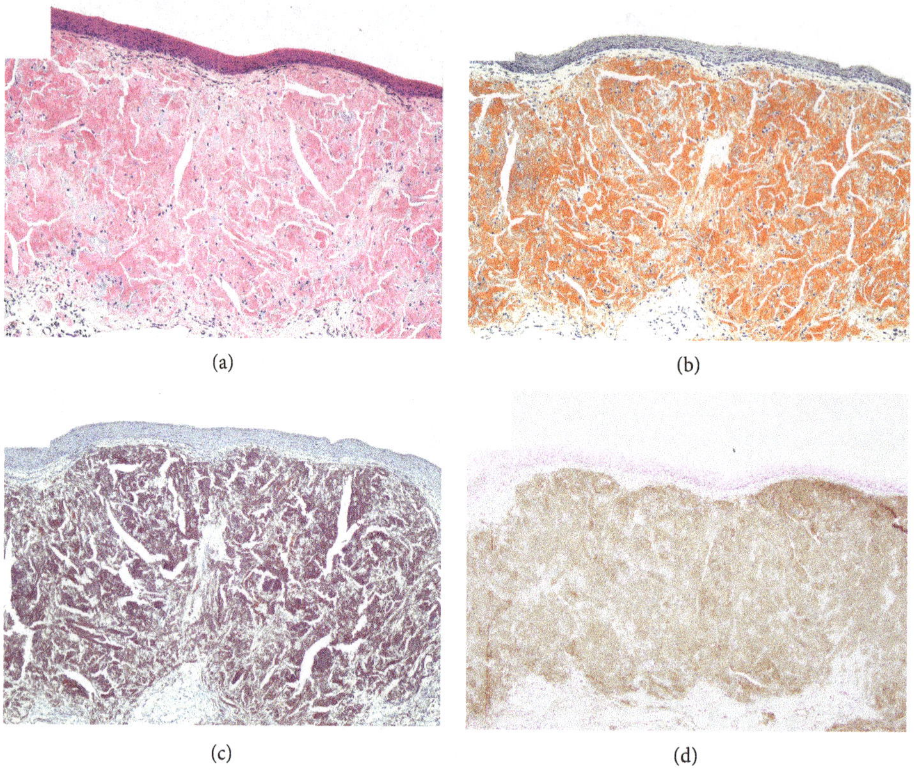

Figure 3: (a) Amorphous extracellular eosinophilic deposits are shown in the subepithelial region (hematoxylin-eosin stain, original magnification ×100). (b) Extracellular deposits show positive staining with direct fast scarlet (DFS) (original magnification ×100). (c) Extracellular deposits show positive staining with potassium permanganate- ($KMnO_4$-) DFS stain (original magnification ×100). (d) Staining for β2-microglobulin is also positive (original magnification ×100).

(Figures 3(b)–3(d)). The pathological diagnosis was amyloidosis, strongly suggestive of DRA. At the 6-month follow-up, no significant change in systemic DRA was seen, including tongue symptoms.

3. Discussion

Recent experimental findings have documented a direct cellular toxicity of β2m fibrils, but the mechanisms underlying β2m fibrillogenesis remain incompletely understood [6]. This syndrome can also be observed in end-stage renal diseases patients undergoing peritoneal dialysis and even in patients with chronic renal failure before the initiation of dialytic therapy, suggesting that HD is not a direct cause, but that accumulation of β2m or some β2m-associated molecules in the body is a common pathogenesis [7]. Although a high plasma concentration of β2m is associated with the development of DRA, other factors have been clearly incriminated, such as older age at dialysis onset and longer dialysis vintage or suspected effects such as proinflammatory effects of bioincompatible dialysis techniques [6].

DRA can be classified into two stages: initial and late. The initial stage recognizes osteoarticular DRA, and the late stage shows extra-articular DRA [8]. Oral amyloidosis belongs to the late stage, developing later than other DRAs. Cases of oral amyloidosis are thus uncommon. In oral DRA, the tongue is the most frequent site [8]. In addition to DRA, oral amyloid deposition can occur in primary amyloidosis, secondary amyloidosis, and localized amyloidosis. In general, with any amyloidosis, the tongue initially presents with whitish-yellow, relatively hard papules and nodules of varying amounts and sizes. Occasionally, functional disturbances of the tongue and dysgeusia are observed. In advanced cases, the tongue shows macroglossia, and eating disorders, respiratory disorders, and dysphagia may arise [3, 8]. Distinguishing DRA from other causes of amyloidosis may be difficult on macroscopic examination. In the present case, although tuberculosis could have been a cause of amyloidosis, the histological findings and dialysis history confirmed DRA by the identification of β2m. As the deposit was fairly localized on the ventral surface of the tongue tip, this might be an early symptom of DRA of the tongue.

Development of DRA is known to occur in almost 100% of cases within 15 years and is also related to the type of membrane and dialysate used. In this case, DRA was identified more than 25 years after starting dialysis. Over the last two decades, the prevalence and severity of DRA appear to have decreased significantly, although recent large-scale epidemiological studies show that DRA continues to be used [6]. Improved dialysis technology has definitely played a role in delaying the onset of disease [6]. In particular, the use of cellulosic low-flux membranes with different biocompatibilities was deeply involved in the retention of β2m [9]. This patient has recently been using a high-flux membrane. In addition, control of the clinical situation involves a regimen using a Lixelle adsorptive column, which uses porous cellulose beads (mean diameter, 460 μm), the surface of which is covered with hydrophobic hexadecylalkyl chains in connection with a dialyzer [10, 11]. The use of ultrapure dialysate and the type of dialyzer membrane also help prevent the deposition of substances such as β2m [12].

Oral DRA previously has been estimated to occur in 20% of patients [8]. However, opportunities to observe oral DRA have been rare. This may also be due to decreases in DRA. In this case, oral DRA was found after more than 35 years of dialysis history.

Importantly, no current dialytic modality seems able to fully prevent DRA, and some patients have not received dialysis under proper dialysis conditions. Therefore, although the onset of DRA is delayed, DRA can still arise [6].

The differential diagnoses include various diseases that form a mass on the tongue and diseases that present as macroglossia. However, not so many diseases show a rugged mass with whitish-yellow coloration like dialysis amyloidosis. Lipomas and verruciform xanthoma are yellowish but are soft and do not feel rugged. In addition, lipomas may present with multiple nodules, and verruciform xanthoma may display a granular appearance [13]. Biopsy is evidently required to confirm the diagnosis, and the history of dialysis is extremely important for the diagnosis of DRA.

No curative treatments are yet available for DRA. In case of DRA of the tongue, palliative surgical reduction may be performed in cases with severe complications [3]. Preventing the development of DRA may require the implementation of improved dialysis technology, including biocompatible high-flux membranes and ultrapure dialysate [9].

In conclusion, DRA has not disappeared altogether. General dentists and oral surgeons should be aware that long-term dialysis can cause oral amyloidosis of the tongue.

References

[1] S. Dolgos, A. Hartmann, J. Bollerslev, P. Vörös, and L. Rosivall, "The importance of body composition and dry weight assessments in patients with chronic kidney disease," *Acta Physiologica Hungarica*, vol. 98, no. 2, pp. 105–116, 2011.

[2] S. Sahathevan, B. H. Khor, H. M. Ng et al., "Understanding development of malnutrition in hemodialysis patients: a narrative review," *Nutrients*, vol. 12, no. 10, p. 3147, 2020.

[3] B. Picciani, C. Gornic, K. S. Cunha et al., "Lingual amyloidosis associated to long-term hemodialysis: two case reports," *Special Care in Dentistry*, vol. 38, no. 6, pp. 434–437, 2018.

[4] R. Scarpioni, M. Ricardi, V. Albertazzi, S. De Amicis, F. Rastelli, and L. Zerbini, "Dialysis-related amyloidosis: challenges and solutions," *International Journal of Nephrology and Renovascular Disease*, vol. 9, pp. 319–328, 2016.

[5] H. Z. Amin, S. Mori, N. Sasaki, and K. Hirata, "Diagnostic approach to cardiac amyloidosis," *The Kobe Journal of Medical Sciences*, vol. 60, no. 1, pp. E5–E11, 2014.

[6] L. Labriola and M. Jadoul, "Dialysis-related amyloidosis: is it gone or should it be?," *Seminars in Dialysis*, vol. 30, no. 3, pp. 193–196, 2017.

[7] S. Kaneko and K. Yamagata, "Hemodialysis-related amyloidosis: is it still relevant?," *Seminars in Dialysis*, vol. 31, no. 6, pp. 612 618, 2018.

[8] K. Matsuo, M. Nakamoto, C. Yasunaga, T. Goya, and K. Sugimachi, "Dialysis-related amyloidosis of the tongue in long-term hemodialysis patients," *Kidney International*, vol. 52, no. 3, pp. 832–838, 1997.

[9] J. Hoshino, K. Yamagata, S. Nishi et al., "Significance of the decreased risk of dialysis-related amyloidosis now proven by results from Japanese nationwide surveys in 1998 and 2010," *Nephrology, Dialysis, Transplantation*, vol. 31, no. 4, pp. 595–602, 2016.

[10] S. Furuyoshi, M. Nakatani, J. Taman, H. Kutsuki, S. Takata, and N. Tani, "New adsorption column (Lixelle) to eliminate β2-microglobulin for direct hemoperfusion," *Therapeutic Apheresis*, vol. 2, no. 1, pp. 13–17, 1998.

[11] K. Tsuchida, Y. Takemoto, K. Sugimura, R. Yoshimura, K. Yamamoto, and T. Nakatani, "Adsorption of endotoxin by beta2-microglobulin adsorbent column (Lixelle): the new approach for endotoxinemia," *Therapeutic Apheresis*, vol. 6, no. 2, pp. 116–118, 2002.

[12] G. Lonnemann and K. M. Koch, "β2-Microglobulin amyloidosis: effects of ultrapure dialysate and type of dialyzer membrane," *Journal of the American Society of Nephrology*, vol. 13, Supplement_1, pp. S72–S77, 2002.

[13] P. Tamiolakis, V. I. Theofilou, K. I. Tosios, and A. Sklavounou-Andrikopoulou, "Oral verruciform xanthoma: report of 13 new cases and review of the literature," *Medicina Oral, Patología Oral y Cirugía Bucal*, vol. 23, no. 4, pp. e429–e435, 2018.

16

Cooccurrence of Talon's Cusp with Dens Invaginatus in the Maxillary Lateral Incisor: A Case Report with Review of Literature

Snehashish Ghosh,[1] Safal Dhungel,[2] Bhawana Subedi,[3] and Subi Pradhan[4]

[1]*Department of Oral Pathology, College of Medical Sciences, Bharatpur, Nepal*
[2]*Department of Oral and Maxillofacial Surgery, College of Medical Sciences, Bharatpur, Nepal*
[3]*Department of Oral Medicine and Radiology, College of Medical Sciences, Bharatpur, Nepal*
[4]*College of Medical Sciences, Bharatpur, Nepal*

Correspondence should be addressed to Snehashish Ghosh; drsnehashishop@gmail.com

Academic Editor: Sreekanth Kumar Mallineni

Morphogenic developmental anomalies are common in maxillary lateral incisors, but simultaneous occurrence of two developmental anomalies in a single tooth is relatively uncommon. In this case report, we present a case of cooccurrence of the talon's cusp with dens invaginatus in the left lateral incisor tooth. Early diagnosis and prompt treatment of such cases are important to prevent any untoward consequences.

1. Introduction

Talon's cusp is an additional entity, projecting from the lingual surface/cingulum area of a maxillary or mandibular anterior tooth. It is an anomalous structure resembling an eagle's talon, so the name talon's cusp has evolved. It is composed of coronal hard and soft tissue structures similar to a normal tooth. It blends smoothly with the tooth except there is a deep developmental groove where the cusp blends with the sloping lingual tooth surface [1]. The first case of the talon's cusp was identified by Mitchell [2].

Sicher and Bhaskar [3] proposed that a disturbance in the morphodifferentiation could lead to the development of the talon's cusp, whereas Hattab et al. [4] thought that the talon's cusp might be a result of outward folding of the inner enamel epithelium with concurrent focal hyperplasia of the dental papilla. It could be one of the presenting features of Mohr syndrome, Rubinstein-Taybi syndrome, and Sturge-Weber syndrome [5–8]. Some authors consider talon's cusp as a hamartoma also [9].

Various clinical problems like attrition, compromised aesthetics, displacement of the involved tooth, interference of tongue space, increased susceptibility to dental caries, and occlusal disharmony could be associated with the talon's cusp [10, 11].

Dens invaginatus/dens in dente is a developmental anomaly that arises as a result of infolding in the surface of the crown/root. Increased localized external pressure, focal growth retardation, and focal growth stimulation in certain areas of the tooth bud are the possible causes of this condition. Siraci et al. and Lwin et al. contemplated an initial contortion followed by the subsequent protrusion of the fragment of the enamel organ could lead to the formation of enamel-lined infolding at the cingulum area even at the incisal tip [10, 12].

It is seen in the order in maxillary lateral incisors, central incisors, canine, premolar, and molar teeth. Usually, it is unilateral, but when occurring in the maxillary central, it could be bilateral [12]. An analogous form of invagination occasionally occurs in the roots of teeth [10]. It results from an infolding of Hertwig epithelial root sheath and takes its origin within the root after development is complete. There is no gender predilection for this condition [12, 13].

Radiographically, the involved tooth may depict an infolding of enamel and dentin reaching towards the pulp cavity or even rarely extending to the root apex.

Histopathologically, hypomineralized enamel is noted at the site of invagination, making that site vulnerable for the development of dental caries and penetration of microorganisms deep into the pulpal area leading to pulpal necrosis and initiation of periapical inflammatory processes [10, 12, 14].

Here in this article, we report a rare case of cooccurrence of the talon's cusp with dens invaginatus in the maxillary lateral incisor.

2. Case Report

A 25-year-old female patient reported to the dental outpatient department of the College of Medical Sciences, Bharatpur, Nepal, with the chief complaint of the fractured tooth in the upper tooth region since 9 yrs. On extraoral examination, the patient had a prognathic mandible with an asymmetric smile, and the midline was shifted towards the right by 2 mm.

Intraoral examination revealed the patient was in the permanent dentition stage with occlusal caries in the upper right back posterior region. She had a class I occlusal relationship. The full mouth intraoral picture is presented (Figure 1). A prominent tubercle in the lingual aspect of the upper left lateral incisor extends from the cingulum area to the incisal edge (Figure 2). This was diagnosed as a talon's cusp. The tooth was discolored, and a crack line was present on the palatal aspect. The patient did not have any problems regarding speech, mastication, and occlusion. The tooth responded well during the cold test and electric pulp test. On both horizontal and vertical percussion, the involved tooth did not show any pain.

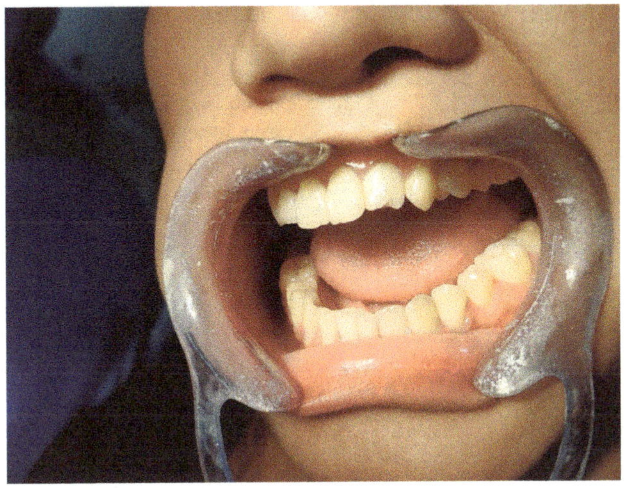

Figure 1: Full mouth intraoral image of the patient.

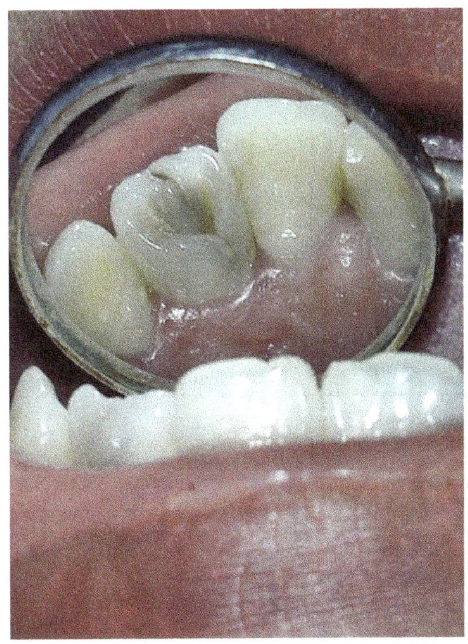

Figure 2: Clinical picture showing talon's cusp with dens invaginatus in maxillary left lateral incisor.

On radiographic evaluation, a shallow V-shaped, tapered radio-opaque structure extending from the cervical third of the crown was noted. A dens invaginatus extending apically beyond the cementoenamel junction was also noted in the same tooth (Figure 3). The apical closure of the tooth was completed. No sign of periapical pathology was witnessed.

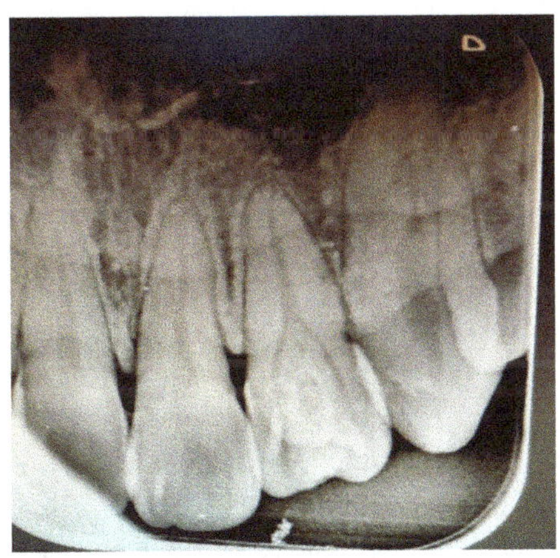

Figure 3: Intraoral periapical radiograph showing talon's cusp with dens invaginatus in maxillary left lateral incisor.

According to clinical and radiographic findings, the case was confirmed to be type II talon's cusp together with type I dens invaginatus. As the anomaly enhances plaque accumulation and makes the tooth vulnerable to dental caries, it was advised to fill the developmental groove with sealant for preventive purposes.

As the condition was asymptomatic, the patient did not want to get any treatment done for the involved tooth. The patient was advised to follow the routine brushing practice and maintain optimum oral hygiene and seek regular dental checkups. The written consent was taken from the patient for the publication of the clinical photographs and the X-ray record.

3. Discussion

Anomalies like talon's cusp, dens invaginatus, and palatogingival groove are fairly seen in lateral incisor, although the exact cause for this remains unknown [15–17]. However, the simultaneous occurrence of two or more anomalies in a single tooth is relatively rare, and here, in

Table 1: Classification of talon's cusp proposed by Hattab et al. [4].

Types	Description
Type I	True talon—distinctive additional cusp projecting from the lingual/cingulum surface of maxillary/mandibular anterior teeth to at least half a distance from the amelocemental junction to the incisal edge
Type II	Semitalon—an additional cusp of 1 mm or more that extends less than half of the distance from the amelocemental junction to the incisal edge, and it blends well with the lingual surface of the teeth.
Type III	Trace talon—prominence/variation in the cingulum, could be conical, bifid, or tubercle-like

Table 2: Classification of dens invaginatus proposed by Oehlers et al. [24].

Types	Description
Type I	Invagination is restricted to the crown up to the cementoenamel junction.
Type II	Invagination extends into the root beyond the cementoenamel junction.
Type IIIa	Invagination extends into the tooth with lateral communication to the periodontal ligament.
Type IIIb	Invagination extends into the tooth with apical communication to the periodontal ligament.

Table 3: Summary of the reported cases of talon's cusp/dens evaginatus with dens invaginatus documented till date.

Serial No.	Author/year	Sex	Primary anomaly	Tooth involved	Associated anomaly	Treatment performed
01	Lorena et al./ 2003 [27]	Male	Talon's cusp	Maxillary left lateral incisor	Dens invaginatus	No treatment
02	Tiku et al./ 2004 [18]	Female	Talon's cusp	Maxillary left lateral incisor	Dens invaginatus	No treatment
03	Mupparapu et al./2004 [28]	Male	Dens evaginatus	Maxillary right lateral incisor	Dens invaginatus	Prophylactic treatment with glass ionomer cement
04	Siraci et al./ 2008 [10]	Female	Talon's cusp	Mandibular right central incisor	Dens invaginatus	Grinding followed by prophylactic sealing with flowable composite
05	Anthonappa et al./2008 [29]	Female	Dens evaginatus	Maxillary right lateral incisor	Dens invaginatus	Prophylactic treatment with glass ionomer cement
06	Vardhan et al./ 2010 [30]	Male	Talon's cusp	Maxillary right and left central and lateral incisor	Dens invaginatus	No treatment
07	Sarraf-Shirazi et al./2010 [31]	Male	Talon's cusp	Maxillary right and left central incisor	Dens invaginatus	Endodontic treatment
08	Yadav et al./ 2011 [15]		Talon's cusp	Maxillary left lateral incisor	Dens invaginatus	Enameloplasty with prophylactic composite resin treatment
09	Nagaveni et al./2011 [32]	Male	Talon's cusp	Mandibular left central incisor	Dens invaginatus	Prophylactic treatment with glass ionomer cement
10	Akers et al./ 2014 [33]	Male	Dens invaginatus	Maxillary left lateral incisor	Dens evaginatus	Endodontic treatment
11	Kasat et al./ 2014 [34]	Female	Talon's cusp	Maxillary left lateral incisor	Dens invaginatus, radicular cyst	Endodontic treatment of the teeth with enucleation of the cyst
12	Babaji /2015 [35]	Male	Dens invaginatus	Supplemental maxillary left central incisor	Dens evaginatus	Extraction as both talon's cusp and dens invaginatus were there on supplemental tooth
13	Lwin et al./ 2017 [12]	Male	Talon's cusp	Maxillary right lateral incisor	Double dens invaginatus	Restoration with pit and fissure sealant
14	Present case	Female	Talon's cusp	Maxillary left lateral incisor	Dens evaginatus	No treatment

this case, we reported the concurrent occurrence of a talon's cusp with dens invaginatus in the maxillary left lateral incisor of the same patient. Talon's cusp reported, in this case, is a "semitalon," according to the classification proposed by Hattab et al. [4], which is mentioned in Table 1.

Studies have shown that the prevalence of talon's cusp varies in different ethnic groups ranging from 0.06% in Mexican children to about 7.7% in Indian children. Mongolians show a higher incidence rate of talon's cusp when compared with Caucasians and Negroes [15–18]. Talon's cusp can occur concurrently with other anomalies like bifid cingulum, dens invaginatus, impacted mesiodens, macrodontia, odontoma, and supernumerary tooth [15, 19–21]. These anomalies can alter the vitality of the pulp and can remain asymptomatic [10, 15] as well and get diagnosed under routine radiographic examination [10, 12, 15] which happened in the present case.

Dens invaginatus carries a significantly increased risk of developing into a pulpal pathology. The invaginated portion communicates with the oral cavity, facilitating the ingress of irritants and microbes into the pulp causing pulpal and periapical pathosis [15, 22]. Its incidence is 0.04 to 10% and is usually detected on a routine roentogenic evaluation [23]. As these pathologies are developmental, the apical root-end closure is questionable if there is pulpal involvement in such a tooth with an open apex [15]. Dens invaginatus reported in this case belongs to the type II variant as per Oehlers classification of dens invaginatus [24], which is mentioned in Table 2. Dens invaginatus might coexist with other developmental anomalies like double teeth, shoveling of the incisor, and multirooted anterior teeth [15, 16, 25, 26]. The documented cases, presenting with the cooccurrence of talon's cusp with dens invaginatus, are summarized in Table 3.

The treatment approach varies from case to case. An asymptomatic talon's cusp without any occlusal interference is left untreated, and vigorous oral hygiene and routine monitoring are good enough, whereas any interference with speech and occlusion requires reduction of the cusp with the application of a desensitizing agent; sometimes intentional endodontic treatment and coverage by full-thickness crown may be required to prevent dental caries and premature tooth loss. The management of dens invaginatus may range from simple oral hygiene instructions, frequent monitoring, and conservative restoration to endodontic treatment, which depends exclusively on the presenting symptoms [10, 12, 15].

The clinical significance of talon's cusp and dens invaginatus is they could be associated with compromised function and esthetics, and as they serve an attachment area for the attachment of food particles, dental plaque, they have a high chance to get affected by the carious process [12, 15]. The message to the clinicians through this case report is that whenever such a case is encountered, early diagnosis and prompt treatment should be performed to restore the function, improve the prognosis, minimize potential complications, and improve the quality of life of the patient.

Based on the research data, both talon's cusp and dens invaginatus are seen unilaterally on the lateral incisors [12]. Although both of these developmental anomalies are not uncommon, based on the knowledge of the authors, the concurrent occurrence of talon's cusp with dens invaginatus in a single tooth has not been reported in the Nepalese population till date.

4. Conclusion

To summarize, talon's cusp and dens invaginatus are the developmental anomalies noted in the anterior teeth. They could be asymptomatic or could be associated with the symptoms mentioned in this case report. Its early detection and prompt intervention can alleviate the symptoms in symptomatic cases, prevent premature tooth loss, enhance esthetics, and overall improve the well-being of the patient.

Consent

Written informed consent was obtained from the patient to publish this report by the journal's patient consent policy.

References

[1] R. Rajendran, *Shafer's Textbook of Oral Pathology*, Elsevier, India, 2009.

[2] W. H. Mitchell, "Case report," *Dental Cosmos*, vol. 36, 1892.

[3] S. Sicher and S. N. Bhaskar, *Orban's Oral Histology and Embryology*, CV Mosby Company, St Louis, Mo, 7th ed. edition, 1972.

[4] F. N. Hattab, O. M. Yassin, and K. S. Al-Nimri, "Talon cusp—clinical significance and management: case reports," *Quintessence International*, vol. 26, no. 2, pp. 115–120, 1995.

[5] D. G. Gardner and S. S. Girgis, "Talon cusps: a dental anomaly in the Rubinstein-Taybi syndrome," *Oral Surgery, Oral Medicine, and Oral Pathology*, vol. 47, no. 6, pp. 519–521, 1979.

[6] E. Goldstein and J. L. Medina, "Mohr syndrome or oral-facialdigital II: report of two cases," *Journal of the American Dental Association*, vol. 89, no. 2, pp. 377–382, 1974.

[7] R. J. Chen and H. S. Chen, "Talon cusp in primary dentition," *Oral Surgery, Oral Medicine, and Oral Pathology*, vol. 62, no. 1, pp. 67–72, 1986.

[8] T. Tsutsumi and H. Oguchi, "Labial talon cusp in a child with incontinentia pigmenti achromians: case report," *Pediatric Dentistry*, vol. 13, pp. 236-237, 1991.

[9] S. Patil, R. S. Rao, and B. Majumdar, "Hamartomas of the oral cavity," *Journal of International Society of Preventive & Community Dentistry*, vol. 5, no. 5, pp. 347–353, 2015.

[10] E. Siraci, H. C. Gungor, and Z. C. Cehreli, "Dens invaginatus and talon cusp co-occurring in a mandibular central incisor: a case report," *Journal of Dentistry for Children*, vol. 75, no. 2, pp. 177–180, 2008.

[11] C. L. Mader, "Talon cusp," *Journal of the American Dental Association*, vol. 103, no. 2, pp. 244–246, 1981.

[12] H. N. Lwin, P. P. Kyaw, and S. W. Thu, "Coexistence of true talon cusp and double dens invaginatus in a single tooth: a rare case report and review of the literature," *Clinical Case Reports*, vol. 5, no. 12, pp. 2017–2021, 2017.

[13] B. W. Neville, D. D. Damm, A. C. Chi, and C. M. Allen, *Oral and Maxillofacial Pathology*, Elsevier, St. Louis, MO, 2015.

[14] M. Hülsmann, "Dens invaginatus: aetiology, classification, prevalence, diagnosis, and treatment considerations," *International Endodontic Journal*, vol. 30, no. 2, pp. 79–90, 1997.

[15] M. Yadav, S. M. Meghana, and S. R. Kulkarni, "Concommitant occurance of dens invaginatus and talon cusp: a case report," *Revista Odonto Ciência*, vol. 26, no. 2, pp. 187–190, 2011.

[16] J. J. Segura and A. Jiménez-Rubio, "Talon cusp affecting permanent maxillary lateral incisors in 2 family members," *Oral Surgery, Oral Medicine, Oral Pathology, Oral Radiology, and Endodontics*, vol. 88, no. 1, pp. 90–92, 1999.

[17] E. A. O'Sullivan, "Multiple dental anomalies in a young patient: a case report," *International Journal of Paediatric Dentistry*, vol. 10, no. 1, pp. 63–66, 2000.

[18] A. Tiku, U. M. Nadkarni, and S. G. Damle, "Management of two unusual cases of dens invaginatus and talon cusp associated with other dental anomalies," *Journal of the Indian Society of Pedodontics and Preventive Dentistry*, vol. 22, no. 3, pp. 128–133, 2004.

[19] P. J. Davis and A. H. Brook, "The presentation of talon cusp: diagnosis, clinical features, associations and possible aetiology," *British Dental Journal*, vol. 160, pp. 84–88, 1985.

[20] E. Natkin, D. L. Pitts, and P. Worthington, "A case of talon cusp associated with other odontogenic abnormalities," *Journal of Endodontia*, vol. 9, no. 11, pp. 491–495, 1983.

[21] S. K. Mallineni, G. K. Panampally, Y. Chen, and T. Tian, "Mandibular talon cusps: a systematic review and data analysis," *Journal of Clinical and Experimental Dentistry*, vol. 6, no. 4, 2014.

[22] S. C. White and M. J. Pharoah, *Dental Anomalies. Oral Radiology: Principles and Interpretation*, Mosby, New York, NY, USA, 5th ed. edition, 2004.

[23] P. V. Abbot, "Labial and palatal "talon cusp" on the same tooth-a case report," *Oral Surgery, Oral Medicine, Oral Pathology, Oral Radiology, and Endodontics*, vol. 85, no. 6, pp. 726–730, 1998.

[24] F. A. Oehlers and Dens invaginatus. II., "Associated posterior crown forms and pathogenesis," *Oral Surgery, Oral Medicine, and Oral Pathology*, vol. 10, no. 12, pp. 1302–1316, 1957.

[25] M. Gul, S. Adnan, and F. Umer, "A variant of the current dens invaginatus classification," *Frontiers in Dentistry*, vol. 17, p. 28, 2020.

[26] M. Ekambaram, C. K. Yiu, and N. M. King, "An unusual case of double teeth with facial and lingual talon cusps," *Oral Surgery, Oral Medicine, Oral Pathology, Oral Radiology, and Endodontology*, vol. 105, no. 4, pp. e63–e67, 2008.

[27] S. C. Lorena, D. T. Oliveira, and E. W. Odellt, "Multiple dental anomalies in the maxillary incisor region," *Journal of Oral Science*, vol. 45, no. 1, pp. 47–50, 2003.

[28] M. Mupparapu, S. R. Singer, and J. H. Goodchild, "Dens evaginatus and dens invaginatus in a maxillary lateral incisor: report of a rare occurrence and review of literature," *Australian Dental Journal*, vol. 49, no. 4, pp. 201–203, 2004.

[29] R. Anthonappa, C. Yiu, and N. King, "A novel combination of *dens evaginatus* and *dens invaginatus* in a single tooth–review of the literature and a case report," *Journal of Clinical Pediatric Dentistry*, vol. 32, no. 3, pp. 239–242, 2008.

[30] T. H. Vardhan and S. Shanmugam, "Dens evaginatus and dens invaginatus in all maxillary incisors: report of a case," *Quintessence International*, vol. 41, no. 2, pp. 105–107, 2010.

[31] A. Sarraf Shirazi, M. Rezaiefar, and M. Forghani, "A rare case of multiple talon cusps in three siblings," *Brazilian Dental Journal*, vol. 21, no. 5, pp. 463–466, 2010.

[32] N. B. Nagaveni, K. V. Umashanikara, B. G. Vidyullatha, S. Sreedevi, and N. B. Radhika, "Permanent mandibular incisor with multiple anomalies - report of a rare clinical case," *Brazilian Dental Journal*, vol. 22, no. 4, pp. 346–350, 2011.

[33] H. F. Akers, C. M. Henderson, and M. A. Foley, "Diagnosis and management of a maxillary lateral incisor exhibiting dens invaginatus and dens evaginatus," *Australian Endodontic Journal*, vol. 40, no. 1, pp. 32–38, 2014.

[34] V. O. Kasat, M. Singh, H. Saluja, and R. Ladda, "Coexistence of two talon cusps and two dens invaginatus in a single tooth with associated radicular cyst-a case report and review of literature," *Journal of Clinical and Experimental Dentistry*, vol. 6, no. 4, 2014.

[35] P. Babaji, "Bilateral supplemental maxillary incisors with both dens invaginatus and dens evaginatus in a non syndromic patient: a rare case report," *Journal of Clinical and Diagnostic Research: JCDR*, vol. 9, no. 1, pp. ZJ01–ZJ02, 2015.

17

Patient Satisfaction with Resin Infiltration Treatment for Masking Noncavitated White Spot Lesions on Anterior Maxillary Teeth: Two Case Reports

Rana A. Alamoudi,[1] Asmaa A. Yaseen,[2] Amjad S. Alharthi,[3] and Sara M. Bagher[1]

[1]*Pediatric Dentistry Department, Faculty of Dentistry, King Abdulaziz University, Jeddah 21589, Saudi Arabia*
[2]*Pediatric Dentistry Resident, Department of Pediatric Dentistry, King Salman Armed Forces Hospital, Tabuk, Saudi Arabia*
[3]*Pediatric Dentistry Resident, Department of Pediatric Dentistry, King Abdulaziz University, Jeddah, Saudi Arabia*

Correspondence should be addressed to Sara M. Bagher; sbagher@kau.edu.sa

Academic Editor: Andrea Scribante

Aim. We assessed patient satisfaction with resin infiltration treatment outcomes for masking postorthodontic treatment noncavitated white spot lesions on anterior maxillary teeth. *Background.* White spot lesions (WSLs) are opaque white areas of demineralization. The lesion may remineralize over time, but the opaque color usually remains, retaining the undesirable tooth color. *Case Description*: Resin infiltration (RI) was administered to two patients with a total of 10 anterior maxillary teeth diagnosed with noncavitated WSLs. Immediately after treatment, patients were asked about their comfort during the RI treatment and their level of satisfaction with treatment outcomes. Two weeks post-treatment, the two patients were asked again about their level of treatment outcome satisfaction and if they thought they needed a second treatment. Both reported that they were comfortable during the treatment and were extremely satisfied with the achieved treatment outcomes immediately and two weeks after the treatment and did not feel that they would need to seek further treatment to reach the desired outcome. *Conclusion.* Resin infiltration is a comfortable, conservative treatment option providing satisfactory outcomes in masking noncavitated WSLs on anterior maxillary teeth after orthodontic treatment. *Clinical Significance.* Resin infiltration is a conservative treatment option to mask noncavitated WSLs after orthodontic treatment.

1. Introduction

Dental caries results from an imbalance between demineralization and remineralization processes after the intake of fermentable carbohydrates [1]. As the microorganisms within the dental plaque biofilm are exposed to fermentable carbohydrates and sugars, an organic acid is produced [2]. This acid dissolves the intercrystalline spaces within the enamel [3], which creates a pathway for the transport of minerals out of the enamel [4].

Caries in enamel is first observed clinically as a noncavitated incipient white spot enamel lesions (WSLs). The surface zone of the WSLs acts as a barrier to bacterial invasion and remains highly mineralized, while the lesion's body loses its minerals [5] and the pores become filled with water or air [6]. Therefore, WSLs appear clinically as opaque white areas of demineralization [7].

Orthodontic fixed appliance increases the likelihood of unsatisfactory oral hygiene, leading to dental plaque adherence to the appliance surfaces. They also limit the ability of saliva, lips, tongue, and cheeks to self-cleanse, which increases the risk of WSL development [8, 9]. Poor oral hygiene, increased the treatment duration, and lack of fluoride supplement use during the orthodontic treatment are risk factors identified to increase the risk of WSL development [10].

Therefore, patient education, oral hygiene instruction, and patient compliance are the most significant prophylactic measures against the formation of WSLs [11]. Professional prophylactic cleaning and routine use of fluoride-containing mouthwash have also been recommended to prevent WSLs formation during fixed orthodontic treatment [12].

The treatment options of post-orthodontic treatment WSLs range from very conservative (natural remineralization) to more invasive (tooth preparation and restoration) procedures, based on the severity of the lesion [13]. Conservative methods for remineralization usually include proper oral hygiene measures, which requires patient's compliance and involves multiple applications of fluorides, and/or casein phosphopeptide-amorphous calcium phosphate containing products [14, 15]. Recently, a few studies reported that the use of biomimetic hydroxyapatite containing toothpaste forms a coating on the enamel surface, promotes superficial enamel repair, and aids in preventing secondary caries around restorations [16, 17, 18].

More invasive treatment modalities include bleaching, microabrasion, resin infiltration (RI), resin restoration, and indirect restoration [19]. Gentle tooth bleaching for WSLs together with the incorporation of nano-bioactive glass ionomer, nano-hydroxyapatite, and nano-amorphous calcium phosphate into the bleaching agents can reduce the negative side-effects associated with bleaching [20]. Microabrasion is a more invasive procedure that bleaching for the treatment of superficial WSLs and includes both chemical and mechanical processing of the enamel surface [6]. Finally, RI is a minimally invasive treatment modality that involves the utilization of strong acid that opens the enamel tubules, which permits a low-viscosity resin to penetrate and replace the air or water in the pores and improves the refractive index of the affected enamel to resemble normal enamel, enhancing lesion appearance immediately [21, 22].

Multiple studies evaluated the esthetic effect of RI in managing postorthodontic treatment WSLs and reported that RI treatments is very effective in camouflaging post-orthodontic treatment WSLs immediately after application [23–26]. But only one study evaluated patients' satisfaction with the RI treatment outcomes [25]. Therefore, the purpose of this report was to assess patient satisfaction with resin infiltration treatment outcomes for masking postorthodontic treatment noncavitated white spot lesions on anterior maxillary teeth.

2. Case Presentation

The two patients were referred by the Orthodontic Department at King Abdulaziz University Faculty of Dentistry (KAUFD) after completing their orthodontic treatment with the chief complaint of WSLs in the labial surfaces of their upper anterior teeth. At KAUFD, patients receiving orthodontic treatments are always encouraged to maintain proper oral hygiene instructions and to use fluoride-containing toothpaste and mouthwash during their treatment and after the debonding. The dental records of patients who finished their orthodontic treatment within the last two weeks were reviewed. Five healthy patients diagnosed with postorthodontic treatment WSLs were identified and contacted by phone. Three of them answered the phone and agreed to attend a scheduled appointment to discuss the treatment options for their post-orthodontic treatment WSLs. Two of them were interested in the RI treatment for their postorthodontic treatment WSLs and were examined clinically by a trained dentist using the International Caries Detection and Assessment (ICDAS) method, which was created to differentiate between the different stages of carious lesions (pit and fissures, and smooth surface) using visual and tactile techniques [28]. For smooth surface lesions, the ICDAS score was 1 if the enamel surface of the anterior maxillary teeth appeared sound, but a white or brown lesion was visible after prolonged air drying. If there was a distinct visual change in the enamel and the lesion appeared white or brown, the ICDAS score was 2. Only WSLs with ICDAS scores of 1 or 2 received RI treatment. Fluorosis was not detected (using Dean's fluorosis index), nor was amelogenesis imperfecta (according to the Witkop classification) [29] on any anterior maxillary teeth of the two patients.

The first patient was a 16-year-old female with four teeth (maxillary central and lateral incisors) diagnosed clinically with noncavitated WSLs (ICDAS scores of 2), and the second was a 23-year-old male with six teeth (maxillary central incisors, lateral incisors, and canines) diagnosed clinically with noncavitated WSLs (ICDAS of 2). Both patients finished their orthodontic treatment three months prior to RI application. They were nonsmokers and reported brushing and flossing their teeth at least once daily during their orthodontic treatment. Neither patient was diagnosed with WSLs determined to have ICDAS scores >2 on their anterior maxillary teeth.

Before the treatment, the patients were asked to report on a numeric scale of 1 to 5, the extent to which they were uncomfortable or annoyed by the WSLs on their anterior maxillary teeth that appeared after orthodontic treatment. A score of 1 was defined as being comfortable and not annoyed at all, and 5 represented extremely uncomfortable and annoyed. Both patients reported feeling extremely annoyed (score = 5) by the WSLs on their anterior teeth.

The noncavitated WSLs were treated with RI (Icon, DMG America; Englewood, NJ, USA) by the same dentist according to the following protocol: (1) the facial surfaces of the affected teeth were cleaned with a rubber cup and plain pumice, then rinsed and dried for 30 seconds; (2) teeth were isolated with a rubber dam, and then 15% hydrochloric acid gel (Icon Etch) was placed on the affected teeth for two minutes, rinsed with water, and air-dried for 30 seconds; (3) ethanol (Icon Dry) was brushed on and dried for 30 seconds; (4) teeth were then visually inspected to determine whether the whitish opaque discoloration lesions had diminished significantly and if the discoloration was not concealed, the previous steps were repeated; (5) once the desired result was achieved, RI was applied to the teeth surfaces for three minutes, and cotton roll was used to remove excess resin material. The teeth were flossed and light-cured for 40 seconds according to the manufacturer's instructions. A second layer of resin was applied for one minute following the same previous steps. Finally, the teeth surfaces were polished using a spiral polishing wheel. The pre- and post-RI treatment outcomes of the first and second cases are shown in Figures 1 and 2, respectively.

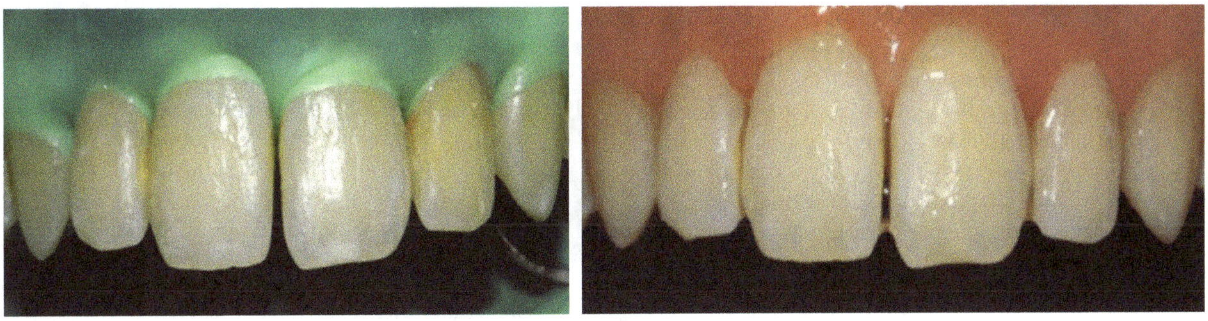

(a) (b)

FIGURE 1: (a) Case 1, pretreatment. (b) Post-treatment with resin infiltration.

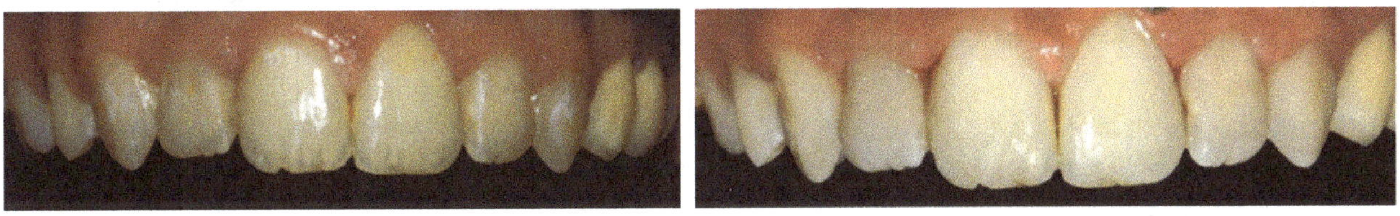

(a) (b)

FIGURE 2: (a) Case 2, pretreatment. (b) Post-treatment with resin infiltration.

Immediately after the RI procedure, both patients were asked whether they felt comfortable during the treatment, their level of satisfaction with the treatment outcomes and if they would recommend this treatment to others. Both reported that they were comfortable during the treatment and extremely satisfied with the achieved treatment outcomes. Moreover, both reported that they would recommend this treatment to others.

Two weeks post-treatment, the patients were contacted by phone and asked again about their level of satisfaction with the treatment outcomes and if they were considering a second treatment visit. Both were extremely satisfied with the achieved treatment outcomes and reported that the outcomes had improved since immediately after the treatment. Furthermore, they did not feel they would need to seek further treatment to reach the desired outcomes.

3. Discussion

High patient satisfaction with RI treatment outcomes in masking noncavitated WSLs on anterior maxillary teeth after orthodontic treatment was reported by both presented cases. WSLs are considered one of the major side effects of orthodontic treatment [30, 31], especially in maxillary lateral incisor, maxillary canine, and central incisors, respectively [32].

A study conducted by Kim et al. [33] to evaluate clinically the effectiveness of RI in masking WSLs after orthodontic treatment. The time lapse between the orthodontic bracket debonding and RI treatment for the included WSLs was 21 months. They reported immediately after the RI application; most of the lesions were completely masked but others were only partially masked or unchanged [33]. This was explained by the fact that the esthetic effect of RI is more effective in active and shallow lesions compared to deeper and inactive lesions with thinker outer protective layer. Therefore, it was recommended to do the RI treatment as soon as possible after bracket removal to avoid lesion progression and the loss of the surface integrity [6, 33]. In our cases the RI treatment was provided a few weeks after the removal of the orthodontic brackets while the lesions were still active and shallow.

The esthetic effect of RI in managing postorthodontic WSLs was reported to be stable 2 [23], 6 [24], and 12 months after the treatment [25, 26]. In the presented cases, patient's satisfaction with the treatment outcomes was done immediately after the treatment and two weeks later. Further follow-up for a longer duration is recommended to ensure that the level of patients' satisfaction with the treatment outcomes is maintained.

A recent study by Solinas et al. [17] reported that the application of biomimetic nanohydroxyapatite for the treatment of incisor and molar hypomineralization for six months in a 4-year-old patient resulted in a significant decrease in the hypersensitivity and improved the enamel appearance for the maxillary incisors. Further studies to evaluate the effect of biomimetic nanohydroxyapatite are recommended in hope that more invasive treatment options can be avoided.

Hughes and Roseberg [27] evaluated patient satisfaction with the esthetic changes resulting from RI treatment of WSLs associated with orthodontic treatment. Before the treatment, patients reported that their smile was extremely important, and that WSLs bothered them. Immediately after treatment, patients were satisfied with the achieved outcomes [27], consistent with our two case reports.

It was also previously reported that combining home bleaching and RI for treating teeth in different stages of fluorosis improves patient confidence and satisfaction with their appearance [34]. Another recent *clinical study showed that patients were highly satisfied* with the RI procedure duration for the treatment of fluorosis lesions [35].

This report demonstrates that RI can be considered an effective and reliable treatment option for masking noncavitated WSLs due to its deep penetration. We recommend that future studies include longer follow-up periods examining the long-term success and relapse rate of RI as a conservative treatment option for noncavitated WSLs.

4. Conclusions

Resin infiltration is a comfortable, conservative treatment option that provides satisfactory outcomes in masking noncavitated WSLs on anterior maxillary teeth after orthodontic treatment.

Additional Points

Resin infiltration is an effective, conservative treatment option to mask noncavitated WSLs after orthodontic treatment.

References

[1] J. D. Featherstone, "The continuum of dental caries evidence for a dynamic disease process," *Journal of Dental Research*, vol. 83, 1_suppl, p. 39, 2004, Spec No C:C39-42.

[2] F. Manji, O. Fejerskov, N. J. Nagelkerke, and V. Baelum, "A random effects model for some epidemiological features of dental caries," *Community Dentistry and Oral Epidemiology*, vol. 19, no. 6, pp. 324–328, 1991.

[3] E. A. Kidd and O. Fejerskov, "What constitutes dental caries? Histopathology of carious enamel and dentin related to the action of cariogenic biofilms," *Journal of Dental Research*, vol. 83, 1_suppl, p. 35, 2004, Spec No C:C35-38.

[4] L. Holmen, A. Thylstrup, B. Ogaard, and F. Kragh, "A scanning electron microscopic study of progressive stages of enamel caries in vivo," *Caries Research Journal*, vol. 19, no. 4, pp. 355–367, 1985.

[5] L. M. Silverstone, "Structure of carious enamel, including the early lesion," *Oral Science Reviews*, vol. 3, pp. 100–160, 1973.

[6] G. C. Heymann and D. Grauer, "A contemporary review of white spot lesions in orthodontics," *Journal of Esthetic and Restorative Dentistry*, vol. 25, no. 2, pp. 85–95, 2013.

[7] G. J. Mount, "Defining, classifying, and placing incipient caries lesions in perspective," *Dental Clinics of North America*, vol. 49, no. 4, pp. 701–723, 2005.

[8] R. G. Rosenbloom and N. Tinanoff, "Salivary Streptococcus mutans levels in patients before, during, and after orthodontic treatment," *American Journal of Orthodontics and Dentofacial Orthopedics*, vol. 100, no. 1, pp. 35–37, 1991.

[9] I. Van Dijken, S. Persson, and S. Sjöström, "Presence of Streptococcus mutans and lactobacilli in saliva and on enamel, glass ionomer cement, and composite resin surfaces," *Scandinavian Journal of Dental Research*, vol. 99, no. 1, pp. 13–19, 1991.

[10] K. Khalaf, "Factors affecting the formation, severity and location of white spot lesions during orthodontic treatment with fixed appliances," *Journal of Oral and Maxillofacial Surgery*, vol. 5, no. 1, article e4, 2014.

[11] M. Khoroushi and M. Kachuie, "Prevention and treatment of white spot lesions in orthodontic patients," *Contemporary Clinical Dentistry*, vol. 8, no. 1, pp. 11–19, 2017.

[12] C. L. Davidson and I. S. Bekke-Hoekstra, "The resistance of superficially sealed enamel to wear and carious attack *in vitro*," *Journal of Oral Rehabilitation*, vol. 7, no. 4, pp. 299–305, 1980.

[13] M. K. Eltayeb, Y. E. Ibrahim, I. A. El Karim, and N. M. Sanhouri, "Distribution of white spot lesions among orthodontic patients attending teaching institutes in Khartoum," *BMC Oral Health*, vol. 17, no. 1, p. 88, 2017.

[14] F. Bergstrand and S. Twetman, "A review on prevention and treatment of post-orthodontic white spot lesions - evidence-based methods and emerging technologies," *Open Dentistry Journal*, vol. 5, no. 1, pp. 158–162, 2011.

[15] A. Bahoum, L. Bahije, and F. Zaoui, "Les déminéralisations amélaires en orthodontie. Utilisation raisonnée du fluor dans la prévention et le traitement [Enamel demineralization in orthodontics. Systematic use of fluoride in prevention and treatment]," *Schweizer Monatsschrift für Zahnmedizin*, vol. 122, no. 10, pp. 937–947, 2012.

[16] M. Lelli, A. Putignano, M. Marchetti et al., "Remineralization and repair of enamel surface by biomimetic Zn-carbonate hydroxyapatite containing toothpaste: a comparative in vivo study," *Frontiers in Physiology*, vol. 5, p. 333, 2014.

[17] G. Solinas, V. Grabesu, M. Lattari, R. Strinna, N. Arnould, and A. A. Amodeo, "Management of a hypomineralisation of the enamel by applying a remineraliser based on zinc hydroxyapatite (microRepair)," *Case Reports in Dentistry*, vol. 2021, Article ID 5291858, 9 pages, 2021.

[18] A. Butera, M. Pascadopoli, S. Gallo et al., "SEM/EDS evaluation of the mineral deposition on a polymeric composite resin of a toothpaste containing biomimetic Zn-carbonate hydroxyapatite (microRepair®) in oral environment: a randomized clinical trial," *Polymers*, vol. 13, no. 16, p. 2740, 2021.

[19] S. M. Hammad, M. El Banna, I. El Zayat, and M. M. Abdel, "Effect of resin infiltration on white spot lesions after debonding orthodontic brackets," *American Journal of Dentistry*, vol. 25, no. 1, pp. 3–8, 2012.

[20] M. Khoroushi, H. Mazaheri, T. Saneie, and P. Samimi, "Fracture toughness of bleached enamel: effect of applying three different nanobiomaterials by nanoindentation test," *Contemporary Clinical Dentistry*, vol. 7, no. 2, pp. 209–215, 2016.

[21] S. Paris and H. Meyer-Lueckel, "Masking of labial enamel white spot lesions by resin infiltration a clinical report," *Quintessence International*, vol. 40, no. 9, pp. 713–718, 2009.

[22] M. C. Peters, "Strategies for non invasive demineralized tissue repair," *Dental Clinics of North America*, vol. 54, no. 3, pp. 507–525, 2010.

[23] S. V. Senestraro, J. J. Crowe, M. Wang et al., "Minimally invasive resin infiltration of arrested white-spot lesions: a randomized clinical trial," *Journal of the American Dental Association*, vol. 144, no. 9, pp. 997–1005, 2013.

[24] M. Knösel, A. Eckstein, and H. J. Helms, "Durability of esthetic improvement following icon resin infiltration of multibracket-induced white spot lesions compared with no therapy over 6 months: a single-center, split-mouth, randomized clinical trial," *American Journal of Orthodontics and Dentofacial Orthopedics*, vol. 144, no. 1, pp. 86–96, 2013.

[25] A. Eckstein, H. J. Helms, and M. Knösel, "Camouflage effects following resin infiltration of postorthodontic white-spot lesions in vivo: one-year follow-up," *Angle Orthodontist*, vol. 85, no. 3, pp. 374–380, 2015.

[26] C. H. Feng and X. Y. Chu, "Efficacy of one year treatment of icon infiltration resin on post-orthodontic white spots," *Beijing Da Xue Xue Bao Yi Xue Ban*, vol. 45, no. 1, pp. 40–43, 2013.

[27] J. Hughes and F. Roseberg, "Patient satisfaction of esthetic with resin infiltration," *New York Medical Journal*, vol. 8, p. 1, 2013.

[28] A. I. Ismail, W. Sohn, M. Tellez et al., "The international caries detection and assessment system (ICDAS): an integrated system for measuring dental caries," *Community Dentistry and Oral Epidemiology*, vol. 35, no. 3, pp. 170–178, 2007.

[29] C. J. Witkop Jr., "Hereditary defects in enamel and dentin," *Prosc First Cong Human Genet Acta Genetica Statist Med*, vol. 7, pp. 236–239, 1957.

[30] S. Paris, H. Meyer-Lueckel, H. Colfen, and A. M. Kielbassa, "Resin infiltration of artificial enamel caries lesions with experimental light curing resins," *Dental Materials*, vol. 26, no. 4, pp. 582–588, 2007.

[31] K. W. Neuhaus, M. Graf, A. Lussi, and C. Katsaros, "Late infiltration of post-orthodontic white spot lesions," *Journal of Orofacial Orthopedics*, vol. 71, no. 6, pp. 442–447, 2010.

[32] E. Tufekci, J. S. Dixon, J. C. Gunsolley, and S. J. Lindauer, "Prevalence of white spot lesions during orthodontic treatment with fixed appliances," *Angle Orthodontist*, vol. 81, no. 2, pp. 206–210, 2011.

[33] S. Kim, E. Y. Kim, T. S. Jeong, and J. W. Kim, "The evaluation of resin infiltration for masking labial enamel white spot lesions," *International Journal of Paediatric Dentistry*, vol. 21, no. 4, pp. 241–248, 2011.

[34] Z. Pan, K. Que, J. Liu et al., "Effects of at-home bleaching and resin infiltration treatments on the aesthetic and psychological status of patients with dental fluorosis: a prospective study," *Journal of Dental*, vol. 91, article 103228, 2019.

[35] F. Zotti, L. Albertini, N. Tomizioli, G. Capocasale, and M. Albanese, "Resin infiltration in dental fluorosis treatment-1-year follow-up," *Medicina*, vol. 57, no. 1, p. 22, 2020.

18

Dedifferentiated Low-Grade Central Osteosarcoma of the Mandible

Kenji Yamagata,[1] Naomi Ishibashi-Kanno,[1] Ryota Matsuoka,[2] Fumihiko Uchida,[1] Satoshi Fukuzawa,[1] and Hiroki Bukawa[1]

[1]*Department of Oral and Maxillofacial Surgery, Institute of Clinical Medicine, Faculty of Medicine, University of Tsukuba, Japan*
[2]*Department of Diagnostic Pathology, Institute of Clinical Medicine, Faculty of Medicine, University of Tsukuba, Japan*

Correspondence should be addressed to Kenji Yamagata; y-kenji@md.tsukuba.ac.jp

Academic Editor: Pia L. Jornet

We present the first, to our knowledge, case of a dedifferentiated low-grade central osteosarcoma (LCOS) of the mandible. A 48-year-old Japanese woman underwent enucleation under general anesthesia after a diagnosis of ossifying fibroma. At the second recurrence, the pathological diagnosis after biopsy was of sarcoma with MDM2(+) and CDK4(+) immunohistochemical staining results. Hemimandibulotomy, supraomohyoid neck dissection, and free-flap reconstruction with a rectus abdominal flap were performed. A retrospective reevaluation of the first specimen with additional immunohistochemical staining for MDM2 and CDK4 yielded a final diagnosis of dedifferentiated LCOS. The patient showed no recurrence or lung metastasis 3 years after the final surgery.

1. Introduction

Low-grade osteosarcoma (LGOS) is rare and includes low-grade central OS (LCOS) and parosteal OS. LCOS represents less than 2% of all OSs reported in the literature [1]. In general, OS of the jaw is a high-grade lesion and relatively rare [2, 3]. The biological behavior of LGOS is more indolent than that of high-grade conventional OS. Microscopically, LGOS is often misdiagnosed as a benign fibrous lesion and is most often confused with fibrous dysplasia. It has been reported that all benign fibrous and fibroosseous lesions and control-group tumors show negative results for *murine double-minute type 2* (MDM2) and/or *cyclin-dependent kinase 4* (CDK4), which are also markers for distinguishing between dedifferentiated LGOS and conventional high-grade OS [4]. Although one case of dedifferentiated parosteal OS of the maxilla has been reported in the literature on the oral and maxillofacial area [5], to our knowledge, LCOS has not been reported to date. We present the first case of this entity, which was retrospectively diagnosed as dedifferentiated LCOS of the mandible based on MDM2 and/or CDK4 immunohistochemical findings.

2. Case Presentation

A 48-year-old Japanese woman who showed radiolucency of the left mandible on panoramic radiography was referred to the Department of Oral and Maxillofacial Surgery, University of Tsukuba Hospital. Her medical history included hypertension and an ovarian cyst. Her face was symmetrical, and slight paresthesia of the lower lip and mentalis was noted. Diffuse elastic hard swelling was observed from the left canine to the second molar. Panoramic radiographs revealed a posterior well-demarcated radiolucent area and an anterior irregular area (Figure 1(a)). A well-enhanced high-signal area measuring 42×13 mm from the center to the left molar of the mandible was observed on T1-weighted magnetic resonance imaging (MRI) (Figure 1(b)). Biopsy was performed, and ossifying fibroma (OF) was diagnosed. The patient underwent enucleation under general anesthesia for OF. The pathological findings included a bundle of spindle cells running across each and storiform patterns. Randomly formed woven bone was observed. There was no atypia, and few mitoses were observed (2–3/50 high-power fields; HPFs).

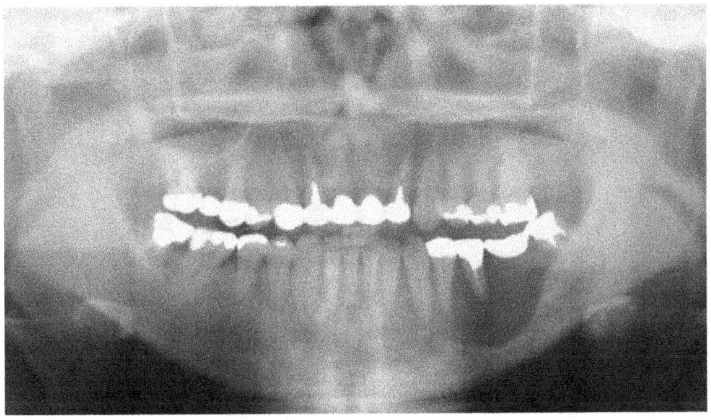

(a)

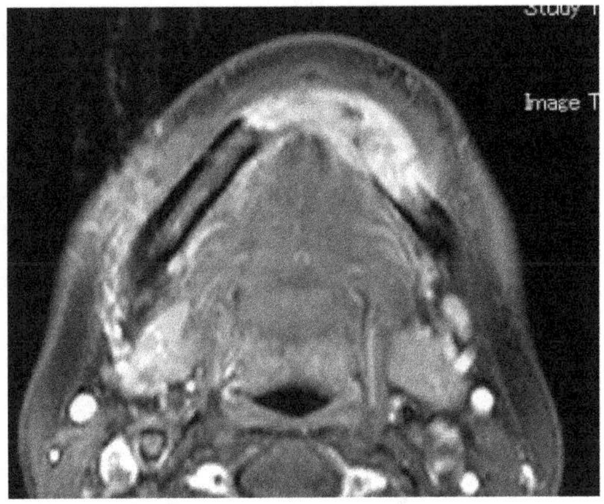

(b)

FIGURE 1: (a) Panoramic radiograph revealing a posterior well-demarcated radiolucent area and anterior irregular area. (b) Magnetic resonance images (T1 weighted) showing a tumor in the midline to the left side of the mandible with a high-signal mass measuring 42 × 13 mm.

Retrospective immunohistochemical staining revealed MDM2(+), CDK4(-), and a Ki-67 index of 2–3% (Figure 2).

Primary recurrence occurred 1 year and 3 months after the first enucleation. A soft tissue mass-like granuloma appeared in the left molar area intraorally. The biopsy indicated granulation tissue with spindle cells. Panoramic radiography revealed an increase in the radiolucent area to the right side of the mandible. Bilateral mandibulectomy and reconstructive surgery with fibula were performed, and the spindle cell-like fibroblast tumor cells were found to be pathologically complicated and thick, forming irregular eosinophilic osteoid. The tumor had destroyed the cortex of the mandible, and the surgical margin was free. The nuclei were swollen and mildly oval. The atypia was mild, and 3 mitoses/50 HPFs were observed. The retrospective immunohistochemical staining findings were MDM2(+), CDK 4(-), and a Ki-67 index of 15%.

Four years and 8 months after reconstructive surgery, a rapidly growing mass was observed in the left posterior part of the mandible (Figure 3(a)). A 39 × 64 × 59 mm highly enhanced mass expanding from the left mandible to the parapharyngeal space was observed on short-term inversion recovery MRI (Figure 3(b)). The pathological diagnosis after biopsy was of sarcoma with MDM2(+) and CDK4(+) immunohistochemical staining results. Hemimandibulotomy of the reconstructed mandible and supraomohyoid neck dissection with a titanium plate and free flap reconstruction with a rectus abdominal flap were performed under general anesthesia (Figure 3(c)). Pathologically, the spindle-like tumor cells were arranged in thick fascicles with severe atypia around the tumor borders and more than 100 mitoses/50 HPFs. Severe hyalinization was also observed. There was no osteoid or necrotic tissue. The results of immunohistochemical staining were as follows: α-SMA(+), desmin(-), h-caldesmon(-), pankeratin(-), S-100(+: sporadic), CD34(-), β-catenin(-), MDM2(+), CDK4(+), and Ki-67 (40%–50%) (Figure 4).

Retrospective reevaluation of the previous specimen with additional immunohistochemical staining for MDM2, CDK4, and Ki-67 was performed, and a final diagnosis of dedifferentiated LCOS (pT1N0, stage IIA: UICC 8th) was made. Postoperative chemotherapy and radiotherapy were not performed because of patient refusal. There was no recurrence or lung metastasis, and the patient's status has remained uneventful for 3 years after the final surgery.

3. Discussion

LGOS is rare and subdivided into parosteal OS and LCOS. Parosteal OS comprises a surface tumor representing 4%–5% of all OSs; it usually develops in the posterior surface of the distal femur in the third decade and in 15% to 43% of cases dedifferentiates into high-grade OS [6]. Only one report has described a dedifferentiated parosteal OS in the oral and maxillofacial region [5]. Conversely, LCOS accounts for 1%–2% of all OSs in the second to third decades and is mainly seen in the metaphysis of the long bones, e.g., the attachment of the tibia and femur. Involvement of the jawbone and axial and small tubular bones is rare. Very rarely, dedifferentiation can occur, resulting in conventional high-grade OS [6, 7]. To the best of our knowledge, previous reports describing dedifferentiated LCOS only involved the fibula and iliac region [8, 9]; our case was the first of dedifferentiated LCOS of the jaw.

Triantafillidou et al. [10] previously reported the clinical characteristics of OF, which is a fibroosseous tumor affecting the jaw and is composed of proliferating fibroblasts and osseous products that include bone and cementum-like material. OF is a slow-growing tumor of the jaw, and small or well-demarcated early tumors are treated with curettage or enucleation. In contrast, aggressive tumors that show rapid enlargement are treated with radical resection [10]. Wagner et al. reported that among all fibrous-osseous lesions, only fibrous dysplasia seems to be associated with a considerably increased risk of malignant transformation [11]. Our case was initially diagnosed as OF, distinguished from fibrous dysplasia, because the tumor was clinically well circumscribed and could be partially separated from normal bone during surgery. However, diagnosis in the absence of MDM2 and CDK4 immunohistochemical staining results

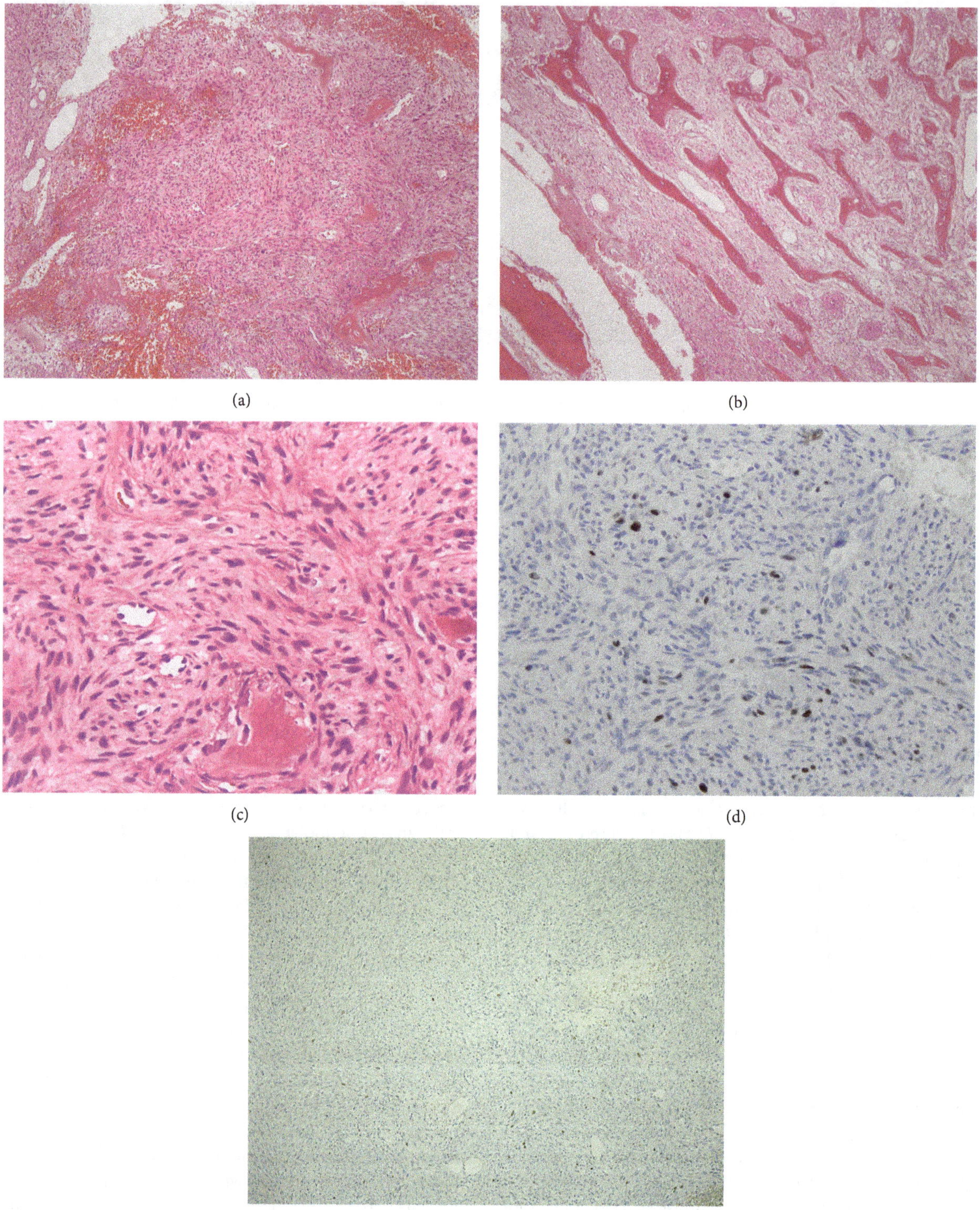

Figure 2: (a) Hematoxylin and eosin staining of the first enucleation (×100). (b) Hematoxylin and eosin staining after the first enucleation (×100). (c) Hematoxylin and eosin staining after the first enucleation (×200). The bundle of spindle cells runs across, and a storiform pattern is observed. Randomly formed woven bone is also observed. There is no atypia, and few mitoses are observed (2–3/50 high-power fields). (d) Immunohistochemical staining. The tumor is positive for MDM2(+). (e) Immunohistochemical staining: Ki-67 index of 2–3%.

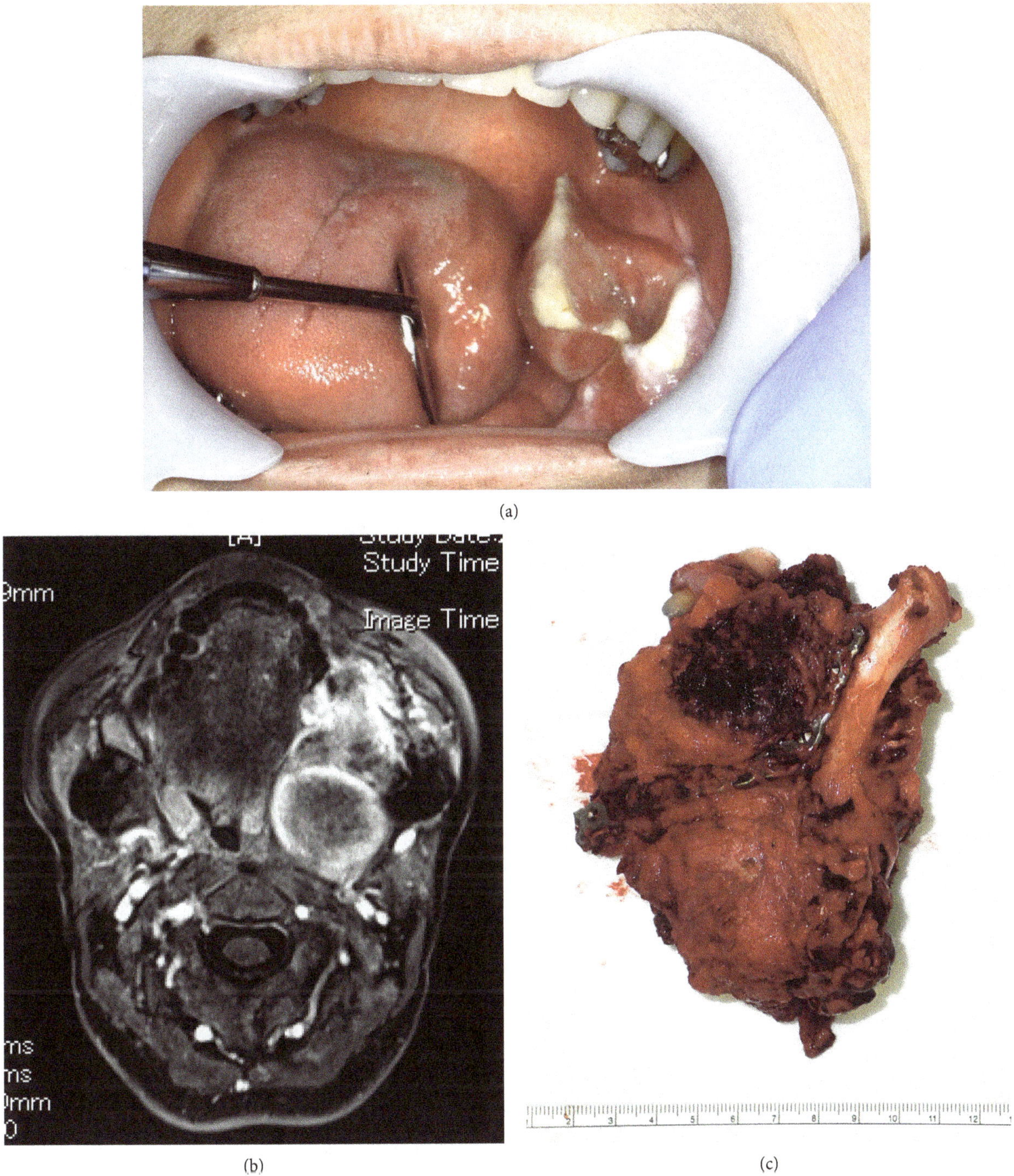

Figure 3: (a) Oral findings for the recurrent tumor. A growing mass is observed at the left posterior part of the mandible showing rapid growth approximately 6 years after the first enucleation. (b) Magnetic resonance image (short-term inversion recovery) depicting a 39 × 64 × 59 mm highly enhanced mass expanding from the left mandible to the parapharyngeal space. (c) The resected specimen.

may cause difficulty in distinguishing these tumors from fibrous-osseous lesions. The first enucleated specimen revealed MDM2(+) and CDK4(-) findings, and the decalcification may have weakened the immunohistochemical staining detection ability. Finally, our case was diagnosed as LCOS based on the clinical course, pathological morphology, and MDM2 and CDK4 immunohistochemical staining findings.

LCOS is also more likely to be misdiagnosed and inappropriately treated with an intralesional procedure because of overlap of its pathological characteristics with those of benign bone tumors [12]. Our patient was initially diagnosed with OF and underwent a resection procedure for benign tumors. However, 4 years and 8 months later, a clinically malignant tumor appeared, and OS was diagnosed following biopsy. Pathologically, during the three surgeries, Ki-67 changed from 2–3% to 15% and then to 40–50%. A previous study reported that all benign fibrous and fibroosseous lesions are negative for MDM2 and CDK4 [4]. In our

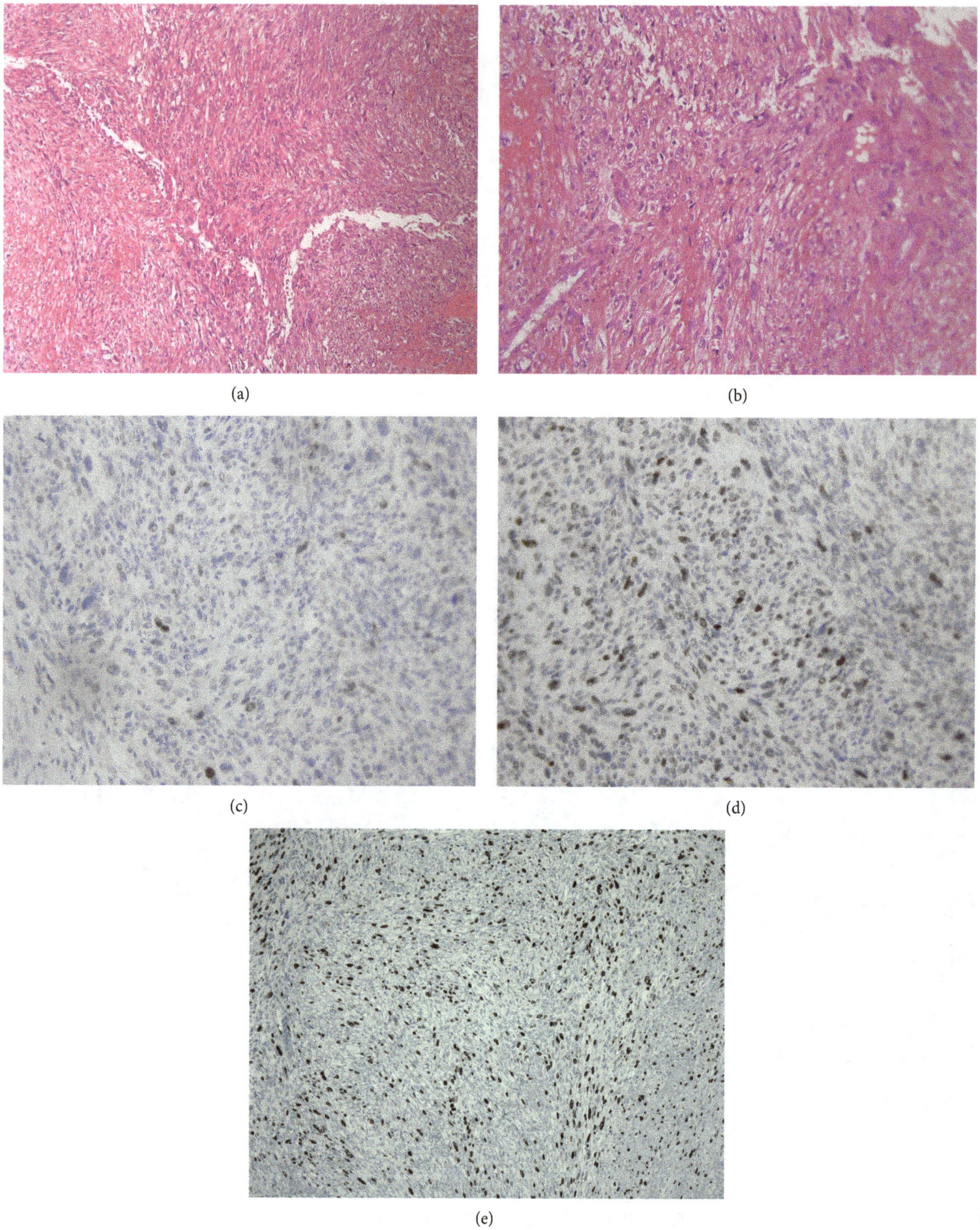

FIGURE 4: (a) Hematoxylin and eosin staining (×100). (b) Hematoxylin and eosin staining (×200). The spindle-like tumor cells appear to have formed thick fascicles with severe atypia around the tumor borders. The cells show more than 100 mitoses/50 high-power fields. There is no osteoid or necrotic tissue. (c) Immunohistochemical staining: positive results for CDK4. (d) Immunohistochemical staining: positive results for MDM2. (e) Immunohistochemical staining: Ki-67 index of 40%–50%.

case, MDM2 changed from a minor component to a positive one at the first enucleation. Based on these results, the initial diagnosis of OF was retrospectively corrected to a diagnosis of LCOS, and the tumor was finally diagnosed as dedifferentiated LCOS.

Dujardin et al. reported that MDM2 and/or CDK4 immunoreactivity was present in 89% of LGOS specimens. Although dedifferentiated LGOS and conventional high-grade OS involve different oncogeneses, they share histological features. Therefore, dedifferentiated LGOS is histologically indistinguishable from conventional OS. MDM2 and CDK4 are also markers for distinguishing between dedifferentiated LGOS and conventional high-grade OSs [4]. Although the prognosis of LGOS is excellent, with 5-year survival rates of 90% with complete resection, in cases of dedifferentiated LGOS, chemotherapy is administered, and the prognosis is similar to that of conventional OS [6]. Toki et al. compared dedifferentiated LGOS with conventional OS, and the 5-year overall survival rates in the dedifferentiated and conventional OS groups were 85.7% and 77.1%, respectively. Dedifferentiated LGOS had a poorer response to a standard chemotherapy regimen than conventional OS, while the clinical outcomes were not markedly different [13]. The prognosis of dedifferentiated LGOS is associated with the timing of synchronous or metachronous dedifferentiation, or the histological amount of dedifferentiated areas remains. Low-grade components are inherently resistant to chemotherapy [13]. Therefore, standard chemotherapy may not be effective for dedifferentiated LGOS. Although our patient did not receive chemotherapy because of her refusal, there was no recurrence or lung metastasis 3 years after the final surgery.

References

[1] A. F. N. M. S. Diniz, J. A. A. Filho, R. C. G. Alencar et al., "Low-grade central osteosarcoma of the mandible: a case study report," *Oral Surgery, Oral Medicine, Oral Pathology, Oral Radiology, and Endodontics*, vol. 103, no. 2, pp. 246–252, 2007.

[2] N. D. Pardhe, A. Jamdade, M. Bajpai, N. Kashyap, and N. Mathur, "Giant osteosarcoma of the mandible," *Journal of College of Physicians and Surgeons Pakistan*, vol. 27, no. 9, pp. S117–S119, 2017.

[3] M. Bajpai, N. Pardhe, B. Chandolia, and M. Arora, "Osteogenic sarcoma of mandible," *Journal of College of Physicians and Surgeons Pakistan*, vol. 27, pp. S26–S27, 2017.

[4] F. Dujardin, M. B. Binh, C. Bouvier et al., "MDM2 and CDK4 immunohistochemistry is a valuable tool in the differential diagnosis of low-grade osteosarcomas and other primary fibro-osseous lesions of the bone," *Modern Pathology*, vol. 24, pp. 624–637, 2011.

[5] H. Miyashita, K. Yoshida, T. Soma et al., "Dedifferentiated parosteal osteosarcoma of the maxilla: a case report and review of the literature," *Journal of Medical Case Reports*, vol. 12, no. 1, p. 235, 2018.

[6] R. Sciot, "MDM2 amplified sarcomas: a literature review," *Diagnostics*, vol. 11, p. 496, 2021.

[7] A. Yoshida, M. A. Bredella, M. Gambarotti, and V. P. Sumathi, "Low-grade central osteosarcoma," in *Soft Tissue Bone Tumors*, pp. 400–402, International Agency for Research on Cancer, Lyon, France, 2020.

[8] S. Kenan, D. T. Ginat, and G. C. Steiner, "Dedifferentiated high-grade osteosarcoma originating from low-grade central osteosarcoma of the fibula," *Skeletal Radiology*, vol. 36, pp. 347–351, 2007.

[9] M. Toya, Y. Yamada, R. Yokoyama et al., "Dedifferentiated low-grade central osteosarcoma with extensive cystic change initially treated as a simple bone cyst," *Pathology, Research and Practice*, vol. 216, no. 4, article 152832, 2020.

[10] K. Triantafillidou, G. Venetis, G. Karakinaris, and F. Iordanidis, "Ossifying fibroma of the jaws: a clinical study of 14 cases and review of the literature," *Oral Surgery, Oral Medicine, Oral Pathology, Oral Radiology*, vol. 114, pp. 193–199, 2012.

[11] V. P. Wagner, R. Carlos, M. J. Romañach, M. A. Lopes, P. M. Speight, and P. A. Vargas, "Malignant transformation of craniomaxillofacial fibro-osseous lesions: a systematic review," *Journal of Oral Pathology & Medicine*, vol. 48, pp. 441–450, 2019.

[12] D. G. Jeon, J. S. Koh, W. H. Cho et al., "Clinical outcome of low-grade central osteosarcoma and role of CDK4 and MDM2 immunohistochemistry as a diagnostic adjunct," *Journal of Orthopaedic Science*, vol. 20, no. 3, pp. 529–537, 2015.

[13] S. Toki, E. Kobayashi, A. Yoshida et al., "A clinical comparison between dedifferentiated low-grade osteosarcoma and conventional osteosarcoma," *The Bone & Joint Journal*, vol. 101-B, no. 6, pp. 745–752, 2019.

19

Forced Eruption: Alternative Treatment Approach to Restore Teeth with Subgingival Structure

Hamid Kermanshah[1,2] **Elmira Najafrad**[1,2] **and Sara Valizadeh**[1,2,3]

[1]*Dental Research Center, Dentistry Research Institute, Tehran University of Medical Sciences, Tehran, Iran*
[2]*Restorative Dentistry Department, School of Dentistry, Tehran University of Medical Sciences, Tehran, Iran*
[3]*Oral Biological and Medical Sciences Department, University of British Columbia, Faculty of Dentistry, Vancouver, BC, Canada*

Correspondence should be addressed to Sara Valizadeh; valizadeh_s@sina.tums.ac.ir

Academic Editor: Andrea Scribante

The management of teeth with deep caries, fracture, or perforation in the cervical third of the root is an integral part of dental practice. Orthodontic extrusion preserves the natural root system and may convert the tooth indicated for extraction into useful tooth with good prognosis and a low risk of failure. Orthodontic tooth eruption can be an alternative to treatment such as surgical crown lengthening, especially in esthetic areas, and provides more favorable conditions for prosthodontic coronal restorations by guaranteeing proper sealing and esthetics and preserving periodontal tissue health. The aim of this case report was to explain a multidisciplinary approach that successfully preserve and treat the teeth with subgingival carious lesion. This innovative method is cost-effective and can be easily done with the equipment available in any office.

1. Introduction

Dentistry is currently making significant strides in meeting the ever-increasing dental and esthetic demands of the community and patients [1, 2]. This has challenged the deep-rooted treatment approaches and values of dentistry, including preserving natural teeth and the root system as long as clinically possible [3].

Esthetic advances in implantology pave the way for successfully and predictably replacing missing teeth, contributing to a "rush-to-implant "mentality, to the detriment of the self-preservation value for patients and the profession [4].

Studies have shown that in 90% of cases, the maxillary anterior facial bone wall thickness is <1 mm, and in 50%, it is <0.5 mm [5, 6]. As a result, thin facial bone walls mainly composed of bundle bone are susceptible to resorption after tooth extraction. Therefore, caution should be exercised when implants are placed in thin gingival biotypes, in which the post-extraction bone is prone to resorb at a high rate, especially in the esthetic zone [7].

In fractured or severely decayed teeth, especially in teeth with previous endodontic treatment, many dentists recommend that a severely damaged/broken endodontically treated tooth should be replaced by an implant [8].

In many cases, dentistry falls short of restoring the normal periodontal architecture, despite novel technologies and biomaterials, soft and hard tissue grafting techniques, and advances in implantology. These shortcomings give rise to sub-optimal esthetic outcomes, including loss of interdental papillae or marginal gingival heights not aligned esthetically with adjacent teeth [1, 9].

Orthodontic tooth extrusion has been advocated instead of sacrificing the natural root system [2, 7]. If this technique is applied correctly, it gives rise to the preservation of the natural root system and the associated periodontal structure and architecture, and the patient can enjoy years of additional service. It can also preserve adjacent supporting tooth structures and the choice for reconstruction with implants [9, 10].

Surgical extrusion is an alternative to extraction for teeth with crown-root fractures, cervical root fractures, and subgingival caries. It is based on the concept of relocating the affected area of a tooth to a supragingival position, leaving sound tooth structure exposed to improve tooth restorability, and providing space for the reestablishment of the biological width. It is widely accepted that the success of surgical extrusion mainly depends on an atraumatic extraction method with as little damage as possible to the cementoblast layer on the root surface; otherwise, progressive root resorption or ankylosis and marginal bone loss or tooth mobility will occur.

Orthodontic root extrusion was first introduced by Heithersay and Ingber [11] to preserve the biologic width, expose sound tooth structure for optimal placement of restorative margins, and achieve esthetics [12].

Orthodontic extrusion is not possible in these situations: unfavorable axial tooth position, compromised periodontal health, short roots that lead to inadequate crown-to-root ratio, and wide internal root form [13].

Orthodontic tooth eruption is the preferred treatment modality to avoid the negative consequences of surgical crown lengthening, especially in esthetic areas. It is an interdisciplinary treatment requiring the expertise of endodontists, periodontists, orthodontists, and restorative dentists [14].

Some of the advantages of orthodontic forced eruption are improved bone level, low cost, and less time; however, poor esthetic outcomes during treatment and the need for more patient cooperation are the disadvantages of this technique [15].

This paper describes two cases with orthodontic extrusion of one and four teeth and the multidisciplinary management of such teeth with subgingival margins.

2. Case Reports

2.1. Case 1. A 48-year-old female patient whose chief complaint was the replacement and esthetic appearance of her upper right lateral incisor, canine, and premolar teeth was referred for treatment to the Restorative Department, Faculty of Dentistry, Tehran University of Medical Sciences, Iran.

The teeth had been endodontically treated one month earlier. The patient's medical history was noncontributory. Clinical examination revealed an extensively damaged crown with thin mesial and palatal walls in the lateral incisor, a too short labial wall in canine, buccal and palatal walls in the first premolar, and palatal wall in the second premolar. The rest of the tooth structures were located 2–3 mm below the gingival margin (Figures 1 and 2).

There was no tenderness on percussion or palpation. The periodontal condition of the teeth was normal with no pockets. The teeth had mobility within the normal limits (Grade 1) without any noticeable swelling. The radiographic examination confirmed that the roots had been endodontically treated without pathosis (Figures 3 and 4).

After analyzing factors such as the height of the smile line, patient's age, root anatomy, and financial resources, with the patient's consent, the teeth were decided to be treated through extrusion to allow the fabrication of crowns

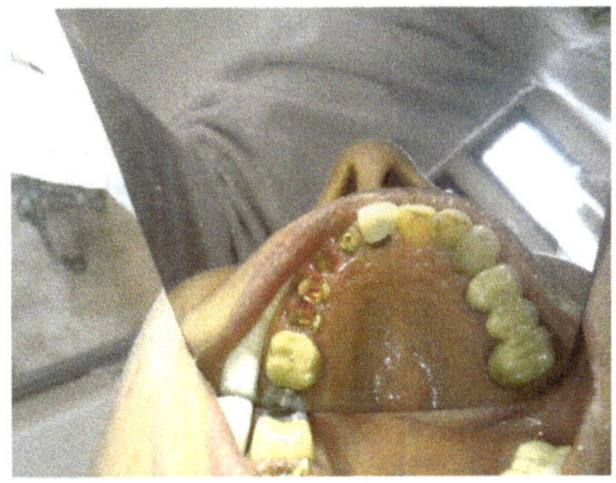

FIGURE 1: Occlusal view of central, lateral, canine, and premolars.

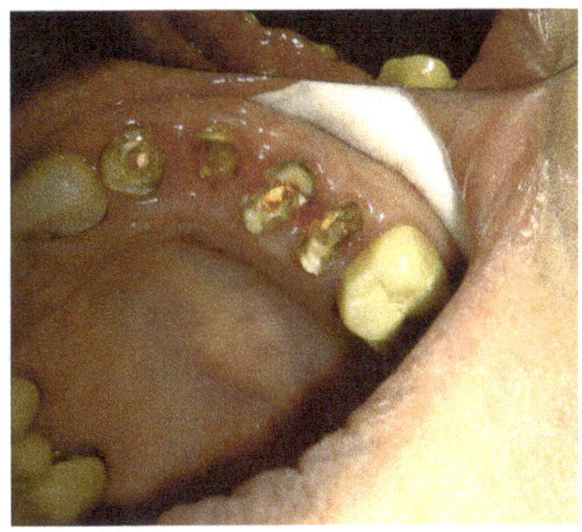

FIGURE 2: Occlusal and palatal view of central, lateral, canine, and premolars.

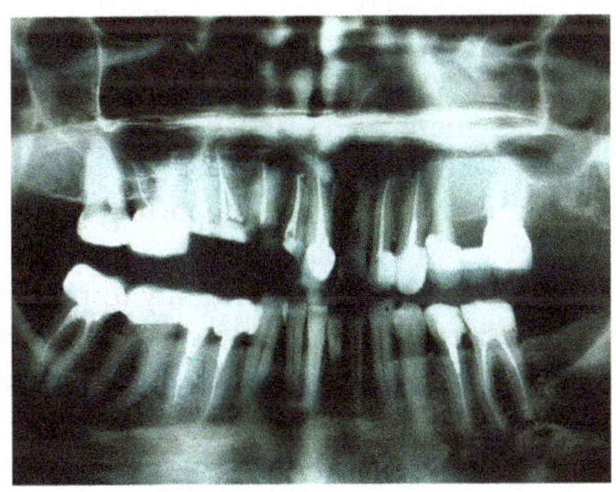

FIGURE 3: Panoramic radiographic view of patient's teeth.

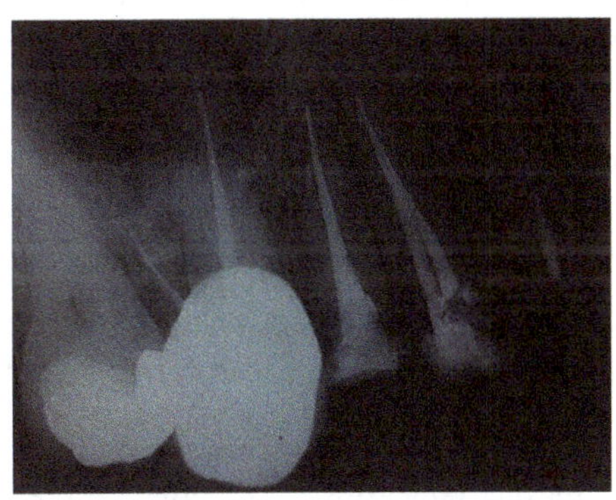

FIGURE 4: Periapical radiographic view of patient's teeth.

for these teeth to achieve improved esthetics and adequate biological width.

The estimated crown-root ratio and the remaining tooth structure were considered. Then, extrusion of approximately 4 mm for canine and 3 mm for the rest of the teeth was deemed adequate for achieving sufficient biologic width and a ferrule for the final restoration.

A fixed appliance was used in this case. After providing oral hygiene instructions (OHI) and implementing prophylactic measures, the carious lesions were eliminated. Because of the inadequate tooth structure remaining in the canine, approximately 5 mm of gutta-percha was removed from the root canal. A hook was fabricated with a piece of SS round wire (Dentarum, Inspringen, Germany), measuring 1 mm in diameter, with several artificial notches on its body for improved retention following cementation. The hook was cemented in the canine root canal with zinc phosphate cement (Harvard, Dahlwitz-Hoppegarten, Germany). For the rest of the teeth, after composite resin build-up, a composite resin bottom was bonded at the gingival area of their remaining buccal wall.

Also, an archwire was shaped conforming to the upper arch and fixed on the buccal surface of the teeth, extending from the first upper right molar to the upper left lateral incisor and covered by flowable composite resin. The wire was adjusted so that it did not interfere with protrusive and excursive movements. An elastic thread was passed between the hook and the archwire. The distance between the hooks and wire was determined, and the elastics were connected to the hooks on the provisional crown, curling around the supporting wire (Figures 5 and 6). The elastic thread was replaced with a shorter one every seven days until predetermined extrusion was achieved. The patient was instructed on how to use fresh elastics daily and to wear them continuously.

Periodic evaluations were carried out every two weeks, and movements were measured for two months. After achieving favorable extrusion, the supporting wire and composite resin were removed, followed by a crown-lengthening procedure and circumferential fiberotomy to rearrange gingival, bone, and periodontal fiber levels to conform to the tooth new position (Figures 7 and 8). No active force was applied during a 60-day stabilization period. The extruded tooth was splinted to the adjacent teeth using composite resin to maintain the tooth position achieved by extrusion.

After a two-month maintenance period, the wire was removed, and the interim crown and hooks were trimmed with diamond burs. PFM crowns were fabricated for these four teeth after core preparation (Figures 9 and 10).

The patient was followed periodically for six years. No signs of postoperative gingival inflammation and other periodontal changes were detected.

2.2. Case 2. A 32-year-old male patient was referred to the Restorative Dentistry Department, Faculty of Dentistry, Tehran University of Medical Sciences, Iran, with the chief complaint of a dislodged crown of his upper left central incisor three times. The patient also wanted to change the PFM crowns of maxillary incisors. He reported no other associated symptoms (Figures 11 and 12) The patient's medical

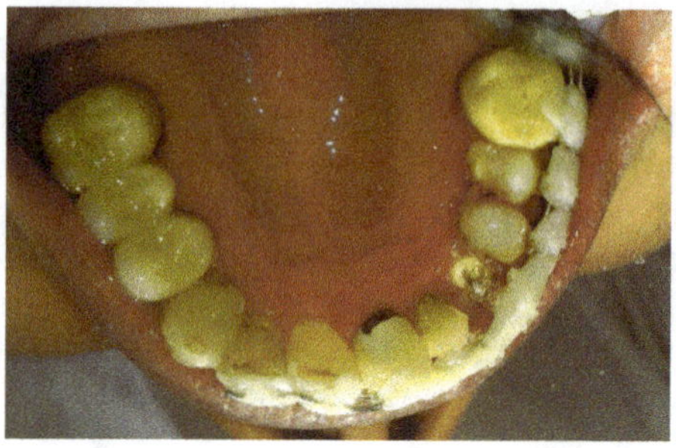

Figure 5: Occlusal view of fixed appliance used for orthodontic extrusion of four teeth.

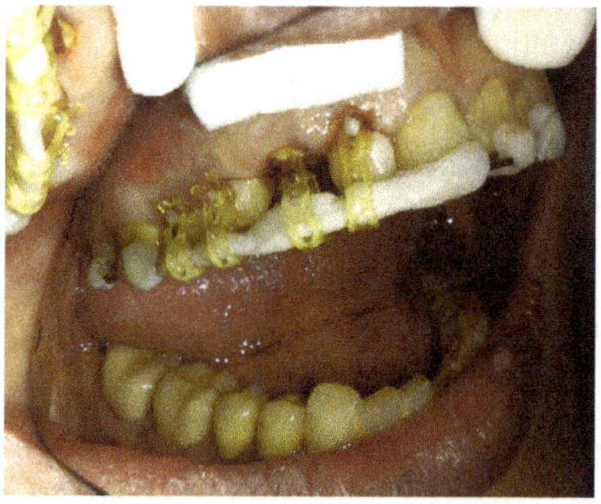

Figure 6: Buccal view of fixed appliance used for orthodontic extrusion of four teeth.

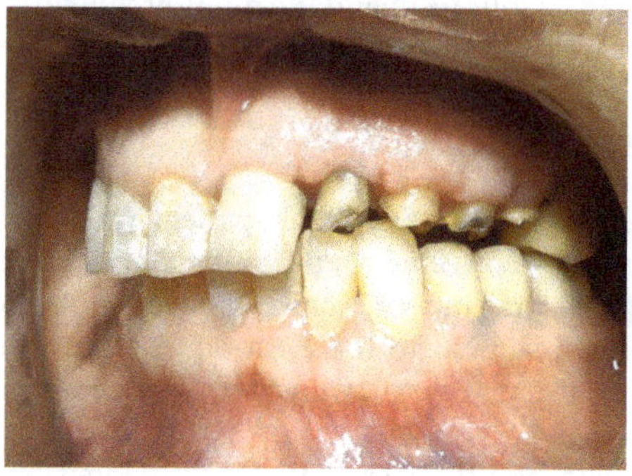

Figure 7: Buccal view of force erupted teeth after crown lengthening.

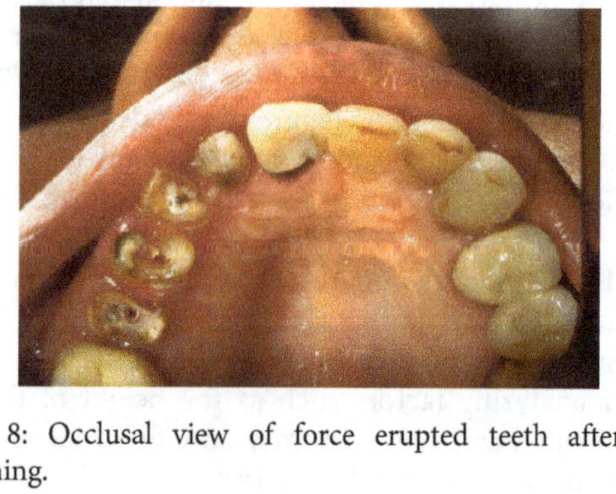

Figure 8: Occlusal view of force erupted teeth after crown lengthening.

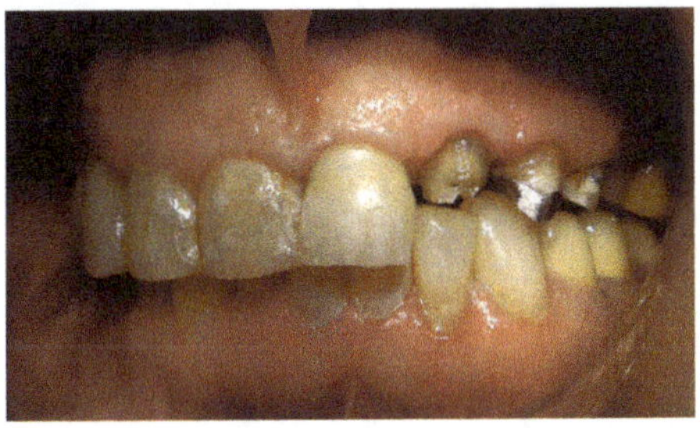

FIGURE 9: Buccal view of core preparation.

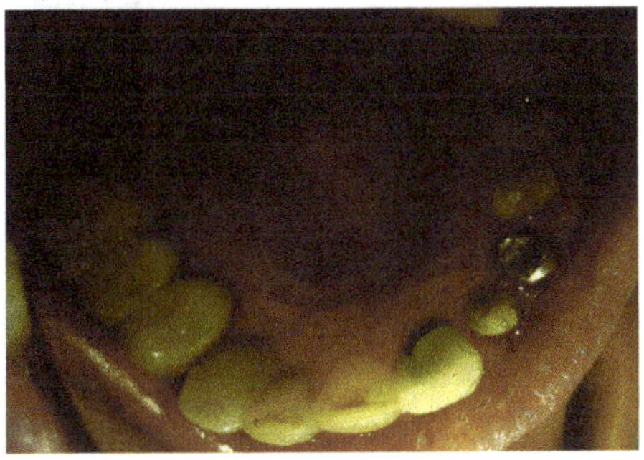

FIGURE 10: Occlusal view of core preparation.

and familial histories were noncontributory, and the extraoral examination results were unremarkable. Clinical examination showed that the tooth structure in the left central incisor was located 2–3 mm below the gingival margin due to extensive decay, with inadequate ferrule to support the crown. Therefore, crown dislodgment had happened many times (Figure 13).

The teeth were asymptomatic and responded negatively to palpation and percussion. There was adequate keratinized gingiva around the tooth, with no inflammation, and the gingival biotype was thin. Periodontal probing depths around the tooth were within the normal range. Radiographic examination showed that the patient's all maxillary incisors were root canal-treated, with custom metal posts and cores; excessive removal of gutta-percha from root canal was noticed in the left central incisor (Figure 14).

A consent form was obtained from the patient for the treatment plan, which consisted of a multidisciplinary approach for plaque control and oral hygiene instructions, orthodontic extrusion and conservative endodontic retreatment of the upper left central incisor, periodontal surgery, and restoration of maxillary incisors.

By considering the estimated crown-to-root ratio and the carious tooth structure in the upper left central incisor, 3–4 mm of extrusion was deemed adequate for achieving sufficient biologic width and ferrule for the final restoration. After removing the carious lesions from the tooth, the previously dislodged post-and-core crown was used to ensure that the anterior region would remain esthetically pleasing during orthodontic forced eruption treatment, with no need to make a temporary crown. The crown was cemented with zinc polycarboxylate cement (Harvard, Dahlwitz-Hoppegarten, Germany); a dentinal pin was then bonded to the most cervical part of the buccal surface of the crown perpendicularly, using composite resin restorative material (Z250: 3 M ESPE, St. Paul, MN, USA) to create a hook for elastic insertion. The wire was made to conform to the upper arch shape using a round 19-gauge rigid stainless steel and bonded to the buccal surface

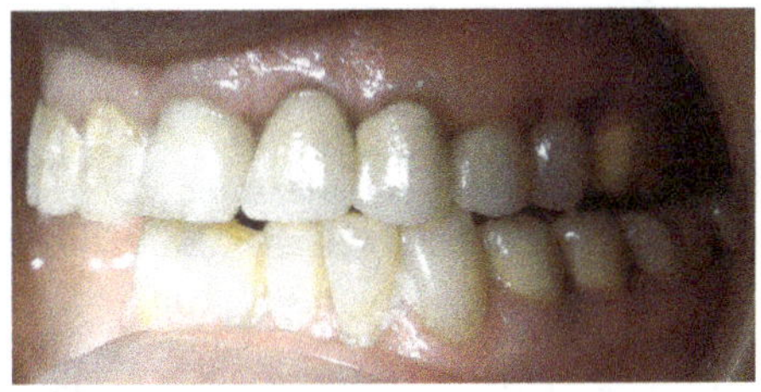

FIGURE 11: Buccal view of PFM crowns for upper left lateral, canine, and premolars.

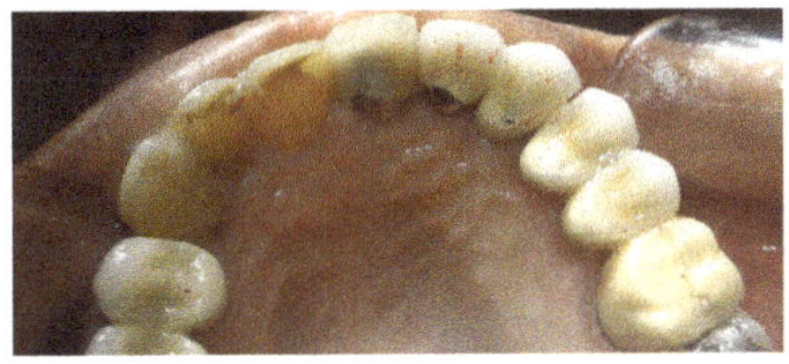

FIGURE 12: Occlusal view of PFM crowns for upper left lateral, canine, and premolars.

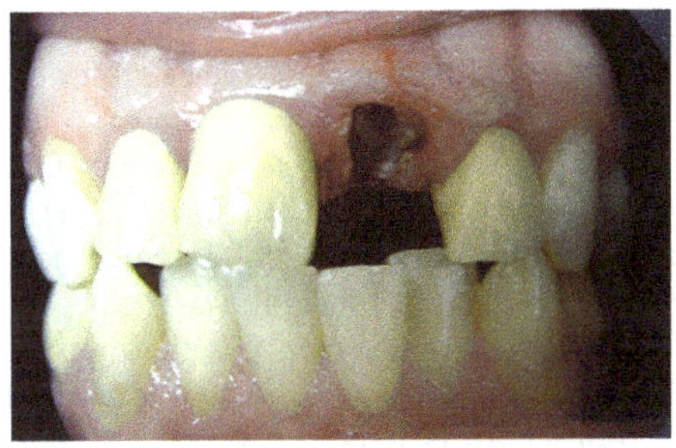

FIGURE 13: Frontal view of incisor teeth.

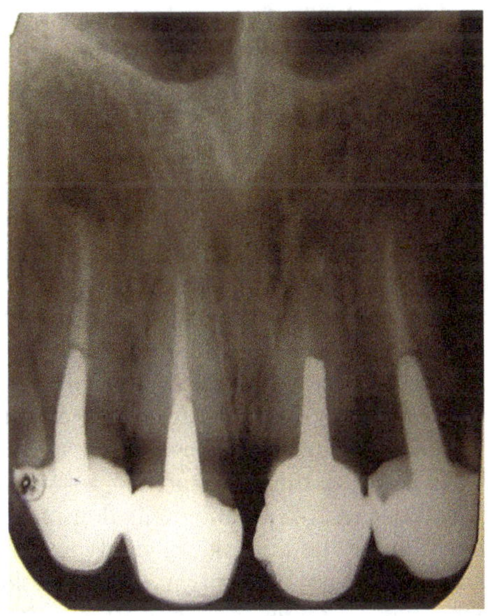

FIGURE 14: Radiographic view of patient's teeth.

of adjacent teeth (the right canine to the left canine) using the composite material. An elastic thread was passed between the pin and the wire (Figure 15).

A 30-g force was applied, measured using a Dontrix gauge (13). The elastic thread was changed every seven days until the predetermined extrusion was achieved. The extrusion was completed in two months (Figure 16). Endodontic retreatment was undertaken immediately after the stabilization period (3–4 weeks). A clinical examination showed that the root canal treatments of other incisors were satisfactory enough to carry out the restorative procedure. Crown lengthening was undertaken to restore gingival contours properly. After a healing period of 4 weeks, a ferrule of 2 mm was achieved. Cast post-and-core of the left central and definitive coronal restorations (pressed/metal crowns) were then fabricated for all incisors (Figures 17 and 18).

The patient was followed for five years, and the treatment outcome was favorable (Figure 19).

3. Discussion

Extensive caries or crown fractures might create a difficult situation for restoration placement. The significant problem is the lack of adequate coronal ferrule and a compromised biological width. Tooth extrusive movements entail the application of tractional forces throughout the periodontium to induce the marginal apposition of crestal bone [16].

Increased alveolar crest height was achieved through slow orthodontic tooth movements. If the tooth remaining structure is below the alveolar bone and free gingival margin, and if the root length is sufficient to provide support for a coronal restoration, the root can be treated endodontically, followed by orthodontic extrusion. Forced eruption provides more favorable conditions for prosthodontic coronal restorations by guaranteeing proper sealing and esthetics and preserving periodontal tissue health [17]. A histological evaluation by Simon et al. indicated that extrusion of endodontically treated teeth did not pose any apparent problems. They reported that the alveolar process moves in the occlusal direction as the tooth is extruded, followed by bone deposition at the alveolar crest and the interradicular area [18].

The cases reported here consisted of teeth with subgingival carious lesions that were successfully treated using a multidisciplinary approach. Among the treatment options for such cases, such as extraction followed by implant rehabilitation, orthodontic extrusion was deemed the best choice. Implant rehabilitation in such cases often involves surgical procedures to improve the hard and soft tissue profiles of implant recipient sites. Systematic evaluation of interproximal and buccal bone and the amount and type of soft tissue available at the implant site might determine long-term esthetic outcomes. The pink and white esthetic scores (PES and WES) are tools that objectively evaluate implant restorations in the esthetic zone and describe the patient's appraisal of their treatment outcomes [19]. A gingival thickness of ≥2 mm was deemed a thick tissue biotype, and a gingival thickness of <1.5 mm was deemed a thin tissue biotype. The prevalence of thin gingival biotype is 43% in the maxillary incisor area [20, 21]. The PES/WES scores of patients

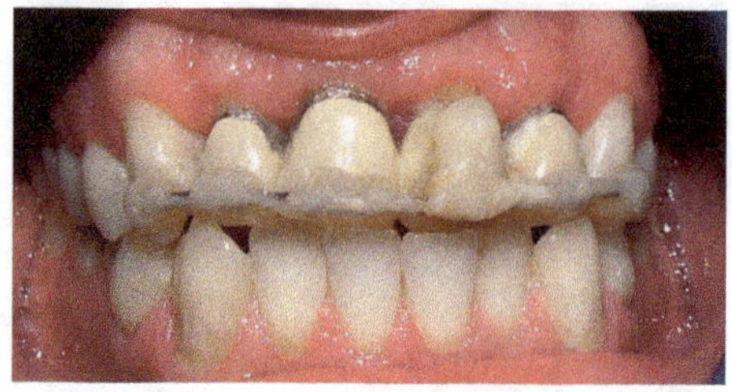

FIGURE 15: Extrusion with 19-gauge stainless steel arch wire.

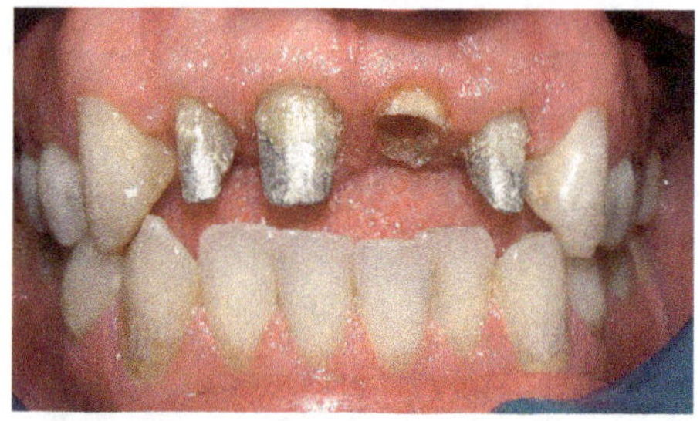

FIGURE 16: After extrusion and remove of other incisors crowns elastic force.

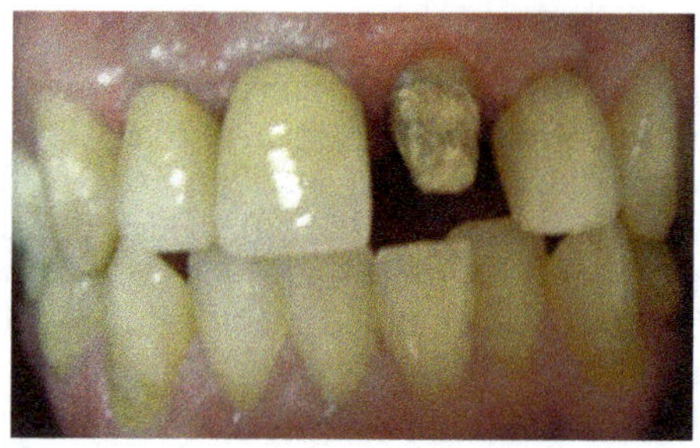

FIGURE 17: Preparation of cast post.

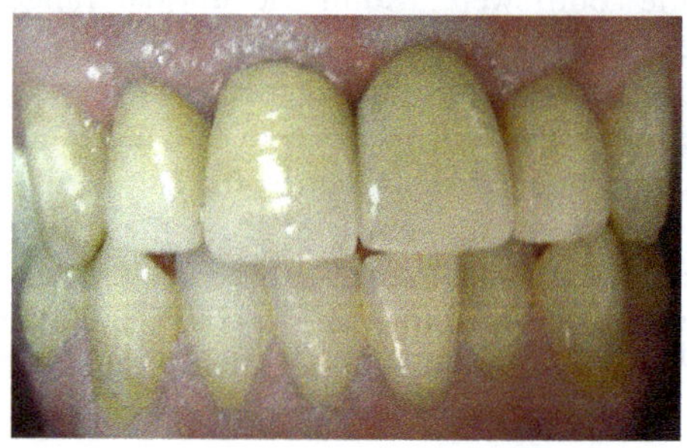

FIGURE 18: Placement of crowns.

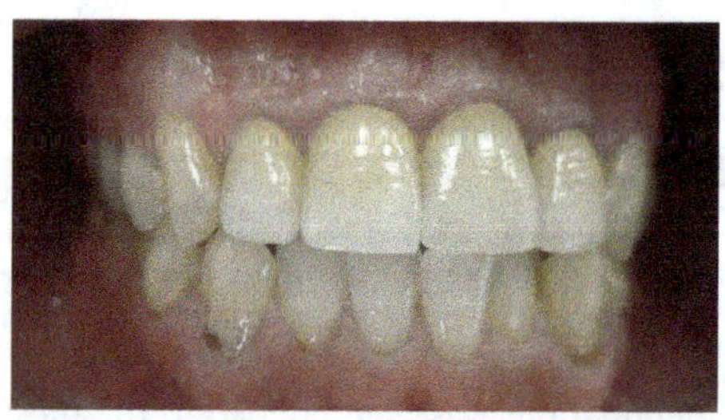

FIGURE 19: Clinical view after 5 years follow-up.

with a thick gingival biotype are significantly higher than those with a thin gingival biotype. A thin gingival biotype might fail to reach the clinically acceptable PES level [22, 23]. Peri-implant soft tissue stability depends on the gingival biotype as a significant parameter for the esthetic outcome of the implant restoration in the esthetic zone [24]. The gingival tissue's potential to cover any underlying material is of utmost importance for achieving aesthetic outcomes, especially in implant, regenerative, and restorative procedures, where subgingival metallic restorations are used [25]. During the restoration of maxillary central incisors, it is important to preserve or reconstruct the interdental papillae. Orthodontic extrusion enhances the quality and quantity of the papilla [26].

The simplified forced eruption technique described has several advantages over other methods; because orthodontic band and bracket are not required, with bonded brackets, there is a necessity to align the anteriors, and time will be lost as a result. Furthermore, reciprocal forces of intrusion might act on the adjacent teeth. In this method, using dentinal pin on the buccal surface of the tooth instead of using a hook inside the root canal has led to overcome the problem of short distance between the hook and the wire to place the elastics; in addition, we will not have occlusal interferences in the palatal surface of the tooth. Therefore, this method can be easily done with the equipment available in any office.

One point that should be considered is that one of the most common ways to prevent caries during orthodontic treatment is to use topical fluoride products such as fluoride varnish and mouthwash. These substances lead to the formation of fluorhydroxyapatite in enamel prisms, which are more resistant to acid attacks and can interfere with the bonding procedures of the composite to the enamel. Therefore, it is recommended that there be more than 15 days delay between the application of topical fluoride products and the bonding procedure to the enamel to achieve the optimal bond strength [27].

Whatever appliance is used, the patient must be seen every 1 to 2 weeks to reduce the occlusal surface of the tooth being extruded, control inflammation, and monitor progress. During the eruptive phase, the application of gel with postbiotics can be useful to prevent gingivitis following plaque accumulation, which can lead to attachment loss and tissue destruction due to the presence of periopathogenic bacteria [28].

The patient's age, the distance the tooth is to be moved, and the PDL viability determine the time required for forced eruption [29]. The extrusion rate used in these cases was similar to that recommended by another author [17]. After two months of extrusion, 3–4 mm of the roots were exposed at an average speed of 0.5 mm/week, while other authors reported an average extrusion rate of 1 mm/week [11, 30]. Slow extrusion requires a 15-g force for the delicate root of a lower incisor tooth, with a 60-g force for a molar tooth. According to some authors, the maximum force for a slow movement should not exceed 30 g [31, 32]; however, rapid extrusion is accomplished by applying forces >50 g. Therefore, extended retention periods are necessary for stabilizing the tooth for the remodeling and adaptation of the periodontal structures to the new tooth position [33]. In these cases, a 30-g force was exerted.

Pressed/metal crowns were used for final restorations. Pre- and postoperative comparisons revealed excellent esthetic results. Moreover, compared to all-ceramic restorations, which require a shoulder finish line, this treatment was considered more conservative. The application of toothpaste and mouthwash containing paraprobiotics-based agents would be an effective protocol for the home maintenance of oral health [34].

4. Conclusion

Orthodontic extrusion or forced eruption is a conservative treatment modality to restore fractured or extensively damaged teeth at a subgingival level to preserve the natural tooth and maintain periodontal architecture.

Additional Points

Key Clinical Message. The forced eruption is an appropriate method for preserving teeth with large destruction of submarginal tissue if case selection was done precisely.

Consent

All authors declare that they agree for publishing this paper in this journal.

Authors' Contributions

Hamid Kermanshah conceived the idea and performed the treatment. Sara Valizadeh and Elmira Najafrad wrote the manuscript, were involved in the project management, and collected the data. The authors alone are responsible for the content and writing of the paper.

References

[1] R. A. Levine, "Forced eruption in the esthetic zone," *The Compendium of Continuing Education in Dentistry*, vol. 18, pp. 795–803, 1997.

[2] R. C. Mandel, W. C. Binzer, and J. A. Withers, "Forced eruption in restoring severely fractured teeth using removable orthodontic appliances," *The Journal of Prosthetic Dentistry*, vol. 47, no. 3, pp. 269–274, 1982.

[3] T. J. Salinas, "A three-unit FPD vs. single tooth implant restoration: what is the standard of care?," in *Annual meeting of the academy of prosthodontics*, Boston, MA, 2003.

[4] F. W. Benenati and J. H. Simon, "Orthodontic root extrusion: its rationale and uses," *General Dentistry*, vol. 34, no. 4, pp. 285–289, 1986.

[5] A. L. Januario, W. R. Duarte, M. Barriviera, J. C. Mesti, M. G. Araujo, and J. Lindhe, "Dimension of the facial bone wall in

the anterior maxilla: a cone-beam computed tomography study," *Clinical Oral Implants Research*, vol. 22, no. 10, pp. 1168–1171, 2011.

[6] C. Vera, I. J. De Kok, D. Reinhold et al., "Evaluation of buccal alveolar bone dimension of maxillary anterior and premolar teeth: a cone beam computed tomography investigation," *The International Journal of Oral & Maxillofacial Implants*, vol. 27, no. 6, pp. 1514–1519, 2012.

[7] V. Chappuis, M. G. Araújo, and D. Buser, "Clinical relevance of dimensional bone and soft tissue alterations post-extraction in esthetic sites," *Periodontology 2000*, vol. 73, no. 1, pp. 73–83, 2017.

[8] D. F. Murchison and R. S. Schwartz, "The use of removable appliances for forced eruption of teeth," *Quintessence International*, vol. 17, no. 8, pp. 497–501, 1986.

[9] D. Ziskind, E. Sharon, Z. Hirschfeld, and A. Becker, "Analysis of lateral tooth movement during forced orthodontic eruption," *The Journal of Prosthetic Dentistry*, vol. 84, no. 4, pp. 462–466, 2000.

[10] J. H. Simon, W. H. Kelly, D. G. Gordon, and G. W. Ericksen, "Extrusion of endodontically treated teeth," *Journal of the American Dental Association (1939)*, vol. 97, no. 1, pp. 17–23, 1978.

[11] J. S. Ingber, "Forced eruption: part II. A method of treating nonrestorable teeth—Periodontal and restorative considerations," *Journal of Periodontology*, vol. 47, no. 4, pp. 203–216, 1976.

[12] B. Bielicka, M. Bartkowiak, E. Urban, and M. Tomasz, "Holistic approach in the management of subgingivally fractured premolar tooth: case report," *Dental and Medical Problems*, vol. 45, pp. 211–214, 2008.

[13] S. R. Fidel, R. A. Fidel-Junior, L. M. Sassone, C. F. Murad, and R. A. Fidel, "Clinical management of a complicated crown-root fracture: a case report," *Brazilian Dental Journal*, vol. 22, no. 3, pp. 258–262, 2011.

[14] A. R. Singh and R. Verma, "Crown lengthening vs forced eruption," *Orthodontic Journal of Nepal*, vol. 1, no. 1, pp. 52–55, 2011.

[15] K. Sirisha, Y. R. Shankar, N. S. Yalavarthy, and K. Suneetha, "Management of crown root fractures: a novel technique with multidisciplinary approach," *Journal of Dr. NTR University of Health Sciences*, vol. 2, no. 1, pp. 72–77, 2013.

[16] S. S. Patil, A. S. Panicker, A. Hindlekar, S. R. Srinidhi, A. Dhumal, and K. Vhora, "Forced orthodontic extrusion for anterior traumatized teeth by a simplistic approach," *Journal of Dental and Allied Sciences*, vol. 3, no. 2, p. 111, 2014.

[17] B. Bielicka, M. Bartkowiak, E. Urban, and M. Tomasz, "Clinical Case," *Dental and Medical Problems*, vol. 45, no. 2, pp. 211–214, 2008.

[18] J. H. Simon, J. B. Lythgoe, and M. Torabinejad, "Clinical and histologic evaluation of extruded endodontically treated teeth in dogs," *Oral Surgery, Oral Medicine, Oral Pathology*, vol. 50, no. 4, pp. 361–371, 1980.

[19] A. R. Jones and W. Martin, "Comparing pink and white esthetic scores to layperson perception in the single-tooth implant patient," *The International Journal of Oral & Maxillofacial Implants*, vol. 29, no. 6, pp. 1348–1353, 2014.

[20] N. Claffey and D. Shanley, "Relationship of gingival thickness and bleeding to loss of probing attachment in shallow sites following non-surgical periodontal therapy," *Journal of Clinical Periodontology*, vol. 13, no. 7, pp. 654–657, 1986.

[21] K. H. Zawawi and M. S. Al-Zahrani, "Gingival biotype in relation to incisors' inclination and position," *Saudi Medical Journal*, vol. 35, no. 11, pp. 1378–1383, 2014.

[22] M. A. Altay, A. Sindel, H. A. Tezerişener, N. Yıldırımyan, and M. M. Özarslan, "Esthetic evaluation of implant-supported single crowns: a comparison of objective and patient-reported outcomes," *International Journal of Implant Dentistry*, vol. 5, no. 1, 2019.

[23] C. Angkaew, P. Serichetaphongse, S. Krisdapong, M. M. Dart, and A. Pimkhaokham, "Oral health-related quality of life and esthetic outcome in single anterior maxillary implants," *Clinical Oral Implants Research*, vol. 28, no. 9, pp. 1089–1096, 2017.

[24] W. R. Proffit, H. W. Field Jr., J. L. Ackerman, L. J. Bailey, and J. F. Camilla Tulloch, *Contemporary Orthodontics*, Mosby, St Louis, 3rd ed edition, 2000.

[25] R. S. Manjunath, A. Rana, and A. Sarkar, "Gingival biotype assessment in a healthy periodontium: transgingival probing method," *Journal of Clinical and Diagnostic Research: JCDR*, vol. 9, no. 5, pp. ZC66–ZC69, 2015.

[26] G. L. Ribeiro, J. V. Maciel, P. J. da Silva, and O. M. Tanaka, "Forced eruption for all four maxillary incisors prior to implant rehabilitation," *European Journal of General Dentistry*, vol. 1, no. 2, pp. 99–103, 2012.

[27] G. Cossellu, V. Lanteri, A. Butera, N. Laffi, A. Merlini, and G. Farronato, "Timing considerations on the shear bond strength of orthodontic brackets after topical fluoride varnish applications," *Journal of Orthodontic Science*, vol. 6, no. 1, pp. 11–15, 2017.

[28] A. Butera, S. Gallo, M. Pascadopoli, D. Taccardi, and A. Scribante, "Home oral care of periodontal patients using antimicrobial gel with postbiotics, lactoferrin, and Aloe barbadensis leaf juice powder vs. conventional chlorhexidine gel: a split-mouth randomized clinical trial," *Antibiotics*, vol. 11, no. 1, 2022.

[29] J. Y. Kan, K. Rungcharassaeng, J. L. Lozada, and G. Zimmerman, "Classification of sagittal root position in relation to the anterior maxillary osseous housing for immediate implant placement: a cone beam computed tomography study," *International Journal of Oral & Maxillofacial Implants*, vol. 26, no. 4, pp. 873–876, 2011.

[30] L. J. Oesterle and L. W. Wood, "Raising the root," *The Journal of the American Dental Association*, vol. 122, no. 7, pp. 193–198, 1991.

[31] L. Minsk, "The role of enamel matrix proteins in periodontal regeneration," *Compendium of Continuing Education in Dentistry*, vol. 21, no. 3, pp. 210–2, 214, 2000.

[32] K. Reitan, "Clinical and histologic observations on tooth movement during and after orthodontic treatment," *American Journal of Orthodontics*, vol. 53, no. 10, pp. 721–745, 1967.

[33] L. Bondemark, J. Kurol, A. L. Hallonsten, and J. O. Andreasen, "Attractive magnets for orthodontic extrusion of crown-root fractured teeth," *American Journal of Orthodontics and Dentofacial Orthopedics*, vol. 112, no. 2, pp. 187–193, 1997.

[34] A. Butera, S. Gallo, M. Pascadopoli et al., "Paraprobiotics in non-surgical periodontal therapy: clinical and microbiological aspects in a 6-month follow-up domiciliary protocol for oral hygiene," *Microorganisms*, vol. 10, no. 2, p. 337, 2022.

20

Prosthetic Rehabilitation on Edentulous Patients with Microstomia: About Three Cases

Oumaima Tayari, Jamila Jaouadi, Safa Jemli, Hela Haloui, and Ali Ben Rahma

Complete Removable Prosthodontic Department, Research Laboratory LR12ES11, Faculty of Dental Medicine, University of Monastir, Monastir, Tunisia

Correspondence should be addressed to Oumaima Tayari; oumaimatayari0@gmail.com

Academic Editor: Giuseppe Alessandro Scardina

Limited oral opening is an acquired or congenital abnormal condition that compromises patient esthetics, nutrition, and quality of life. In addition, it may hinder conventional prosthetic procedures of edentulous patients, make it challenging, and present difficulties at all its stages. This clinical report presents different clinical treatment options suitable to be chosen by the prosthodontic carer in the case of reduced oral aperture.

1. Introduction

The reduction of oral opening (microstomia) is a change seen in a minority of patients [1]. It can occur due to electrical, thermal, or chemical burns, maxillofacial trauma, surgical treatment for orofacial neoplasms and reconstruction of lip defects (cleft lips), head and neck radiotherapy, microinvasion of the muscles of mastication or temporomandibular joint (TMJ) dysfunction syndrome, genetic disorders such as partial duplication of chromosome 6q, Hallopeau-Siemens-type recessive dystrophic epidermolysis bullosa, Freeman–Sheldon (whistling face) syndrome, Burton skeletal dysplasia, and diseases such as Plummer–Vinson syndrome or scleroderma and connective tissue diseases such as systemic sclerosis or other systemic disease [2–5].

Due to the restricted mouth opening, patients often face difficulty with eating and sometimes speech. In addition, it is difficult for them to insert and remove the prosthesis [5, 6].

In the other hand, this condition presents a challenge for the clinician through all the prosthetic treatment stages. It may be impossible to make impressions and fabricate dentures using conventional methods, so a modified denture approach, depending on the cause and severity of microstomia, must be employed [7–9].

Literature is abundant with various techniques of prosthodontic management of limited oral opening, and this paper aims at presenting different prosthodontic options for managements of edentulous patients with microstomia.

2. Case Report 1

A 26-year-old male was referred to the Department of Prosthodontics, Faculty of Dental Medicine, University of Monastir, Tunisia, for prosthetic rehabilitation. He was suffering from microstomia resulting of radiotherapy about 12 years ago following cavum carcinoma classified T3N0M0 (Figure 1). The patient had no experience about removable complete prosthesis rehabilitation.

Oral examination revealed a limited maximal mouth opening (MMO) measuring about 21 mm, with tight and inflexible labial tissues (Figures 2(a) and 2(b)).

He presented complete edentulous maxillary and mandibular resorbed ridges.

Restricted oral access made it difficult to make primary impression using classic stock impression trays. Hence, the choice was made to fabricate a mandibular sectional impression tray for each half of the arch by manually molding soft wax to the ridge, intraorally (Figure 3(a)). Then, the sectional special trays were reinforced by the autopoly-

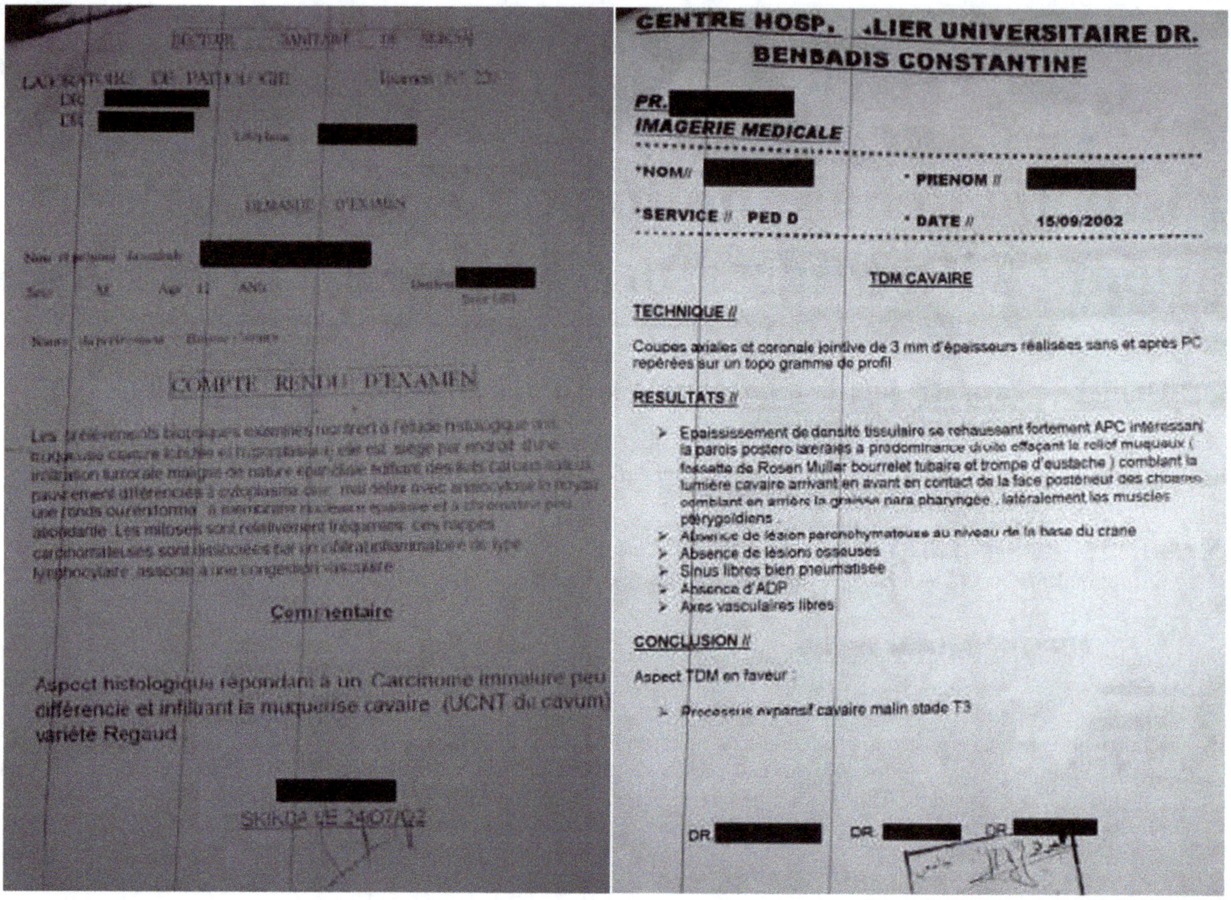

COMPTE RENDU D'EXAMEN

Commentaire

Aspect histologique répondant à un Carcinome immature peu différencie et infiltrant la muqueuse cavaire (UCNT du cavum) variété Regaud

SKIKDA LE 24/07/02

CENTRE HOSP. .LIER UNIVERSITAIRE DR. BENBADIS CONSTANTINE

PR.
IMAGERIE MEDICALE

*NOM// * PRENOM //

*SERVICE // PED D * DATE // 15/09/2002

TDM CAVAIRE

TECHNIQUE //

Coupes axiales et coronale jointive de 3 mm d'épaisseurs réalisées sans et après PC repérées sur un topo gramme de profil

RESULTATS //

- Epaississement de densité tissulaire se rehaussant fortement APC intéressant la parois postero laterales a predominance droite effaçant le relief muqueux (fossette de Rosen Muller bourrelet tubaire et trompe d'eustache) comblant la lumière cavaire arrivant en avant en contact de la face posterieur des choanes comblant en arrière la graisse para pharyngée , latéralement les muscles ptérygoïdiens .
- Absence de lésion parenchymateuse au niveau de la base du crane
- Absence de lésions osseuses
- Sinus libres bien pneumatisee
- Absence d'ADP
- Axes vasculaires libres

CONCLUSION //

Aspect TDM en faveur :

- Processus expansif cavaire malin stade T3

DR. DR. DR.

Figure 1: Histological and CT scan results.

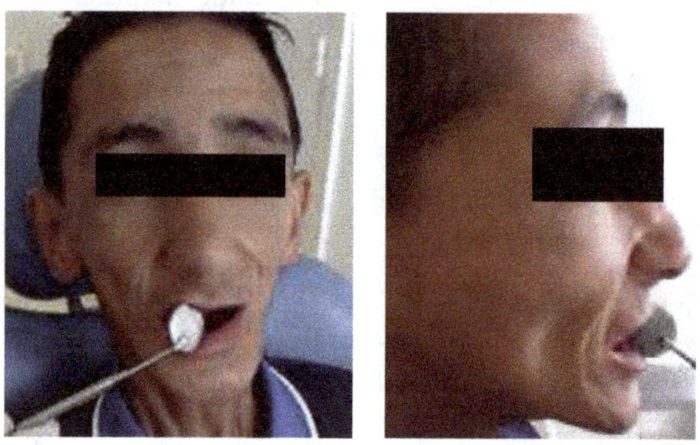

(a) (b)

Figure 2: Preoperative views of the patient with severe limitation of oral aperture. (a) Frontal view; (b) side view.

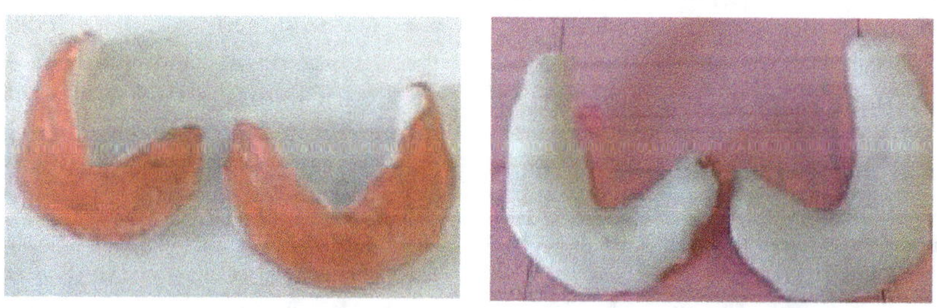

(a) (b)

Figure 3: Sectional special mandibular tray. (a) Under side view (soft wax); (b) upper side view (autopolymerizing resin).

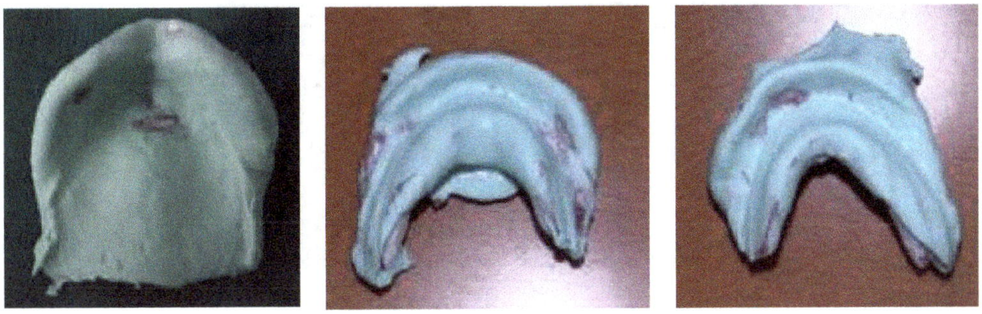

(a) (b) (c)

Figure 4: Primary impressions. (a) maxillary primary impression; (b) Right sectional mandibular impression; (c) left sectional mandibular impression.

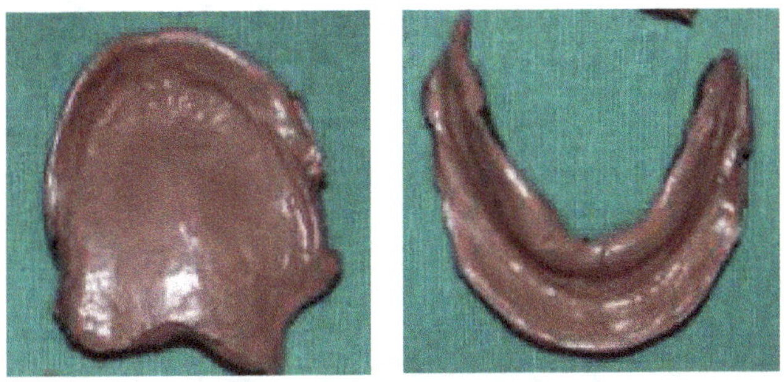

(a) (b)

Figure 5: Final impressions. (a) Maxillary impression; (b) mandibular impression.

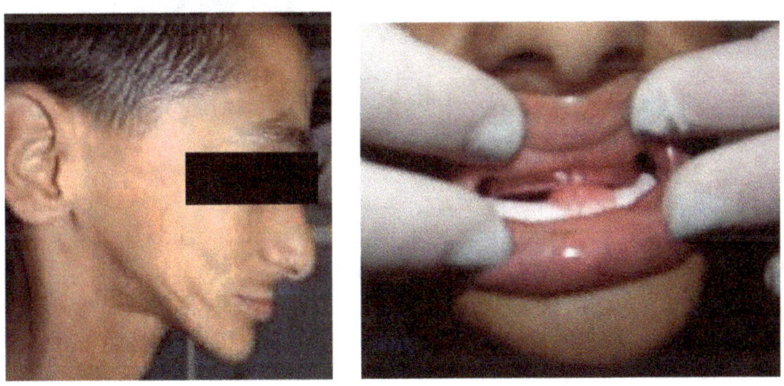

(a) (b)

Figure 6: The maxillomandibular relationship record (OVD, CR). (a) Lateral view with established vertical dimension of occlusion; (b) intraoral view.

merizing acrylic resin extraorally (Figure 3(b)). They were inserted into the patient's mouth in two separated pieces: left and right.

For the maxillary arch, the impression tray was made in one piece as the same manner as the mandibular one.

The preliminary impressions were made with irreversible hydrocolloid impression material (alginate).

The maxillary impression was made on one step (Figure 4(a)).

The two mandibular hemi-impressions were made separately (Figures 4(b) and 4(c)). Recording the anterior ridge, in addition to the corresponding side, by each hemi-impression is an indispensable condition to validate it.

First, the right mandibular hemi-impression was poured with type II dental plaster to obtain the right sectional primary cast. After it was set, and thanks to the central common area of the two hemi-impressions, the left hemi-impression could be positioned on the right sectional cast and poured. It was held with finger pressure until plaster was set ensuring not to displace the first sectional cast seated in the impression. So, we got an entire primary cast.

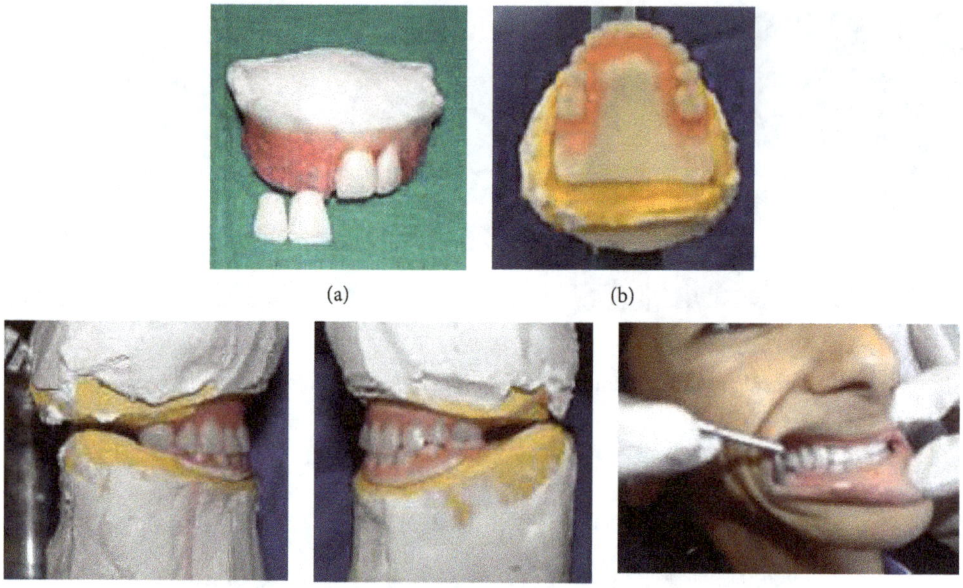

(a) (b)

(c) (d) (e)

FIGURE 7: Teeth arrangement and try-in. (a) Teeth size reshaping; (b) teeth formula reduction (1 premolar and 1 molar); (c) right view; (d) left view; (e) try-in.

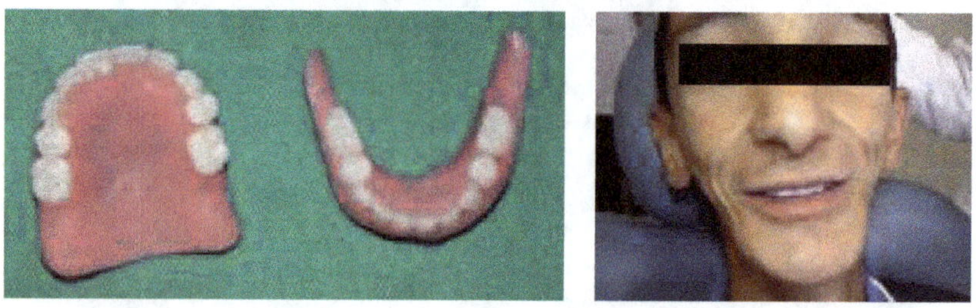

(a) (b)

FIGURE 8: (a) Final dentures; (b) frontal view of the patient after insertion.

For the secondary impression, single custom trays were fabricated for each arch using autopolymerizing acrylic resin. Once placed intraorally, it was carefully positioned onto denture-bearing areas and molded to appropriate contour using functional and manual manipulation. Care was taken during border molding to correctly record the peripheral extension, as the vestibular depth and width were shallow (Figures 5(a) and 5(b)). Final impressions were poured to get final casts.

Mandibular movements become restricted because of facial skin fibrosis, muscular atrophy, and temporomandibular joint damage, which make recording the maxillomandibular relationship problematic. By making the mandibular record base, as possible, shorter and thinner and with patient cooperation, jaw relation record was obtained with the use of occlusion rims oriented to the established vertical dimension of occlusion, the anatomic occlusal plane, and the patient's centric relation (Figure 6(a)). The mandibular wax occlusal rim thus obtained was very short because of the reduction of the vertical prosthetic space which complicated the teeth arrangement (Figure 6(b)).

Because of a lack of teeth in appropriate sizes and shapes, conventional artificial teeth were reshaped to be managed in the available transversal and vertical space (Figures 7(a)–7(d)).

During the try-in stage, the stability and occlusion were verified and the esthetic aspect was accomplished (Figure 7(e)).

After teeth arrangement, complete dentures were fabricated with the usual laboratory procedures using heat polymerized polymethyl methacrylate resin. After bench cooling, the dentures were finished and polished (Figure 8(a)).

At the insertion appointment, the balanced occlusion was adjusted (Figure 8(b)). Oral hygiene instructions and prosthesis insertion and removal were imparted. Routine follow-up appointments were scheduled after a week. The patient was satisfied with the esthetics and functional ability of the dentures.

3. Case Report 2

A 47-year-old edentulous female consulted at the prosthodontic department of the Faculty of Dental Medicine of Monastir, Tunisia. She had extremely unuseful maxillary complete denture (Figure 9(a)).

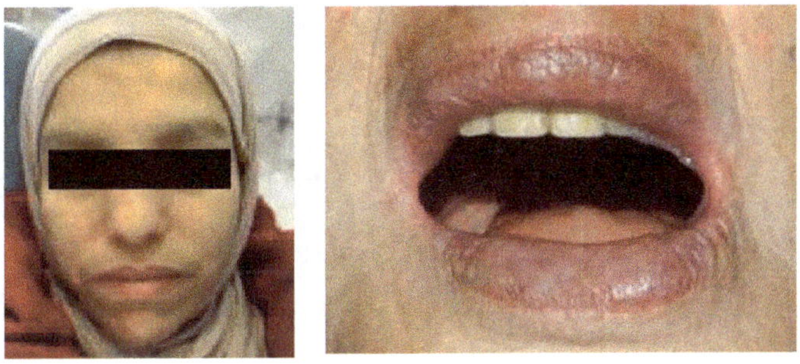

(a) (b)

FIGURE 9: Preoperative view of the patient. (a) Frontal view; (b) maximal mouth opening.

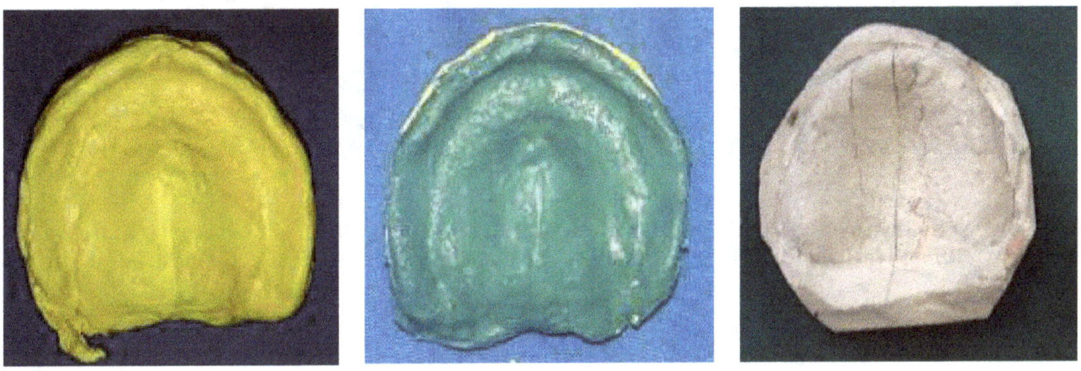

(a) (b) (c)

FIGURE 10: Maxillary preliminary impression. (a) First step of primary impression with putty silicon material; (b) second step of primary impression with light silicone material; (c) primary maxillary cast.

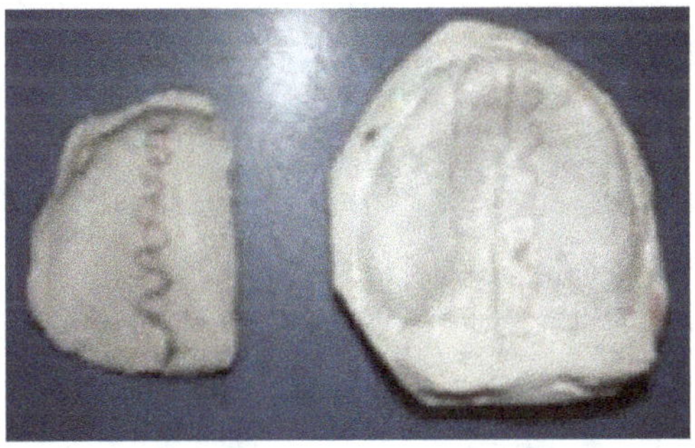

FIGURE 11: Left impression tray segment.

Her lips were stretched, and she had a limited oral opening with a diameter and circumference of approximately 27 mm and 98 mm, respectively, resulting from cervical radiotherapy (Figure 9(b)). Her alveolar crest was sufficiently high, but her buccal and labial mucosas were thin and the saliva quantity and flowability were inadequate.

The treatment plan consisted of fabricating complete dentures with proper extension of the flanges.

With effort, preliminary impressions for both arches were obtained with flexible impression trays: a putty silicon impression material was inserted, and once placed intraorally, it was carefully molded by finger pressure covering the entire important anatomic regions using functional and manual manipulation.

Due to flexibility, the silicone tray could be easily removed (Figure 10(a)).

A light silicone material was injected on the first impression, then, the light body wash impression was made by reinserting the silicone tray in the oral cavity (Figure 10(b)).

The custom trays for the final impressions were fabricated with autopolimerized acrylic resin on each primary stone cast (Figure 10(c)).

For the mandibular impression, the oral opening was sufficient for the custom tray to be inserted on the patient's mouth.

The maxillary custom tray was cut into two unequal sections, so that the labial frenum is recorded accurately in the

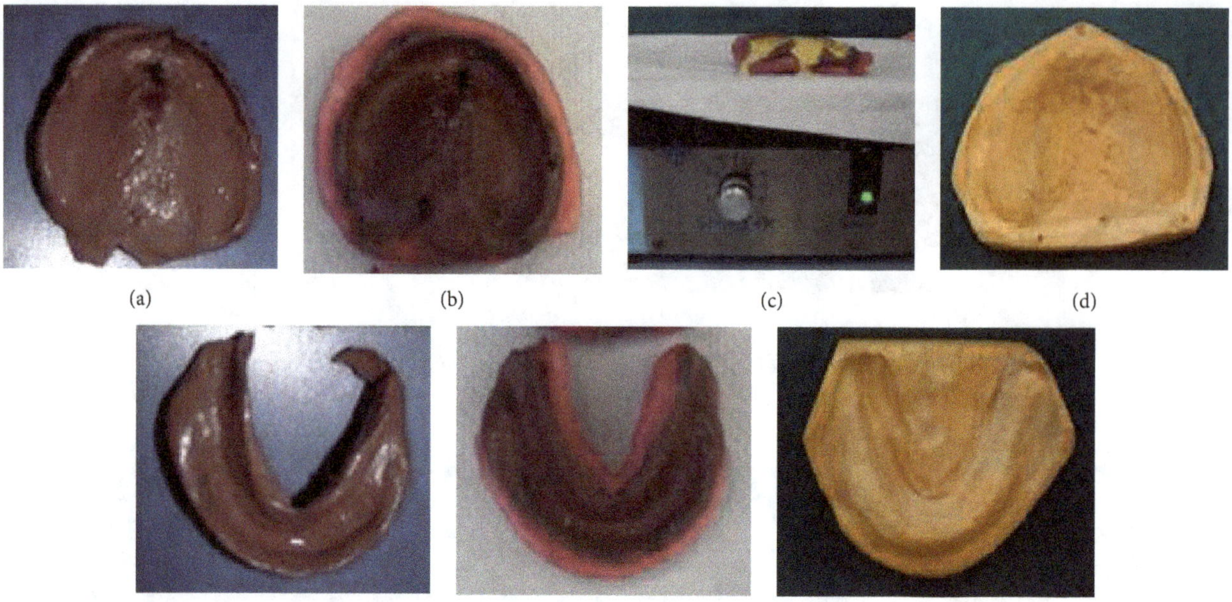

FIGURE 12: Final impression treatments. (a) Joined sectional maxillary impression; (b) maxillary impression coffrage; (c) maxillary impression pouring; (d) maxillary final cast; (e) mandibular final impression; (f) mandibular impression coffrage; (g) mandibular final cast.

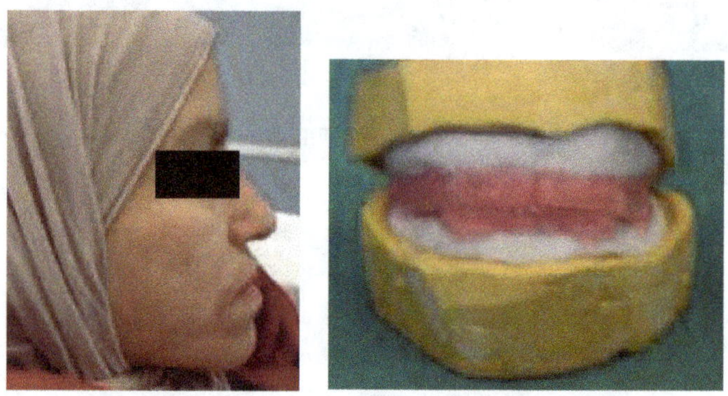

FIGURE 13: Occlusal record. (a) Lateral view with established vertical dimension of occlusion; (b) extraoral view.

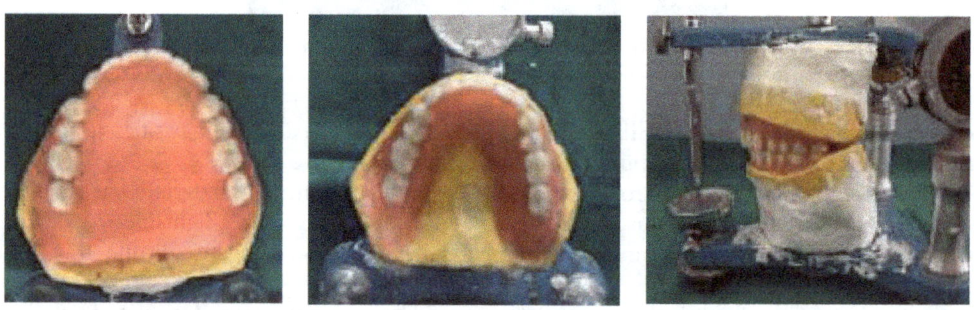

FIGURE 14: Teeth arrangement. (a) Maxillary view; (b) mandibular view; (c) lateral view.

impression. The two segments of the tray are joined using nick and notches (Figure 11). This facilitated the reassembling of the impressions outside the mouth. The insertion and movement to interlock the tray segments should be rehearsed in the mouth prior to the impression procedure.

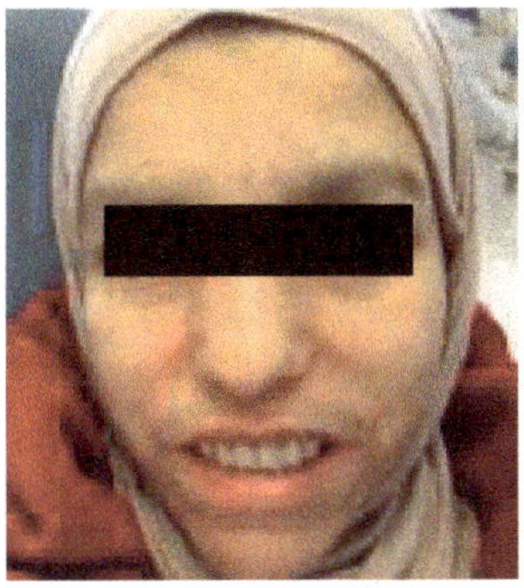

FIGURE 15: The postoperative view of the patient rehabilitated with a set of functional and esthetic complete dentures.

The maxillary impression tray was inserted into the patient's mouth in two separate pieces, left and right. The fit of the borders was evaluated. Then, the peripheral borders of the trays were trimmed so that they were 2 mm shorter than the depth of the vestibule to allow space for the border-molding material. This latter was separately done for each half.

Final maxillary impressions were made by using polysulfide material alternately for the first and second halves of the sectional trays. After the impression paste set, the right and left tray segments were removed separately. The acrylic resin halves were carefully joined extraorally, and minor discrepancies at the seam were filled with soft impression wax (Figure 12(a)).

Final impressions were boxed and gently poured to get final casts (vibrator) (Figures 12(b)–12(g)).

On final casts, record bases were fabricated and occlusion rims were prepared.

After making a centric relation record, transferring the record from the patient to a semiadjustable articulator was done (Figures 13(a) and 13(b)).

Because of the lack of the prosthetic vertical space between the arches, the record bases were removed from the casts and replaced with thin slices of wax that supported the teeth arrangement (Figures 14(a)–14(c)).

The try-in was evaluated to verify jaw relations and teeth arrangement. After patient acceptance, final festooning and flasking of the dentures were completed.

The final dentures were manufactured using similar designs to that of the record bases. The prostheses were deflasked, finished, and polished. The patient was provided with instructions for cleaning, inserting, and removing the prostheses (Figure 15). She was recalled for follow-up visits to check for the maintenance and her adaptability with the new dentures. Initially, the patient felt difficulty in the insertion and removal of denture, but progressively, she became used to.

4. Case Report 3

A 56-year-old edentulous patient presented to our Department of Prosthodontics. He reported esthetic and functional difficulties. Extraoral examination revealed a small

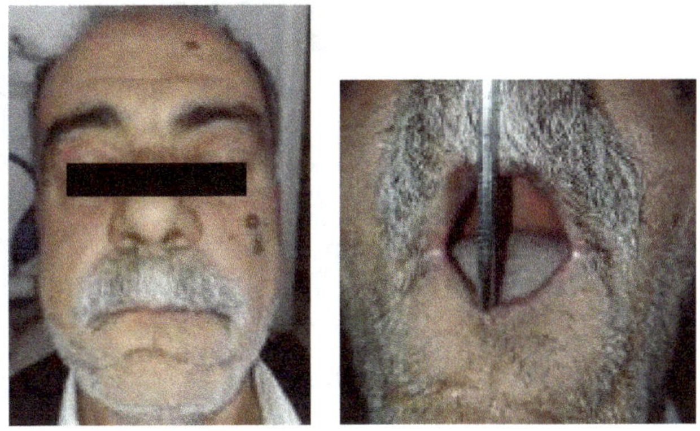

(a) (b)

FIGURE 16: Preoperative view of the patient. (a) Frontal view; (b) maximal mouth opening.

vertical oral aperture measuring 30 mm due to the presence of scars on the coetaneous side of the lower lip after surgical resection of a squamous cell carcinoma complicated by an active mentalis muscle (Figures 16(a) and 16(b)).

Maxillary and mandibular ridges were found to be large and well-formed. And as the patient could insert the mandibular denture into his mouth by rotating it 90 degrees, a conventional design was used.

With some amount of difficulty, conventional procedures for fabricating a set of complete denture were followed until the stage of occlusion record.

After centric relation recording, we found that the lower lip was interposed under the upper occlusal rim although there is a sagittal coincidence of the vestibular side of the two occlusal rims (Figures 17(a) and 17(b)).

So, the buccal side of the mandibular rim was arranged by removing the vestibular wax, trimming the record base, and perforating the occlusal rim (Figures 18(a) and 18(b)) to make a space to the putty silicone material (Figure 18(c)).

The silicone was molded intraorally until having sufficient esthetic aspect and lower labial support. New jaw relation was recorded. The occlusal plane and the midlines were established (Figures 19(a) and 19(b)). The mandibular occlusal rim was placed more buccally than the maxillary rim (Figure 19(c)).

Definitive casts were mounted on a semiadjustable articulator by using the maxillomandibular relationship records. The putty index record would assist the arrangement of artificial anterior teeth (Figure 20).

Before teeth setting, multiple stops were prepared on the exterior surface of the mandibular cast (Figure 21(a)). A buccal key was made with dental stone to mark the buccal inclination of the mandibular incisives and the midline (Figures 21(b) and 21(c)).

In the same way, the arrangement was completed (Figure 21(d)). Thus, it maintains the anatomic relation between the upper and lower lips in rest and function (Figures 22(a) and 22(b)).

After the try-in stage, complete dentures were fabricated.

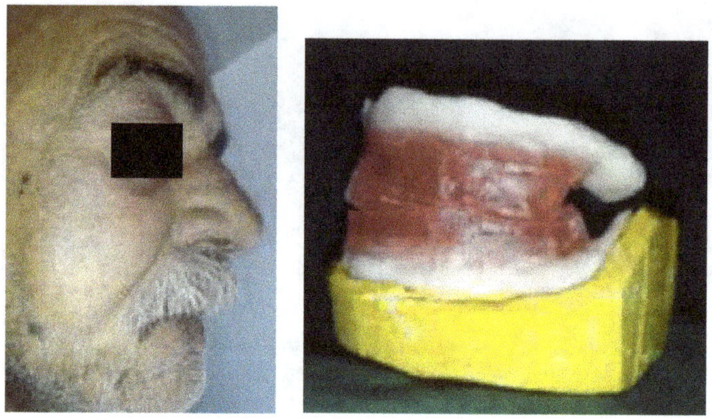

(a) (b)

Figure 17: Occlusal record. (a) Lateral view with established vertical dimension of occlusion; (b) sagittal view of the occlusal rim in centric relation.

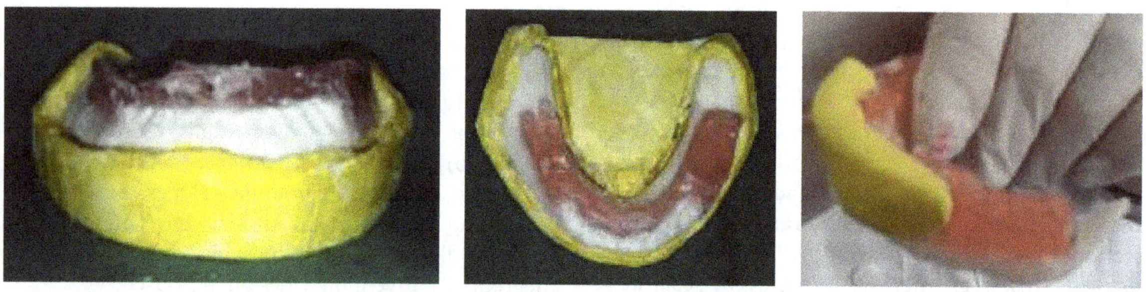

(a) (b) (c)

Figure 18: Mandibular occlusal rim modifications. (a) Frontal view of the modificated record base; (b) upper view of the modificated record base; (c) putty silicone in place.

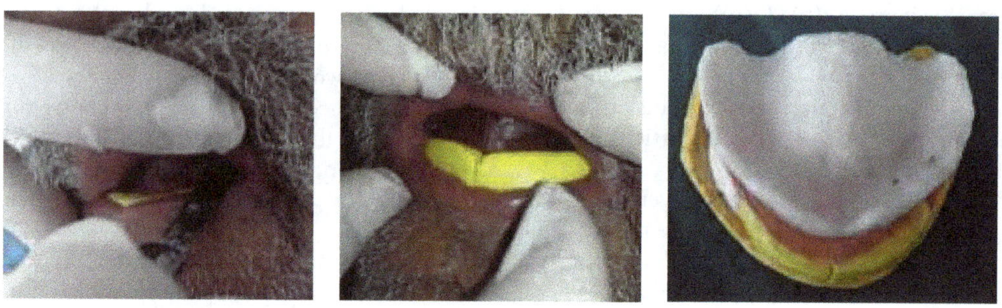

(a) (b) (c)

Figure 19: Second occlusal record. (a) Occlusal plan setting; (b) midline setting; (c) extraoral view.

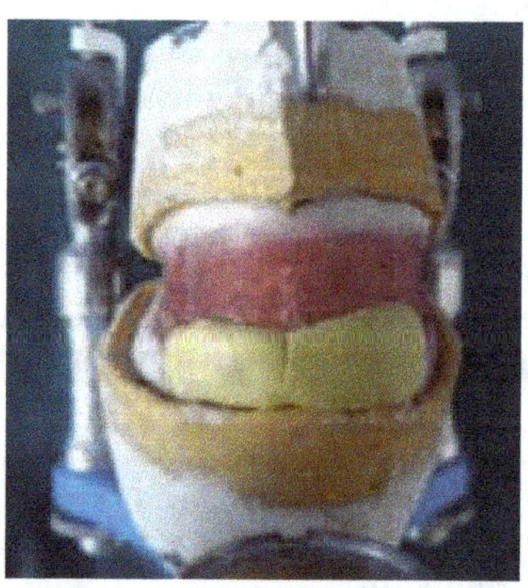

Figure 20: Definitive casts mounted on semiadjustable articulator.

5. Discussion

Maximal oral openings may range from 36 to 77 mm in healthy persons with mean values from several studies within the 50 to 60 mm "normal range" reported by Posselt. Deviations from normal were classified as either "slight" (Class I, 41 to 50 mm), "moderate" (Class II, 31 to 40 mm), or "severe" (Class III, 30 mm or below) microstomia [10].

During prosthodontic rehabilitation, patients who present with nonideal/pathological conditions for replacement of missing teeth, such as limited mouth opening, should be made aware of the limitations of the prosthesis.

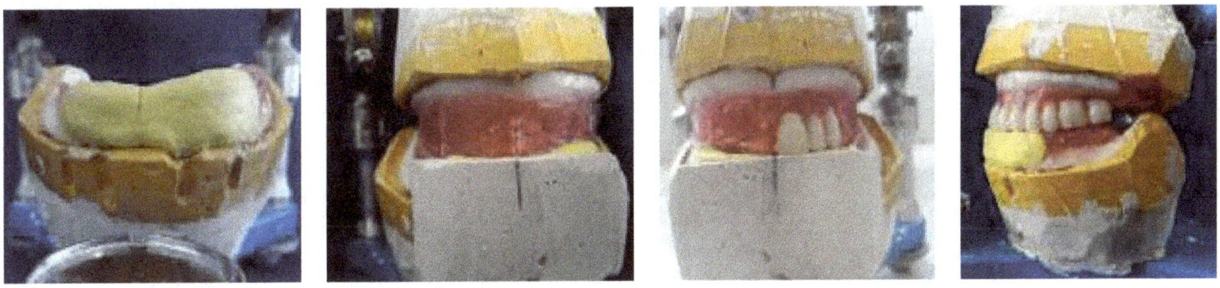

(a) (b) (c) (d)

FIGURE 21: Teeth arrangement. (a) Buccal slots; (b) plaster key; (c) anterior teeth arrangement; (d) upper teeth arrangement.

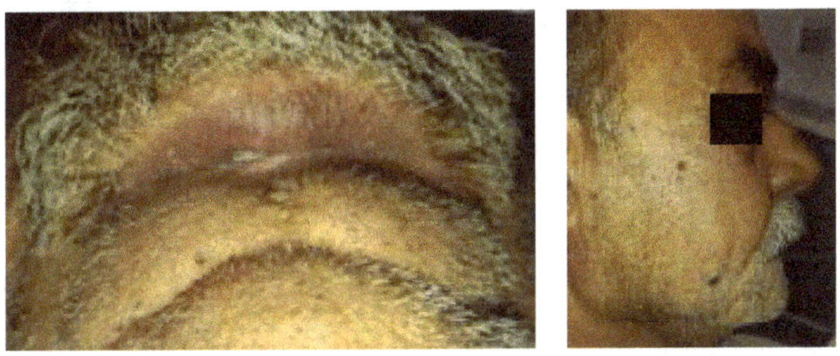

(a) (b)

FIGURE 22: Try-in. (a) Close view of the lips situation; (b) lateral view.

This situation is considered as inconvenient for the patient and challenging for both the dentist and dental technician. Proper treatment planning should be adopted so that a functionally acceptable prosthesis can be fabricated.

So, to plane treatment for a patient with microstomia, it is important to have knowledge about existing complications, alternative methods, and the patient's ability and comfort [11–13].

In some cases, successful prosthetic treatment for patients with microstomia is very difficult without a surgical operation [1].

If not, making complete dentures for them presents difficulties at all stages, from the impressions to the fabrication of the prostheses. It may even be impossible to make it by using conventional methods [2].

Various techniques for making preliminary impressions for patients with microstomia have been presented in the literature. In the treatments described, sectional impression trays and flexible impression trays with semi rigid silicone putty impression material were used. A review of the literature shows that different impression methods and designs have been used in a similar procedure. On the one hand, sectional impression trays are advocated. Mirfazaelian, for example, used orthodontic expansion screws to fabricate sectional trays. Cura et al. used metal pins and an acrylic resin block to attach the sections of the impression trays used. Plastic building screws, hinges, and acrylic resin blocks or locking levers had been proposed to attach the sections of the impression trays. On the other hand, Benetti et al. used an entire flexible plastic tray intended for fluoride application to make the preliminary impression [2, 6, 8].

In addition, the fabrication of complete dentures depends on making accurate final impressions that capture the movable tissues in their functional state. For this purpose, a few methods such as flexible and sectional stock trays have been proposed to obtain optimal final impressions [1, 6].

Some amelioration was done to the sectional tray. For example, on one of the sections, Benetti et al. prepared a stepped butt joint to make a definitive impression [8].

An inconvenience of the method of sectional trays is that it was not possible to remove the custom tray in 1 piece; it could be removed as 2 separate segments. This would be done by fracturing the impression material [8].

In addition, it was believed that the cross-section of the sectional impression paste was not wide enough in the midline and that this would negatively affect the stability of the right and the left tray pieces. Also, the two pieces of the tray were arranged in 2 different planes, which affect the proper approximation of two halves of the tray [14].

With patients suffering from microstomia, when the abnormality of the jaw relations is very marked, various modifications in the artificial teeth arrangement may be necessary to obtain satisfactory results in the functional rehabilitation of complete dentures [11].

Because of a lack of denture teeth in appropriate sizes and shapes, conventional denture teeth would be reshaped to appropriate sizes.

In some cases, occlusal areas of posterior artificial teeth were formed with 0-degree cusps to facilitate eccentric mandibular movements [3].

Another way of overcoming the problem in the arrangement of teeth due to the abnormal jaw relation is by using nonanatomic teeth with flate occlusal surfaces. Thanks to this morphology, achieving a satisfactory occlusal relation with the opposing arch will be easier than with semianatomic or anatomic teeth [11].

During the try-in stage, the stability and occlusion of complete dentures would be verified.

Several techniques and designs have been described in the literature for the fabrication of the definitive denture base. The most common procedure used is sectional or foldable denture. During the follow-up period of these types of prostheses, the patient reported dislodgment of the denture during chewing. In fact, Lego pieces for joining the sectional segments do not provide good stability or interlocking, and the result was unsuccessful [5, 12].

Also, earlier reports have fabricated the maxillary complete denture in two parts which creates the problem of midline diastema (esthetics) as well as problems in phonetics [15].

This technique also has some other disadvantages in the term of longer chair time, additional lab time, and material used for the fabrication of sectional denture [16].

Special recommendations must be given to the patient at the prosthesis delivery appointment about how to insert and remove his denture.

(1) Involve the patient in the technique: he chooses which denture to insert first. It is preferable to place the maxillary denture prior to inserting the mandibular one and inversely on removing.

(2) It is better to repeat inserting and removing prostheses in front of a mirror until he gets acquainted with the new denture manipulation.

(3) The denture must be inserted, tilted, and then turned horizontally (90°) to be in place.

6. Conclusion

Although patients with microstomia presenting for prosthetic rehabilitation pose a challenge to the clinician at all the clinical procedures, they can conservatively be managed by modifying clinical and laboratory procedures. However, in these modifications, care should be taken to avoid compromising the basic principles of providing optimum function and esthetics to the patient. The authors recommend that selection of an appropriate technique should be based on the case requirement and the operator's skills.

References

[1] M. Yenisey, T. Kulunk, S. Kurt, and C. Ural, "A prosthodontic management alternative for scleroderma patients," *Journal of Oral Rehabilitation*, vol. 32, no. 9, pp. 696–700, 2005.

[2] N. Rathi, R. Heshmati, B. Yilmaz, and W. Wilson, "A technique for fabricating a hinged mandibular complete dental prosthesis with swing lock for a patient with microstomia," *The Journal of Prosthetic Dentistry*, vol. 110, no. 6, pp. 540–543, 2013.

[3] F. Mahboub, K. Sadr, F. Heidary, and E. Hosseini, "A simple method for prosthodontic rehabilitation of edentulous patient with epidermolysis bullosa: a clinical case report," *Journal of Dental Research, Dental Clinics, Dental Prospects*, vol. 5, 2011.

[4] K. A. Kumar, V. Bhat, K. C. Nair, and R. Suresh, "Preliminary impression techniques for microstomia patients," *Journal of Indian Prosthodontic Society*, vol. 16, no. 3, 2016.

[5] S. S. Colvenkar, "Sectional impression tray and sectional denture for a microstomia patient," *Journal of Prosthodontics*, vol. 19, no. 2, pp. 161–165, 2010.

[6] K. Singh, N. Gupta, R. Gupta, and D. Abrahm, "Prosthetic rehabilitation with collapsible hybrid acrylic resin and permanent silicone soft liner complete denture of a patient with scleroderma-induced microstomia," *Journal of Prosthodontics*, vol. 23, no. 5, pp. 412–416, 2014.

[7] J. G. Egan and S. A. Swindells, "A novel prosthodontic alternative for patients who are edentulous and have microstomia: a case report," *Special Care in Dentistry*, vol. 32, no. 4, pp. 160–164, 2012.

[8] O. Geckili, A. Cilingir, and T. Bilgin, "Impression procedures and construction of a sectional denture for a patient with microstomia: a clinical report," *The Journal of Prosthetic Dentistry*, vol. 96, no. 6, pp. 387–390, 2006.

[9] A. G. Türk and M. Ulusoy, "A collapsible partial denture for a patient with limited mouth opening induced by scleroderma: a clinical report," *Journal of Prosthodontics*, vol. 24, no. 4, pp. 334–338, 2015.

[10] W. P. Naylor and C. W. Douglass, Eds.E. Mix, "The nonsurgical treatment of microstomia in scleroderma: a pilot study," *Oral Surgery, Oral Medicine, Oral Pathology*, W. P. Naylor and C. W. Douglass, Eds., vol. 57, no. 5, pp. 508–511, 1984.

[11] A. Tambe, S. B. Patil, S. Bhat, and M. M. Badadare, "Cross-arch arrangement in complete denture prosthesis to manage an edentulous patient with oral submucous fibrosis and abnormal jaw relation," *BMJ Case Reports*, vol. 2014, 2014.

[12] M. Hajimahmoudi and A. S. Mostafavi, "A simple and effective method for prosthetic rehabilitation in scleroderma patients: a clinical report," *The International Journal of Prosthodontics*, vol. 27, no. 2, pp. 169–173, 2014.

[13] U. Adali, S. Schober, F. Beuer, and B. C. Spies, "Digital impression-taking facilitates prosthetic rehabilitation of microstomia patients: a case history report," *The International Journal of Prosthodontics*, vol. 32, no. 1, pp. 110–112, 2018.

[14] S. Kumar, A. Arora, and R. Yadav, "Foldable denture: for microstomia patient," *Case Reports in Dentistry*, vol. 2012, Article ID 757025, 3 pages, 2012.

[15] S. K. Dewan, A. Arora, M. Sehgal, and A. Khullar, "Microstomia—a treatment challenge to a prosthodontist," *Journal of Clinical and Diagnostic Research*, vol. 9, no. 4, 2015.

[16] A. Patel, R. Sethuraman, P. Prajapati, and J. R. Patel, "Microstomia: entry made easy in no entry (with sectional tray and sectional denture)," *BMJ Case Reports*, vol. 2013, 2013.

21

Repeated Occurrence and Recurrence of Secondary Oral Solid Cancers after Hematopoietic Stem Cell Transplantation for Leukaemia: Long-Term Follow-Up

Takumi Takahashi,[1] Miki Yamada,[1] Keisuke Sawada,[2] Nami Nakayama,[1] Yosuke Iijima,[1] Shunsuke Hino,[1] Takahiro Kaneko,[1] and Norio Horie[1]

[1]*Department of Oral and Maxillofacial Surgery, Saitama Medical Center, Saitama Medical University, Saitama, Japan*
[2]*Department of Pathology, Saitama Medical Center, Saitama Medical University, Saitama, Japan*

Correspondence should be addressed to Miki Yamada; xiki714@saitama-med.ac.jp

Academic Editor: Tommaso Lombardi

Hematopoietic stem cell transplantation (HSCT) is a common method for patients such as hematologic malignancies. However, HSCT generally has a higher risk of secondary solid cancer development. The aim of this study was to emphasize the need for lifelong follow-up of oral secondary solid cancer. The patient was a male who underwent HSCT for chronic myelogenous leukaemia at the age of 31 years. He underwent ten onsets on oral secondary solid cancers during his subsequent follow-up of more than 20 years. In conclusion, patients after HSCT require lifelong observation of oral secondary solid cancer, which may be accompanied by repeated new and recurrent occurrences.

1. Introduction

Hematopoietic stem cell transplantation (HSCT) is a vital therapeutic method for most patients who have hematologic malignancies such as leukaemia and non-malignant disease such as aplastic anaemia. HSCT has increased steadily over the past three decades worldwide [1–3], and has greatly improved the patient's long-term survival rate. However, HSCT generally has a higher risk of secondary solid cancer development, which became an important cause of late mortality, regardless of the stem cell source [2]. Among the secondary solid cancers, the high-risk cancer includes oropharyngeal cancer, oesophageal cancer, colon cancer, skin cancer and brain/nervous system cancer [1]. In these, oropharyngeal cancer is most frequent, and the incidence rate of oropharyngeal cancer after HSCT ranges from 32 to 92 per 100,000 person-years with a 7- to 16-fold higher risk than the general population [4]. The risk of secondary solid cancers begins to increase around 10 years after transplantation. The rate of secondary solid cancers was 1–6% at 10 years and 6–13% at 15 years [1, 2, 4]. Limited to oral secondary solid cancers, the time from HSCT to the onset of secondary solid oral cancers have been 1–17 years or more, and Mawardi et al. described that mean time was 8 years [5, 6]. The risk of secondary solid cancers continues even 20 years later and the risk of developing of oropharyngeal cancer continues to life-long [1, 4].

Although a relatively large number of oral secondary solid cancers have been reported, including statistical observations, most were merely reporting of first onset and have a short follow-up period [1, 7]. Oral secondary solid cancers can occur and recur in various sites of the oral cavity repeatedly over a long period of time. However, there have been a few reports of long-term follow-up, looking at how often the secondary cancers occur and recur during that time [6, 8–10].

In this study, we report a case of oral secondary solid cancers with ten times repeated occurrence and/or recurrence, which has been followed up for more than 20 years after undergoing HSCT at the age of 31 years in order to emphasize the need for long-term observation of the onset of oral secondary solid cancer.

2. Case Report

In April 2019, a 51-year-old man visited the oral and maxillofacial surgery clinic to continue follow-up of oral examination after HSCT. The patient was previously diagnosed with chronic myelogenous leukaemia in 2000. In September 2000, the patient underwent an allogeneic HSCT from his human leukocyte antigen–matched sister. Immediately after the transplantation, graft-versus-host disease (GVHD) of oral mucosa appeared. However, no prominent symptoms of GVHD other than the oral cavity were observed, and immunosuppressive therapy associated with GVHD was not performed. In addition, no local therapy was given.

After that, the patient could continue to follow up at the previous oral surgery clinic for oral GVHD and underwent surgery for secondary solid cancers of right buccal mucosa and left mandibular gingiva, both of which were diagnosed as squamous cell carcinoma (SCC) in February 2012; left mandibular gingiva in July 2012 (SCC); left mandibular gingiva in September 2012 (SCC); and right upper lip (SCC) in July 2013. Subsequently, biopsies were performed on the left upper lip in November 2017 and on the right side of the dorsum of the tongue in December 2017, both of which were negative for malignancy. After that, regular observations were continued, but due to work, our department took over the flow-up.

His medical history other than that associated with chronic myelogenous leukaemia included hypertension, hyperuricemia, chronic kidney disease, diabetes, and dyslipidemia. Current medications included omega-3-acid ethyl esters (hyperlipidemia), atorvastatin calcium hydrate (hypercholesterolaemia), amlodipine besilate (hypertension), perindopril erbumine (hypertension), febuxostat (hyperuricemia), and insulin aspart (diabetes).

On examination, erythema was observed on the right side and left margin of the tongue, while on the dorsal surface, exophytic masses were found. The left maxillary anterior gingiva showed whitish change (Figure 1(a)). The right buccal mucosa and pharyngeal mucosa showed lichenoid striae with erythema, in which white slightly raised lesions were observed, and white plaque was found posterior to the first molar (Figure 1(b)). On the right side of lower lip, a white lesion with a diameter of 7 mm, with an indistinct border and no induration, was observed (Figure 1(c)). Most of the palate showed erythema. A relatively clear white ridge was observed on the right molar (Figure 1(d)).

After the biopsies, in June, surgical resections were performed. The diagnosis of the left dorsal surface of the tongue and the right buccal mucosa was severe dysplasia, and lower lip was SCC, and the left maxillary palatal gingiva was carcinoma in situ (Figures 2(a)–(d)). In addition, the specimens were immunostained with anti-p16 antibody to search for human papillomavirus (HPV) infection. Histopathologically, HPV infection was negatively diagnosed. In April 2021, a white lesion in the maxillary anterior gingiva became prominent, and a biopsy revealed severe dysplasia, resulting in surgical procedure (Figure 3). To date, no relapse of leukaemia has been observed. The patient has seen recurrence and the development of new lesions, but so far, the early response has been successful. Strict follow-up needs to be continued in the future.

3. Discussion

With improved clinical outcomes of hematologic diseases performed by HSCT, there is rising interest in secondary solid cancers after HSCT. Among them, oropharyngeal region is the most prominent high-risk organ of development of secondary solid cancers [1, 7]. In this study, we presented a case of patient with 10 times repeated new and recurrent oral secondary solid cancers who had been followed up for more than 20 years after HSCT.

Skin and oropharyngeal secondary solid cancer is predominantly squamous cell carcinoma [2]. Various risk factors have been reported for the development of secondary oropharyngeal solid cancers. In these risk factors, chronic GVHD is most important [1, 2, 4, 7]. GVHD is a major cause of morbidity and mortality in patients who undergo HSCT [11]. GVHD is divided into acute and chronic GVHD. Acute GVHD is a reaction of donor immune cells against host tissues, and the three main tissues that acute GVHD affects are the skin, liver, and gastrointestinal tract. Chronic GVHD is a syndrome of variable clinical features resembling autoimmune and other immunologic disorders, and manifestations of chronic GVHD may be restricted to a single organ or site or may be widespread, with profound impact on quality of life. After HSCT, GVHD is estimated to occur in 30–40%, and 25–80% of chronic GVHD patients present with oral symptoms [11]. Mawardi et al. described that 96% of patients with oral secondary solid cancers affected oral chronic GVHD [5].

The symptoms of oral acute GVHD and chronic GVHD may overlap. Diagnostic features of oral chronic GVHD include lichen planus-like changes, characterized by hyperkeratotic white lines and lacy-appearing lesions on the oral mucosa, and distinctive features of chronic GVHD include xerostomia (dryness), mucoceles, mucosal atrophy, ulcers, and pseudomembranes [12]. Symptoms that are common to both acute and chronic GVHD include gingivitis, mucositis, erythema, and pain [12].

The clinical and histological features of chronic GVHD are very similar to those of oral lichen planus. In both diseases, the immune system plays a primary role in the pathogenesis, and the same mechanisms are considered to be associated with malignant transformation. Clinically, it may be difficult to distinguish the secondary solid cancers from chronic GVHD with lichen planus-like changes. The most frequent clinical features presented at diagnosis of the solid cancers were described to be plaques (50%), exophytic masses (39%), and ulcers (28%) [5]. The median interval from the diagnosis of oral chronic GVHD to the diagnosis of oral secondary cancer was six years [5].

Other risk factors of the oropharyngeal cancers included reduced-intensity conditioning regimens associated with

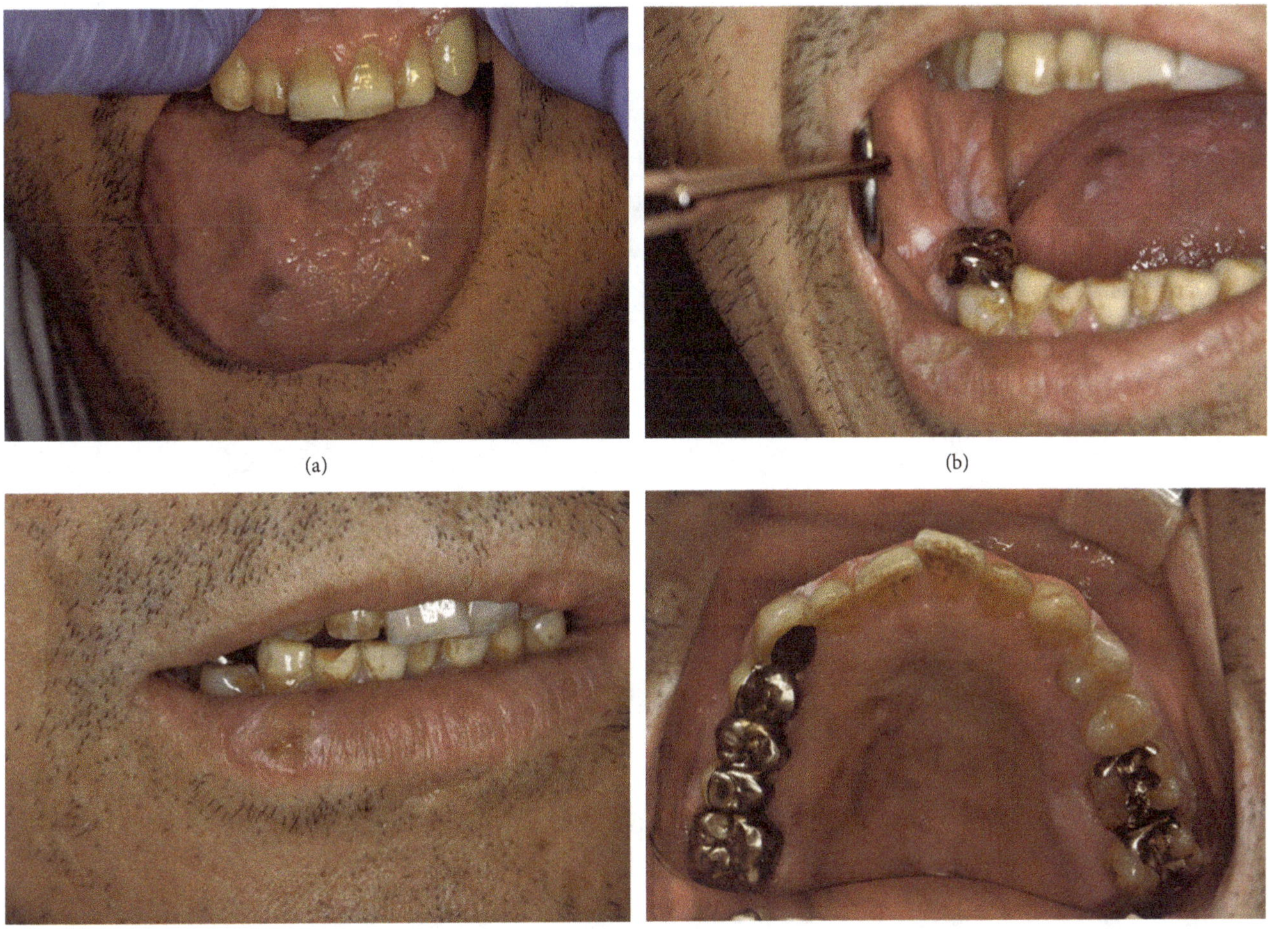

(a) (b) (c) (d)

FIGURE 1: Clinical photographs (April 2019), (a) Erythema is observed on the right side and left margin of the tongue, and exophytic masses are found from the center to the left side of the dorsal surface. The left maxillary anterior gingiva shows whitish change. (b) The right buccal mucosa and pharyngeal mucosa shows lichenoid striae with erythema, in which white slightly raised lesions are observed, and white plaque is found posterior to the molar. (c) The right side of lower lip, a white lesion with a diameter of 7 mm, with an indistinct border, no induration, is observed. (d) Most of the palate shows erythema. A relatively clear white ridge is observed on the right molar (Mirror image).

HSCT, autologous HSCT and hereditary disorders such as Fanconi anaemia in paediatric patients. Limited to oral cancer, long-term immunosuppressive therapy associated with chronic GVHD ≥24 months, conditioning regimens with limited field irradiation, and male gender were risk factors [2, 7]. In immunocompromised patients, oncogenic viruses such as HPV may contribute to oropharyngeal SCC [7]. In this case, as a result of immunostaining, HPV infection was ruled out. It was described that there has been no association between the incidence of secondary solid cancers and donor type or human leukocyte antigen [1, 4].

Secondary oral solid cancers can occur at any site in the oral cavity, but Mawardi et al. stated that the occurrence at the tongue was 56%, being the most predominant site, followed by buccal mucosa, 39% [5]. It needs to be emphasized that secondary oral solid cancers may appear multifocal or recur. Mawardi et al. described that multifocal oral cancers were found in 28% of cases, and localized recurrence was observed in 44% of their cases [5]. However, detailed reports of how many new occurrences and recurrences occurred during the observation period have been rare. To the best of our knowledge, there have been four cases showing the multiple onsets in chronological order, including new occurrences and recurrences, 3 cases with 2 onsets, and 1 case with 6 onsets (Table 1) [6, 8–10]. In the present case, there have been ten onsets in almost 10 years, and there have been no reports of follow-up of oral condition for more than 20 years in detail. According to the concept of field cancerization, secondary oral solid cancers are stated to show repeated onset of new lesions and recurrence [5]. It is important to know that secondary oral solid cancers may develop more than 10 years after HSCT and that they occur repeatedly over the years, in order to examine patients who have undergone HSCT.

As for follow-up, it is predicted that the secondary oral solid cancers will occur for a lifetime, so regular and uninterrupted scrutiny is necessary. Screening every six months may be considered for patients at high risk for developing oropharyngeal cancer [7]. Evaluation for premalignant lesions or oral cancer by a dentist or an oral surgeon is extremely important. The development of secondary solid cancers was likely to be influenced by GVHD-affected sites

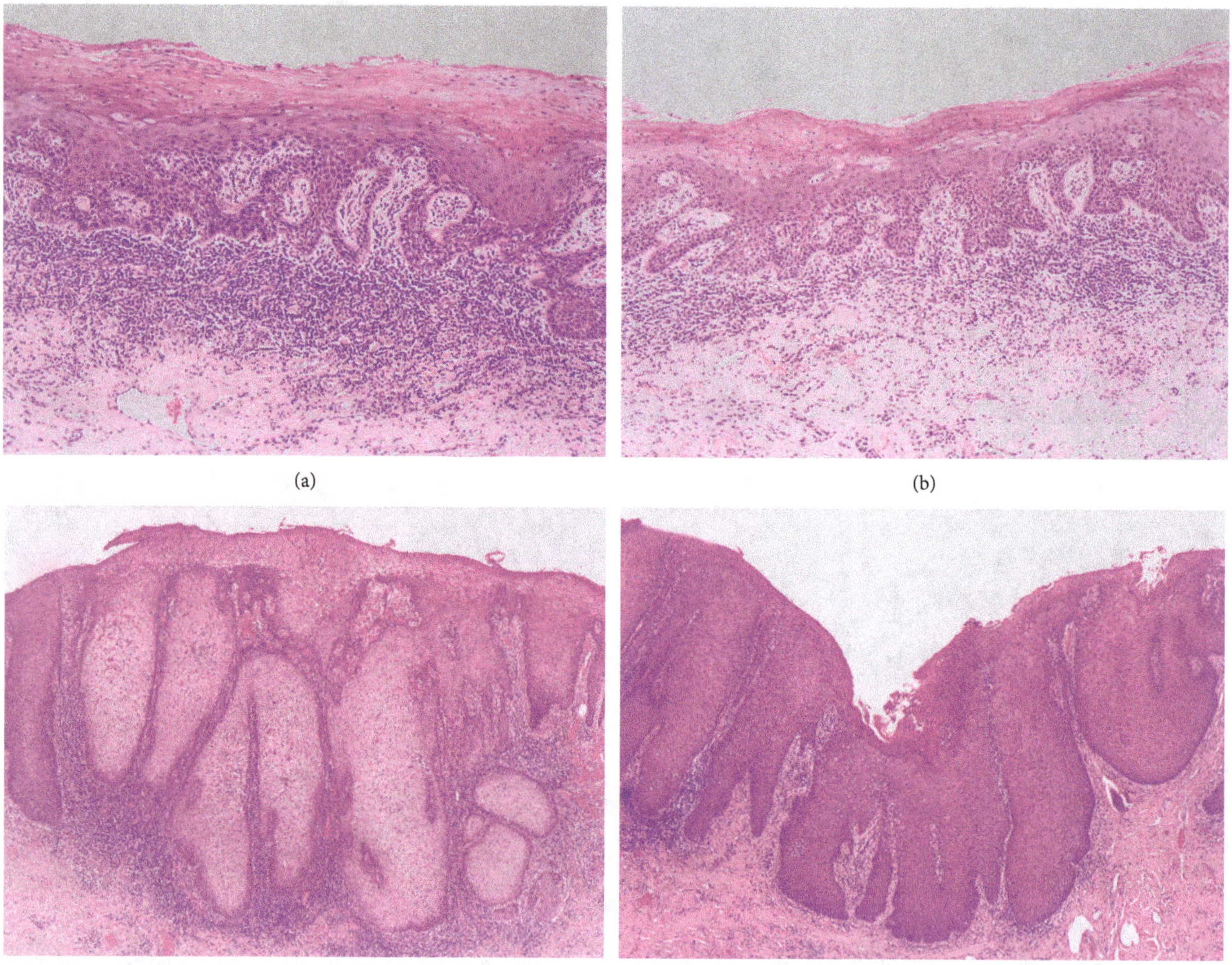

(a) (b) (c) (d)

Figure 2: Photomicrographs of surgical specimens. (a) Specimen of tongue showing severe dysplasia. (b) Specimen of the right buccal mucosa showing severe dysplasia. (c) Specimen of the right side of lower lip showing squamous cell carcinoma. (d) Specimen of the right palatal gingiva showing carcinoma in situ (hematoxylin-eosin stain—original magnification ×100; (a and b), ×40; (c and d) ×40).

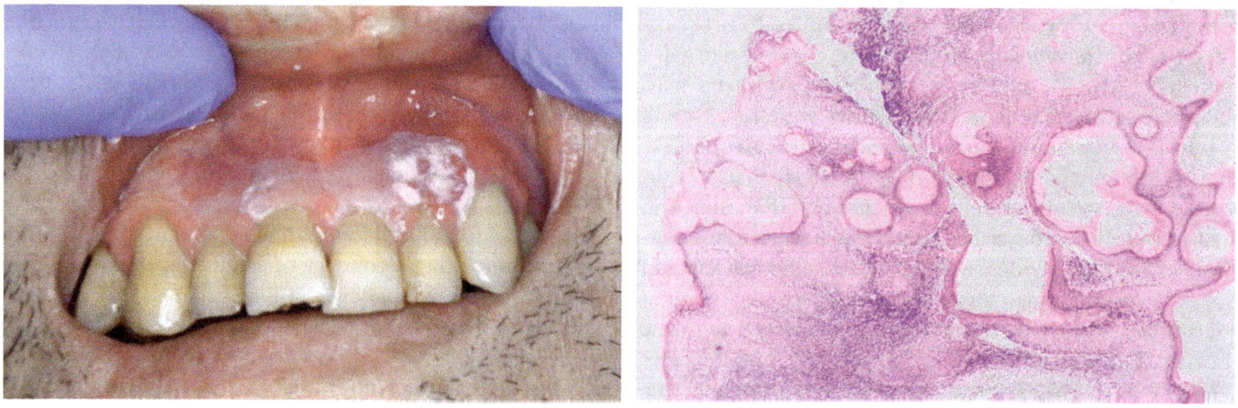

(a) (b)

Figure 3: Clinical photographs (April 2021). (a) Compared to the April 2019 photograph, white lesions in the maxillary anterior gingiva have clearly developed and plaque formation is observed. (b) Surgical specimen shows severe dysplasia (hematoxylin-eosin stain, original magnification ×40).

TABLE 1: Cases of multifocal and recurrence of secondary oral solid cancers after hematopoietic stem cell transplantation.

	Primary disease	Age at the time of HSCT (gender)	Age at the time of initial oral secondary cancer	Site of oral secondary cancer including new occurrences and recurrence (diagnosis[a])	Time after HSCT
Abdelsayed et al. [8]	ALL	22 (M)	24	Left buccal mucosa (CIS)	2 y 5 m
				Left buccal mucosa (mild-to-moderate dysplasia)	2 y 10 m
Kano et al. [9]	CML	33 (F)	45	Tongue (SCC)	12 y 6 m
				Oral cavity (SCC)	13 y 7 m
Zhang et al. [10]	AML	49 (M)	54	Lower lip (CIS)	5 y 1 m
				Lower lip (CIS)	5 y 6 m
Weng et al. [6]	AML	37 (M)	42	Left buccal mucosa (SCC)	5 y
				Right maxillary gingiva (SCC)	5 y
				Left buccal mucosa (SCC)	5 y 3 m
				Right maxillary gingiva (SCC)	7 y
				Right maxillary gingiva (mild dysplasia)	7 y 6 m
				Right buccal mucosa (SCC)	
Takahashi et al. (present study)	CML	31 (M)	44	Right buccal mucosa (SCC)	11 y 5 m
				Left mandibular gingiva (SCC)	
				Left mandibular gingiva (SCC)	11 y 10 m
				Left mandibular gingiva (SCC)	12 y 0 m
				Right upper lip (SCC)	13 y 10 m
				Left dorsal surface of tongue (severe dysplasia)	19 y 1 m
				Right buccal mucosa (severe dysplasia)	
				Right lower lip (SCC)	
				Left maxillary posterior palatal gingiva (CIS)	
				Left maxillary anterior gingiva (severe dysplasia)	21 y 1 m

[a]Including not only squamous cell carcinoma but also carcinoma in situ and dysplasia.
ALL, acute lymphoblastic leukaemia; AML, acute myelogenous leukaemia; CIS, carcinoma in situ; CML, chronic myelogenous leukaemia; HSCT, hematopoietic stem cell transplantation; SCC, squamous cell carcinoma.

[1, 5]. Therefore, scrutiny of patients with chronic GVHD is important.

4. Conclusion

This study reported a patient with repeated new and recurrent secondary oral solid cancers who were followed up for more than 20 years after HSCT. The number of leukaemia survivors with HSCT is expected to increase in the future. In particular, there has been a dramatic increase in the number of transplant recipients who are more than 50 years of age at transplant over the past decade [1]. Dentists and oral surgeons should keep in mind that recipients of HSCT such as survivors of leukaemia need lifelong follow-up for new and recurrent oral secondary solid cancers.

Consent

Written consent was obtained from the patient.

References

[1] Y. Atsuta, R. Suzuki, T. Yamashita et al., "Continuing increased risk of oral/esophageal cancer after allogeneic hematopoietic stem cell transplantation in adults in association with chronic graft-versus-host disease," *Annals of Oncology*, vol. 25, no. 2, pp. 435–441, 2014.

[2] R. E. Curtis, P. A. Rowlings, H. J. Deeg et al., "Solid cancers after bone marrow transplantation," *The New England Journal of Medicine*, vol. 336, no. 13, pp. 897–904, 1997.

[3] M. C. Pasquini, Z. Wang, M. M. Horowitz, and R. P. Gale, "2010 report from the Center for International Blood and Marrow Transplant Research (CIBMTR): current uses and outcomes of hematopoietic cell transplants for blood and bone marrow disorders," *Clinical Transplants*, pp. 87–105, 2010.

[4] J. D. Rizzo, R. E. Curtis, G. Socié et al., "Solid cancers after allogeneic hematopoietic cell transplantation," *Blood*, vol. 113, no. 5, pp. 1175–1183, 2009.

[5] H. Mawardi, S. Elad, M. E. Correa et al., "Oral epithelial dysplasia and squamous cell carcinoma following allogeneic hematopoietic stem cell transplantation: clinical presentation

and treatment outcomes," *Bone Marrow Transplantation*, vol. 46, no. 6, pp. 884–891, 2011.

[6] X. Weng, Y. Xing, and B. Cheng, "Multiple and recurrent squamous cell carcinoma of the Oral cavity after graft-versus-host disease," *Journal of Oral and Maxillofacial Surgery*, vol. 75, no. 9, pp. 1899–1905, 2017.

[7] Y. Inamoto, N. N. Shah, B. N. Savani et al., "Secondary solid cancer screening following hematopoietic cell transplantation," *Bone Marrow Transplantation*, vol. 50, no. 8, pp. 1013–1023, 2015.

[8] R. A. Abdelsayed, T. Sumner, C. M. Allen, A. Treadway, G. M. Ness, and S. L. Penza, "Oral precancerous and malignant lesions associated with graft-versus-host disease: report of 2 cases," *Oral Surgery, Oral Medicine, Oral Pathology, Oral Radiology, and Endodontics*, vol. 93, no. 1, pp. 75–80, 2002.

[9] Y. Kano, H. Ishii, M. Konno et al., "Cells of origin of squamous epithelium, dysplasia and cancer in the head and neck region after bone marrow transplantation," *International Journal of Oncology*, vol. 44, no. 2, pp. 443–450, 2014.

[10] L. Zhang, J. B. Epstein, C. F. Poh et al., "Comparison of HPV infection, p53 mutation and allelic losses in post-transplant and non-posttransplant oral squamous cell carcinomas," *Journal of Oral Pathology & Medicine*, vol. 31, no. 3, pp. 134–141, 2002.

[11] J. Murray, J. Stringer, and D. Hutt, "Graft-versus-host disease (GvHD)," in *The European Blood and Marrow Transplantation Textbook for Nurses*, M. Kenyon and A. Babic, Eds., pp. 221–251, Springer, Cham, 2018.

[12] M. H. Jagasia, H. T. Greinix, M. Arora et al., "National Institutes of Health consensus development project on criteria for clinical trials in chronic graft-versus-host disease: I. the 2014 diagnosis and staging working group report," *Biology of Blood and Marrow Transplantation*, vol. 21, no. 3, pp. 389–401.e.381, 2015.

22

Restoration of a Nonvital Tooth with Fiber Reinforce Composite (Wallpapering Technique)

Sara Valizadeh,[1] Ladan Ranjbar Omrani,[1] Simone Deliperi,[2,3] and Farzaneh Sadeghi Mahounak[4]

[1]Restorative Dentistry Department, School of Dentistry, Tehran University of Medical Sciences, Tehran, Iran
[2]Tufts University School of Dental Medicine, Boston, MA, USA
[3]Private Practice, Cagliari, Italy
[4]Restorative Dentistry Department, School of Dentistry, Shahid beheshti University of Medical Sciences, Tehran, Iran

Correspondence should be addressed to Farzaneh Sadeghi Mahounak; farzaneh.sadeghi.m@gmail.com

Academic Editor: Ali I. Abdalla

Introduction. Reconstruction of endodontically treated tooth (ETT) is one of the greatest challenges in dentistry. Clinical success of fiber reinforcement composite (FRC) restorations in ETT depends on many factors like remaining tooth structure, knowing advantages of adhesive dentistry besides its drawbacks, and the correct use of fibers in combination with resin composite. *Case Report.* This article presents a case in which fibers have been used in composite buildup in order to increase the toughness and strength of the ETT direct restoration. In addition, this technique does not require root canal enlargement to eliminate the risk of root perforation. Also, this one visit treatment can be helpful for patients that could not pay the cost of indirect restoration and/or have no time. *Conclusion.* It seems in selected patients with special considerations, FRC composite restoration is valid alternatives for indirect restoration.

1. Introduction

Without placing the coronal restoration, root canal treatments were not considered complete. Restoration of nonvital teeth is always challenging for dentists.

Appropriate treatment plan selection should be based on remaining tooth structure, cavity wall thickness, tooth position in the arch, and load applied to the tooth [1].

Previously, endodontically treated teeth (ETT) were reconstructed automatically with post and core and full crown. But this treatment plan had many risks like root perforation, sacrificing a considerable amount of sound tooth structure, and tooth fracture [2].

By modern adhesive dentistry, some alternative methods are proposed for ETT restoration in accordance with minimally invasive dentistry. Composite improvements in regard of physical and mechanical properties, besides esthetic appearance, were led to the progressive use of these dental materials and more tooth tissue preservation. This was ideal for patients who could not afford the cost of the indirect restorations [3].

However, the most important drawback of resin composites, which is polymerization shrinkage that produces stresses in the interface of tooth and restoration, has still been existed [4].

There are several methods for compensating these stresses due to the composite shrinkage.

One of them is an incremental technique for composite insertion in the cavity. The other way for controlling stress is light-curing techniques like soft start or ramp mode [5].

Clinicians should keep in mind that composite resin restoration is a rigid material; it lacks toughness but does not lack of strength or stiffness.

Material resistance to rapid propagation of cracks called toughness and it is an inherent material property, which can be used for predicting structural performance [6].

Fiber-reinforced composite (FRC) restoration has been introduced to increase durability in composite restoration, enhance composite stiffness, and provide better force distribution along fibers. FRC development has increased the use of composite resin materials in extensive preparations [7].

Due to the mode of failure of composite and weakened walls in ETT, it is advised to insert fibers against the cavity walls to avoid failure. New techniques and materials help the practitioner to solve old problems from a different perspective and achieve innovative and unique solutions [8].

This article describes a clinical approach in the reconstruction of ETT posterior teeth in two cases by direct fiber-reinforced composite (FRC) restoration, as well as critical discussion of the advantages and disadvantages.

2. Case Report

A 23-year-old male patient presented with an endodontically treated first right upper molar with two weeks delay after completing endodontic therapy. The second case was a 35-year-old female that had root canal therapy on the upper left first molar after 3 weeks delay after RCT (Figure 1). Preapical radiographies of the upper first molar of these two cases after root canal therapy are seen in Figure 2.

Because the whole cavosurface margins were on the enamel, it was explained to the patient that the treatment plan of choice was the placement of an indirect ceramic onlay. Alternatively, because of the intact mesial marginal ridge, a direct cuspal coverage restoration with resin composite could be an option. After discussing the treatment plan with the patient for both direct and indirect restorations and getting an informed consent, fiber-reinforced direct composite (FRCDC) restoration was selected for the upper first molars due to the financial issues.

It was decided to follow the six-step stress-reduced direct composite (SRDC) Protocol from Deliperi et al. [8, 9].

The first step for SRDC protocol is "Analysis of the occlusion" to avoid either overloading or lack of centric stops in occlusal area. So preoperative occlusal analysis was done and showed even distribution of the occlusal load on the whole of residual tissue of tooth #16; thus, we decided not to reduce mesiofacial and mesiopalatal cusps.

The second step is "Cavity Preparation and Caries Removal End Points". Thus existing temporary restoration was removed using #2 and #4 round burs (Tizkavan, Iran). The cavity was prepared in a very conservative manner, being sure to remove all the decayed dental tissue and trying to preserve the remaining sound tooth structure as much as possible according to the basic guidelines for direct minimally invasive dentistry. Residual sharp angles and unsupported enamel were smoothed. No bevels were placed on the occlusal and gingival margins (Figure 3). The main goals of step 2 were to avoid the formation of any sharp line angle

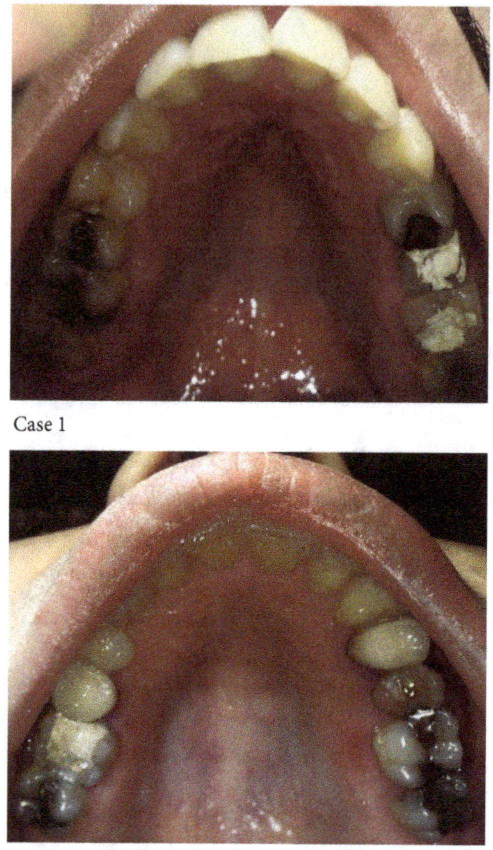

Case 1

Case 2

FIGURE 1: Preoperative view of tooth #16 and #26 with temporary restoration after root canal therapy.

on either the prepared enamel or dentin and to preserve the peripheral rim for bonding.

In the third step, "Analysis of Residual Tooth Structure" was done. Once the preparation was complete, it was determined that the distolingual cusp was unsupported. However, the thickness of the residual facial walls was greater than 2 mm, and the preservation of the entire mesial marginal ridge was sufficient to support an FR-SRDC restoration.

For the fourth step, we "Prepare the Dental Substrate to Achieve a Reliable Bond to Enamel and Dentin". A Tofflemire Matrix Retainer and band were placed around teeth #16 and #26, using a wooden wedge and burnishing the metal matrix provided good adaptation to the gingival margin. Isolation was provided by means of cotton roll and suction. The tooth was etched for 15 seconds using a 37% phosphoric acid (Meta etchant, Bio Med, Korea). The etchant was removed, and the cavity was rinsed with water for 30 seconds, being careful to maintain a moist surface. A two-step etch and rinse ethanol-based adhesive system (adper single bond 2, 3M ESPE, USA) was placed in the preparation and gently air thinned and light cured for 20 seconds using an LED curing light (woodi pecker, China).

For "Control of Polymerization Stresses" in the fifth step, the missing peripheral tooth structure was reconstructed with the 2 mm wedge-shaped composite increments. Filtek Z250 (3M ESPE, USA) microhybrid composite resin was used

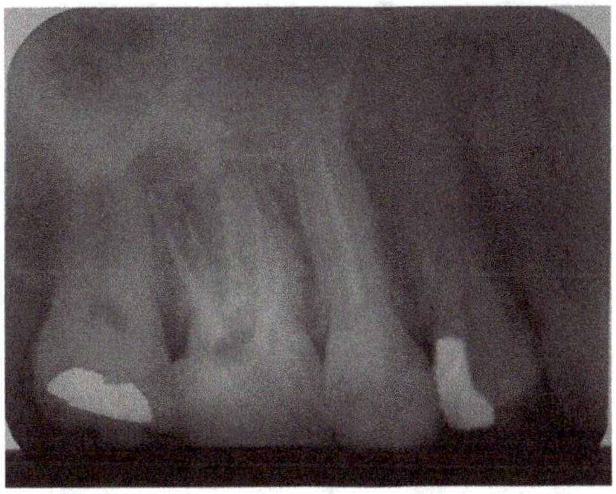

Case 1

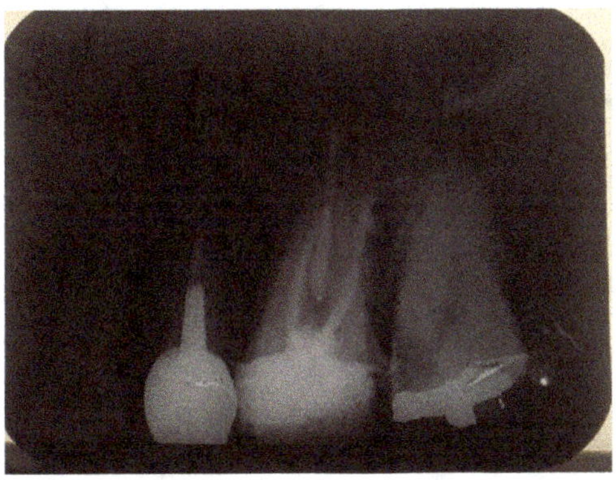

Case 2

FIGURE 2: Preapical radiographic of #16 and #26 teeth after root canal therapy.

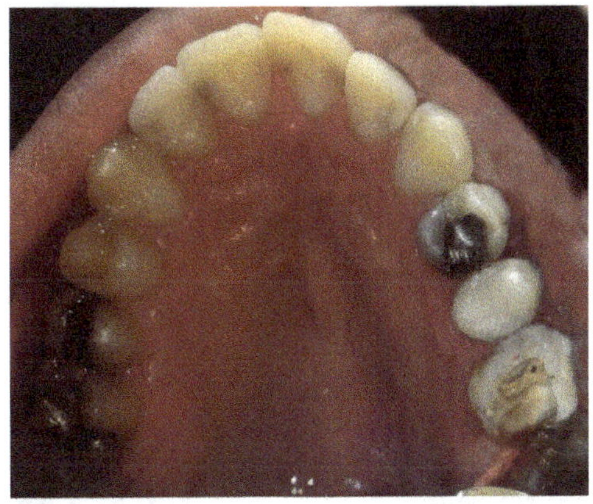

Case 1

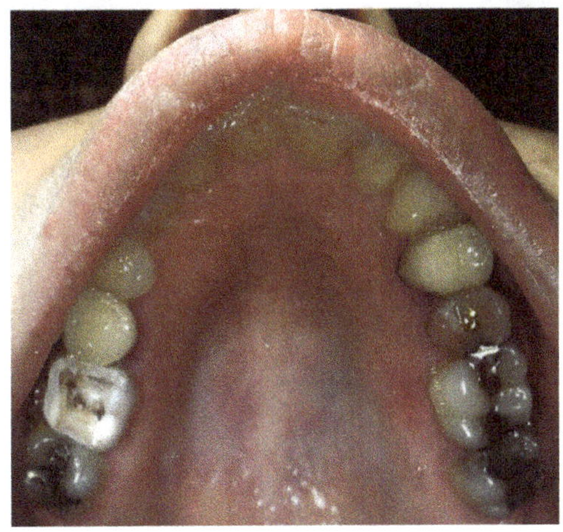

Case 2

FIGURE 3: Occlusal view of #16 and #26 after removing temporary restoration.

to restore the distal marginal ridge (Red Arrow in Figure 4). Filtek Z250 A3 shade was used to build up the cervical third of both the distopalatal and distal surfaces of the tooth. The rest of the distal surface and distopalatal wall was completed using the Filtek Z250 A2 shade in order to make two-third of the reconstruction lighter than the gingival part. Then, matrix retainer, band, and wedges are removed.

(1) The sixth step followed by "Wallpapering Dentin Walls with Polyethylene Fiber Strands" was done by the selecting of the correct length and width of the fibers. For measuring the accurate length of the fiber, a dental probe (Hu-Friedy, Chicago, IL, USA) was used to measure the mesiodistal distance of cavity walls. Two preimpregnated glass fiber (Interlik, Angelus, Brazil) strand pieces (4 mm wide and 11 mm length) were cut. Fibers can be cut with a microtome and low-speed cutting machine but, in this case, they were cut with bistoury and no. 11 blade. The cutting edge of the blade was placed in a perpendicular direction to the fibers and with the almost heavy pressure without very much back and forward movements. Fibers were covered with a very thin layer of a flowable composite (Filtek Bulk Fill, 3M ESPE, USA); prior to insertion into the cavity, they were precontoured c-shaped and then carried into the cavity by cotton plier, and fitted into the cavity walls properly with thin composite spatule, bonded, and cured for 20 seconds. (Blue Arrow in Figure 4). They were placed one after the other as described; if two fibers were placed simultaneously, the adaptation to the cavity wall and exact position may be compromised. At the proximal surfaces, the fiber strands overlapped each other. They were placed to the buccal and palatal wall and their extension to the proximal surface overlapped each other approximately 1 to 1.5 mm

(2) The key point of reducing polymerization shrinkage stress on the residual weakened walls is decreasing the composite volume between the fibers and tooth structure which is gained by tight adaptation of fibers to the tooth structure. 2 fibers were used in this case because it was decided to splint buccal and palatal cusps together. There are some techniques in the literature using fiber strands inside the composite body, but we choose just 2 fibers for cross splinting

After that restoration process, "Dentin and Occlusal Surface Buildup" was done. Due to the stress absorbing effect

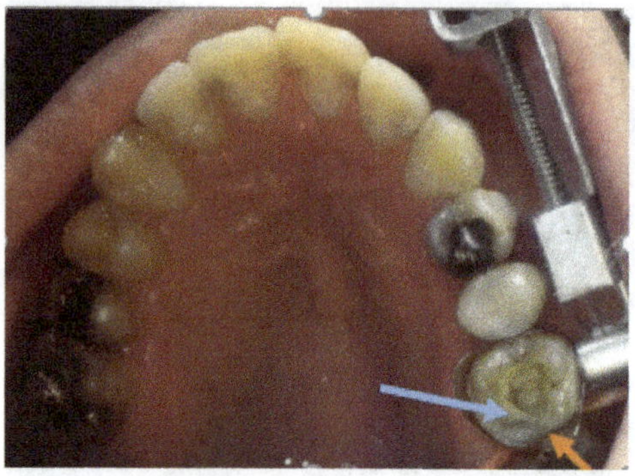

Case 1

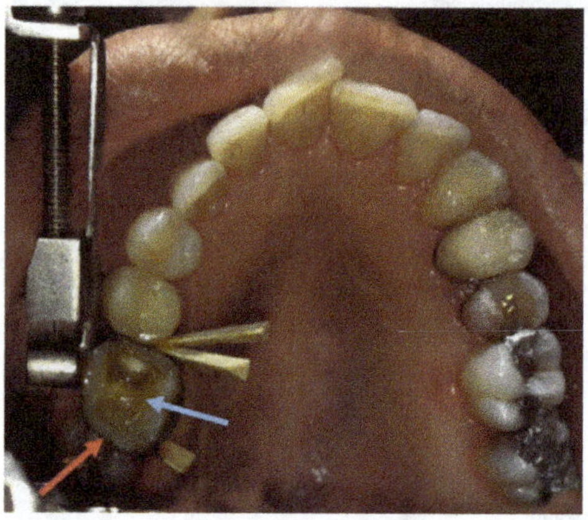

Case 2

FIGURE 4: Peripheral enamel skeleton was built up in the distal part (Red Arrow) using wedge-shaped increments and placing appropriate length fiber in close contact with a palatal cusp (Blue Arrow).

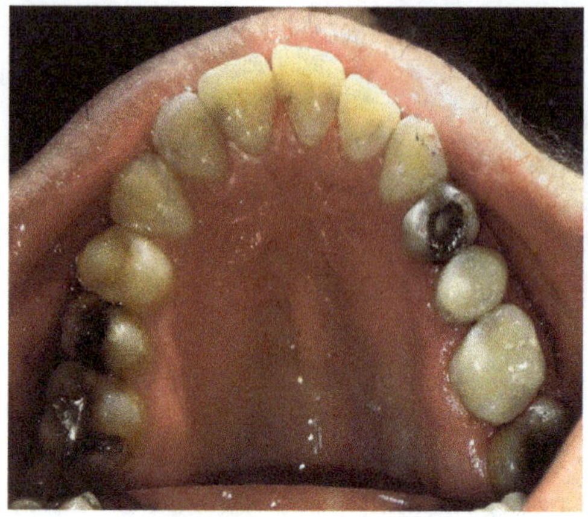

Case 1

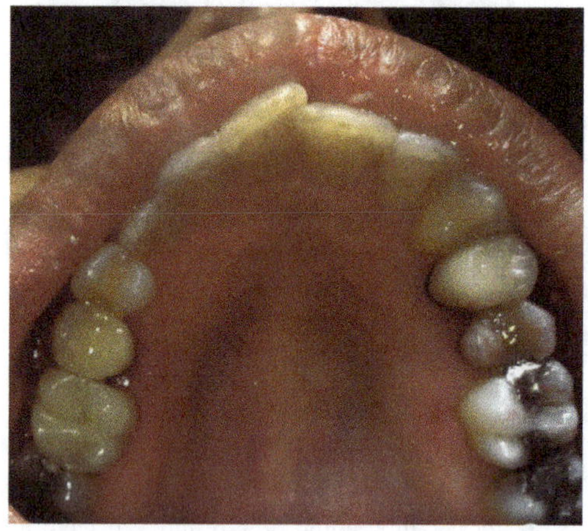

Case 2

FIGURE 5: Composite buildup of #16 and #26 teeth.

of the fiber strands, a 2 mm thick dentin wedge-shaped increments layers of composite resin was placed into contact with the fiber strand in order to decrease the C-factor ratio. Single increments of A2 shade of Filtek Z250 were applied to each cusp separately, achieving the final occlusal morphology (Figure 5). Postcuring done by irradiating the restored tooth through the facial and palatal surface for 30 s each to complete polymerization.

Finishing was done by diamond finishing bur, and polishing was followed by moulets (Shofu dental, Japan).

Finally, "Occlusal Force Equilibration" performed by occlusal adjustment by locating centric stops on the tooth structure and composite resin simultaneously and by the same intensity to prevent excessive forces and also like the adjacent teeth.

3. Discussion

One of the dentistry challenges is the coronal restoration of root filled posterior teeth. The ideal technique for restoration for ETT is still a debate. Loss of dentine structure is the main factor that has an effect on the survival rate of pulpless teeth [10]. Indirect restoration is considered the treatment of choice in endodontically treated teeth (ETT) for many years. Amalgam builds up and post and cores and crown are being replaced by direct composite and glass-fiber posts, in addition to fiber reinforce composite resin and all ceramic crowns are being often chosen because of their superior aesthetic outcome and avoiding problems like root perforation, more loss of sound tooth structure, and invasiveness of such treatments.

This method has advantages like more fracture resistance and less polymerization shrinkage than composite buildup. But in practice, it is not easy to adapt fibers in precise position on cavity walls and also provide complete isolation and also need more chair time.

Amalgam has been used in direct cusp capping of posterior teeth in the past, and studies have been shown an acceptable long-term survival rate for large amalgam restorations [11].

Tooth strengthening is also the purpose of restoration besides tooth repair.

It seems that the reinforcement of residual tooth structure is possible with modern adhesive systems and composite resins [4]. Functional stresses could be better distributed along the interface of bonding. In addition, with the use of bonded restorations, a more sound tooth structure would be preserved and fracture resistance be increased [12]. But several clinical studies are needed to evaluate the bond durability of these restorations over time [9].

Due to the polymerization shrinkage which is the main drawback of direct composite restorations, dentists may encounter many problems in selecting these restorations [13]. However, Stress Reduced Direct Composite (SRDC) technique could be considered as an alternative to indirect restorations [8].

Although resin-based composites (RBCs) were showing loss of anatomical shape and marginal breakdown in the past, they exhibit more wear resistant and better mechanical characteristics now. Current direct composite restoration wear rate is 10 to 15 μm per year [14].

In order to improve the inherent deficiencies of RBCs, the use of fibers in combination with resin composite in restoring ETT that are structurally compromised, consider as a promising treatment [15]. Fiber Reinforced Composite (FRC) restorations would change the dynamics of stresses at the interface of restoration and tooth. Fracture toughness and flexural strength of RBCs increase with fiber insertion. Fiber design makes a network that leads to a rapid crack growth stopping mechanism [16].

In this case, pieces of fibers were used circumferentially in the closest distance of vertical facial and palatal walls of residual tissue of the teeth and the composite buildup. Belli and others showed that fracture strength increased and cusp movement decrease if fibers were placed against the dentinal wall. It was described also that fibers have influenced in lowering C-factor and enhancing microtensile bond strength [17].

The first step in this case composite buildup was making peripheral skeleton in missing distal marginal ridge to transform multisurface to class I cavity. It can help to reach smooth surface restoration without excess in margins [18].

Wedge-shaped increments are essential for compensating stress from polymerization shrinkage. In fact, the goal of multiple wedge-shaped increments technique is decreasing C-factor by trying no more than two bonded cavity walls at a time [8]. The wallpapering technique which uses fibers circumferentially in contact with vertical walls could absorb lateral forces that are created during occlusal vertical loading. Therefore, decrease failures or if failures happen, the damage is not catastrophic and in most cases is reparable. Higher risk for catastrophic failure will exist if the remaining cavity walls become thinner than 2 mm [19].

In a study done by Kuijs and colleagues, it was shown that there is a comparable failure mode in direct and indirect composite resin restorations regarding fracture [20].

Even ceramic restorations have some issues besides being costly and time-consuming than direct composite restorations. Internal fitness and tooth preparation design play an important role in the success of them and also resin cement wear is another concern that occurs in ceramic restorations [21].

Precise evaluation of patients' criteria is mandatory for selecting the wallpapering technique as an acceptable treatment plan. Parafunctional habits and heavy occlusion make this treatment inappropriate [22].

In the following session after one and half year, no recurrent caries, chipping, or fracture was seen. However, more long-term in vitro and clinical studies are necessary for supporting this type of treatment plan.

4. Conclusion

One visit treatment, preservation of sound tooth structure and reduced cost, make RFC restoration an acceptable treatment for ETT reconstruction. It seems that in special cases, minimally invasive treatment could be considered as an alternative for indirect restorations.

Additional Points

Clinical Relevance. Endodontically treated tooth could benefit from proper use of fibers reinforced composite restoration in some special clinical situations. It not only has acceptable performance but also delaying or preventing complex indirect restorations.

References

[1] S. Deliperi, "Direct fiber-reinforced composite restoration in an endodontically-treated molar: a three-year case report," *Operative Dentistry*, vol. 33, no. 2, pp. 209–214, 2008.

[2] S. Deliperi, N. David, D. N. Bardwell, and C. Coiana, "Reconstruction of devital teeth using direct fiber-reinforced composite resins: a case report," *Journal of Adhesive Dentistry*, vol. 7, no. 2, pp. 165–171, 2005.

[3] C. P. Ernst, G. R. Meyer, J. Müller, E. Stender, M. O. Ahlers, and B. Willershausern, "Depth of cure of LED vs QTH light-curing devices at a distance of 7 mm," *The Journal of Adhesive Dentistry*, vol. 6, no. 2, pp. 141–150, 2004.

[4] S. Belli, A. Erdemir, M. Ozcopur, and G. Eskitascioglu, "The effect of fibre insertion on fracture resistance of root filled molar teeth with MOD preparations restored with composite," *International Endodontic Journal*, vol. 38, no. 2, pp. 73–80, 2005.

[5] C. J. Soares, M. d. P. Rodrigues, A. L. Faria-e-Silva et al., "How biomechanics can affect the endodontic treated teeth and their restorative procedures?," *Brazilian Oral Research*, vol. 32, article e76, Supplement 1, 2018.

[6] G. T. Rocca and I. Krejci, "Crown and post-free adhesive restorations for endodontically treated posterior teeth: from direct composite to endocrowns," *The European Journal of Esthetic Dentistry*, vol. 8, no. 2, pp. 156–179, 2013.

[7] S. Deliperi and D. N. Bardwell, "Reconstruction of nonvital teeth using direct fiber-reinforced composite resin: a pilot clinical study," *The Journal of Adhesive Dentistry*, vol. 11, no. 1, pp. 71–78, 2009.

[8] S. Deliperi, D. Alleman, and D. Rudo, "Stress-reduced direct composites for the restoration of structurally compromised teeth: fiber design according to the "wallpapering" technique," *Operative Dentistry*, vol. 42, no. 3, pp. 233–243, 2017.

[9] S. Deliperi, D. N. Bardwell, and D. Alleman, "Clinical evaluation of stress-reducing direct composite restorations in structurally compromised molars: a 2-year report," *Operative Dentistry*, vol. 37, no. 2, pp. 109–116, 2012.

[10] J. A. Skupien, "Endodontically Treated Teeth," *Success and Failure from a Restorative Perspective*, [S.l. : s.n.], 2016, (Doctoral Dissertation).

[11] R. J. Smales and W. S. Hawthorne, "Long-term survival and cost-effectiveness of five dental restorative materials used in

various classes of cavity preparations," *International Dental Journal*, vol. 46, no. 3, pp. 126–130, 1996.

[12] S. Deliperi, "Functional and aesthetic guidelines for stress-reduced direct posterior composite restorations," *Operative Dentistry*, vol. 37, no. 4, pp. 425–431, 2012.

[13] A. Pahlevan, M. H. Tabatabaei, S. Arami, and S. Valizadeh, "Effect of LED and argon laser on degree of conversion and temperature rise of hybrid and low shrinkage composite resins," *The Open Dentistry Journal*, vol. 10, no. 1, pp. 538–545, 2016.

[14] S. Deliperi, "Clinical evaluation of nonvital tooth whitening and composite resin restorations: five-year results," *The European Journal of Esthetic Dentistry*, vol. 3, no. 2, pp. 148–159, 2008.

[15] S. Garoushi, A. Gargoum, P. K. Vallittu, and L. Lassila, "Short fiber-reinforced composite restorations: a review of the current literature," *Journal of Investigative and Clinical Dentistry*, vol. 9, no. 3, article e12330, 2018.

[16] H. Abouelleil, N. Pradelle, C. Villat, N. Attik, P. Colon, and B. Grosgogeat, "Comparison of mechanical properties of a new fiber reinforced composite and bulk filling composites," *Restorative Dentistry & Endodontics*, vol. 40, no. 4, pp. 262–270, 2015.

[17] S. Belli, N. Dönmez, and G. Eskitascioğlu, "The effect of c-factor and flowable resin or fiber use at the interface on micro-tensile bond strength to dentin," *The Journal of Adhesive Dentistry*, vol. 8, no. 4, pp. 247–253, 2006.

[18] R. de Souza Ferreira, G. Carpena Lopes, and L. Narcisco Baratieri, "Direct posterior resin composite restorations: considerations on finishing/polishing. Clinical procedures," *Quintessence International*, vol. 35, no. 5, pp. 359–366, 2004.

[19] S. Deliperi and D. N. Bardwell, "An alternative method to reduce polymerization shrinkage in direct posterior composite restorations," *The Journal of the American Dental Association*, vol. 133, no. 10, pp. 1387–1398, 2002.

[20] R. H. Kuijs, W. M. M. Fennis, C. M. Kreulen, F. J. M. Roeters, N. Verdonschot, and N. H. J. Creugers, "A comparison of fatigue resistance of three materials for cusp-replacing adhesive restorations," *Journal of Dentistry*, vol. 34, no. 1, pp. 19–25, 2006.

[21] R. E. Campos, P. V. Soares, A. Versluis, O. B. de O Júnior, G. M. B. Ambrosano, and I. F. Nunes, "Crown fracture: Failure load, stress distribution, and fractographic analysis," *The Journal of Prosthetic Dentistry*, vol. 114, no. 3, pp. 447–455, 2015.

[22] S. Deliperi and D. N. Bardwell, "Direct cuspal-coverage posterior resin composite restorations: a case report," *Operative Dentistry*, vol. 31, no. 1, pp. 143–150, 2006.

23

Conservative Therapy of External Invasive Cervical Resorption with Adhesive Systems: A 6-Year Follow-Up Case Report and Literature Review

Riccardo Aiuto,[1] Gianluca Fumei,[2] Erica Lipani,[3] Daniele Garcovich,[3] Mario Dioguardi,[4] and Dino Re[1]

[1]*Department of Biomedical, Surgical and Dental Sciences, Istituto Stomatologico Italiano, University of Milan, Milan, Italy*
[2]*Department of Restorative Dentistry and Endodontics, University of Insubria, Varese, Italy*
[3]*Department of Dentistry, Universidad Europea de Valencia, Valencia, Spain*
[4]*Department of Clinical and Experimental Medicine, University of Foggia, Foggia, Italy*

Correspondence should be addressed to Erica Lipani; erica.lipani@outlook.it

Academic Editor: Hamdi Cem Gungor

The diagnosis and treatment of external invasive cervical resorption (EICR) could be a challenging clinical situation even for the most experienced dentists. It is a fairly rare lesion and a poorly understood phenomenon, and its insidious and aggressive nature can lead to tooth loss. Even in the era of dental implants, trying to save a compromised tooth is imperative for any clinician. This report presents a case of an upper central incisor with a class II Heithersay EICR in which treatment was performed using a multidisciplinary approach and the defect was restored with resin composite. The surgery in which the defect was exposed and repaired was followed by an endodontic treatment and the placement of a fiber-reinforced post. In this case, the use of modern materials, such as resin composites, allowed not only the avoidance of tooth extraction but also the achievement of satisfactory aesthetic results. The 6-year follow-up demonstrated the success of therapy and the resolution of clinical symptoms. This case report highlights the importance of early detection of EICR and how composite resins could provide an effective and aesthetic restauration of the defect, which favors the health of the surrounding gingival tissue.

1. Introduction

Root resorption is characterized by the loss of tooth hard tissues; this process can be physiological if it occurs during teething, but it is a pathological if it occurs in the permanent dentition, producing irreversible damage and/or potential tooth loss [1]. Root resorption may be classified, according to the location on the root surface, into external resorption (if it starts from the periodontal tissue) and internal resorption (if it starts from the pulp tissue). Furthermore, external root resorption can also be divided into superficial resorption, external inflammatory resorption, external invasive cervical resorption (EICR), external replacement resorption, and transient apical breakdown [2].

EICR is a clinical term used to describe a rare condition whose prevalence ranges from 0.02 to 2.3% [3] but often leads to tooth loss as a result of its insidious and asymptomatic nature [4]; the lesion may become symptomatic in advanced cases when pulp tissue is involved [5].

The lesion is characterized by a cervical location and an invasive nature. The resorptive process begins on the surface of the root below the epithelial attachment, namely, the connective tissue attachment zone [6]. Several clinical classifications were introduced to assist the clinician in treatment planning. The Heithersay classification [7] was the first to be developed, but despite its great usefulness, it relied on a two-dimensional radiograph that cannot guarantee a detailed assessment of a three-dimensional lesion. Patel et al. has

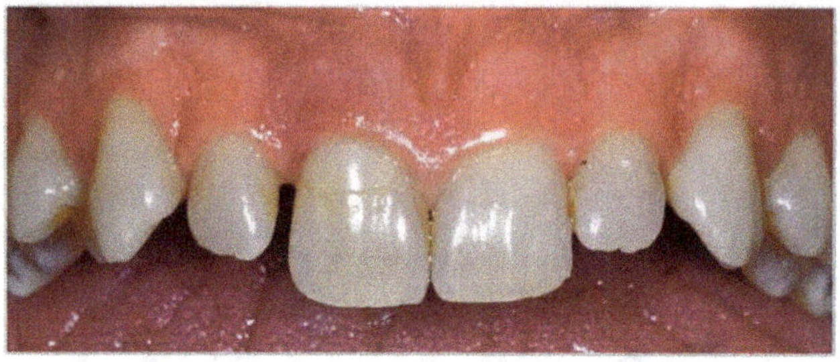

Figure 1: Preoperative clinical condition.

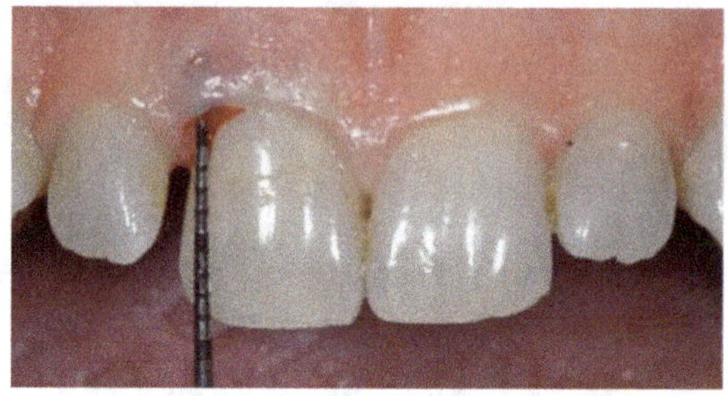

Figure 2: Bleeding on probing exam.

recently introduced a three-dimensional classification [8]. This new classification aims to provide a more accurate estimate of the preoperative EICR condition using cone beam computed tomography (CBCT) imaging.

The etiology of EICR is complex and unclear; several factors are potentially involved, such as a history of trauma, intracoronal bleaching, orthodontic treatment, and periodontal root planning or scaling [3].

A correct diagnosis of EICR, based on a clinical and radiological examination, is an essential prerequisite for its successful treatment. Several materials have been proposed in the literature to restore the defect. In the past, in these cases, amalgam [9] and glass ionomer [7] were widely used. Currently, an approach based on biocompatible materials is preferred, such as MTA (Dentsply-Tulsa Dental, Johnson City, TN, USA) [10] or Biodentine (Septodont, Saint-Maur-des-Fossés, France) [11], and materials with high aesthetic properties, such as composite resins [12]. In the last few years, there has been a growing interest in the treatment of EICR, perhaps due to the increased use of CBCT in endodontics or also due to the aggressive and invasive nature of this type of lesion. This case report aims to illustrate the effects of a multidisciplinary approach and the use of composite resin as a restorative material in EICR.

2. Case Report

A 38-year-old male who attended the University Department of the Istituto Stomatologico Italiano (ISI) referred a slight pain during brushing of the upper left central incisor (1.1). The patient reported a good level of general health, and a detailed anamnesis did not report a history of trauma or other relevant problems. During clinical examination, a class V composite restoration was observed in the cervical third of 1.1. In the same area, the presence of bleeding on probing (Figures 1 and 2) indicated a relevant gingival inflammation. The tooth was negative to the pulp sensitivity thermal test.

To confirm suspicion of EICR, a radiographic examination was also realized; first of all, a periapical radiograph was performed and showed the presence of a radiolucent lesion in the coronal third of the root of 1.1, in its distal portion (Figure 3(a)). However, in this case, CBCT imaging was essential to assess the stage of the lesion and which structures were compromised (Figure 3(b)). 3D images revealed that the lesion had already penetrated close to the coronal pulp, but it appears that there was no communication. Considering the clinical and radiological findings, the resorptive defect was classified as a Heithersay class II.

Due to the importance of saving a natural tooth and the aesthetic value of a central incisor, all treatment options were discussed with the patient, and finally, the external approach was chosen. That included a surgical phase, endodontic treatment, and finally replacement of the previous restoration. The informed consent form was obtained from the patient prior to the beginning of treatment.

The main phases of the clinical procedure are reported as follows.

2.1. First Session: Surgical Step. The complexity of this pathology requires the use of an operating microscope and the exposition of the defect by a surgical flap. After administering local anesthesia (articaine 4% with epinephrine 1 : 100,000, Pierrel, Capua, Italy), a full thickness flap was performed (Figure 4(a)). Once the defect was exposed, the resorptive granulation tissue was accurately removed, and the site was debrided and cleaned with surgical straight handpieces (Ultimate Power+, B.A. International, Fiumana, Italy) and with a round tungsten carbide ball bur. Once hemostasis was managed, isolation with a liquid rubber dam was obtained (Figure 4(b))), and common steps were followed for composite restoration.

First, a dentin etching was performed for 15 seconds with 37% phosphoric acid, and a two-step bonding system (Scotchbond Universal Adhesive, 3M Company, St. Paul, MN, USA) was applied and light cured for 40 seconds. Subsequently, the defect was filled and restored with flowable composite (Filtek™ Universal Restorative, 3M Company, St. Paul, MN, USA), and the restoration was accurately finished and polished (Figure 4(c))). Finally, the flap was repositioned with interrupted 4\0 silk suture (Perma-Hand™, Ethicon Inc., Johnson & Johnson Company, Somerville, NJ, USA; Figure 4(d)). Ice application was recommended, and a twice-daily oral rinse with 0.20% chlorhexidine was prescribed during the 7 days after surgery.

2.2. Second Session: Endodontic Step. Due to the negative pulp response, endodontic treatment was required. In this appointment, soft tissue healing was checked, sutures were removed, and root canal therapy was performed.

First, local anesthesia (articaine 4% with epinephrine 1 : 100,000, Pierrel) was administered, and a rubber dam (Nic Tone, Manufacturera Dental Continental S.A. De C.V., Zapopan, Mexico) isolation was placed (Figure 5(b))

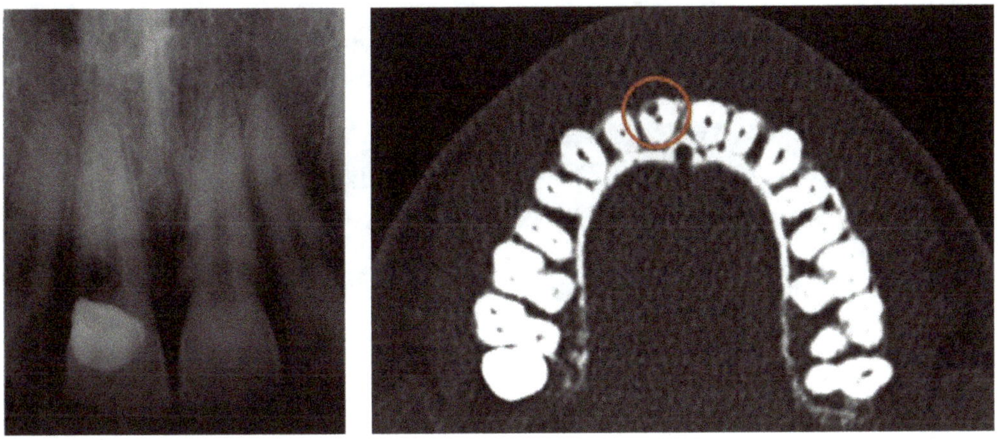

(a) (b)

FIGURE 3: (a) Preoperative periapical X-ray and (b) preoperative CBCT.

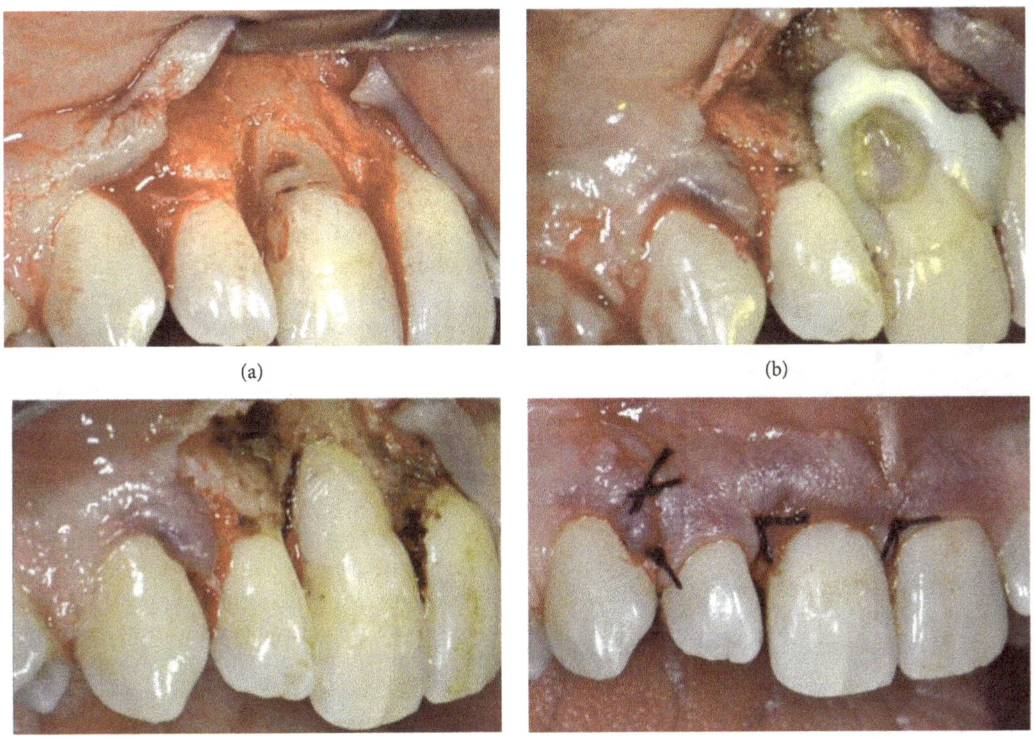

(a) (b) (c) (d)

FIGURE 4: Phases of surgery: (a) defect exposition by surgical flap, (b) isolation by liquid rubber dam, (c) composite restoration of the defect, and (d) repositioning and suture of the flap.

with a 9 clamp (Ivory®, Kulzer Nordic AB, Helsingborg, Sweden) fixed on tooth 1.1. The cleaning and shaping of the root canal were carried out with a rotary file (ProTaper Gold, Dentsply Maillefer, Ballaigues, Switzerland), 5% NaOCl irrigation (NICLOR 5, OGNA, Muggiò, Milan, Italy), and 17% EDTA (OGNA, Muggiò).

In Figure 5(a), it is possible to appreciate the characteristic grey color of a necrotic pulp tissue. After drying the canal with paper points, the root canal was filled with a 40# ProTaper Gold master cone and cement (AH Plus®, Dentsply Sirona, Lancaster, A, USA) using the continuous wave of condensation technique. Once the canal was definitely filled, the post space was realized, and a fiber-reinforced post was subsequently inserted. Postoperative X-ray was performed (Figure 6).

2.3. Third Session: Restorative Step. The patient was recalled after 3 months. On clinical examination, the periodontal probing revealed healthy periodontal tissues, without bleeding and a probing depth of less than 3 mm. The class V restoration was replaced, on the patient's request. Rubber dam

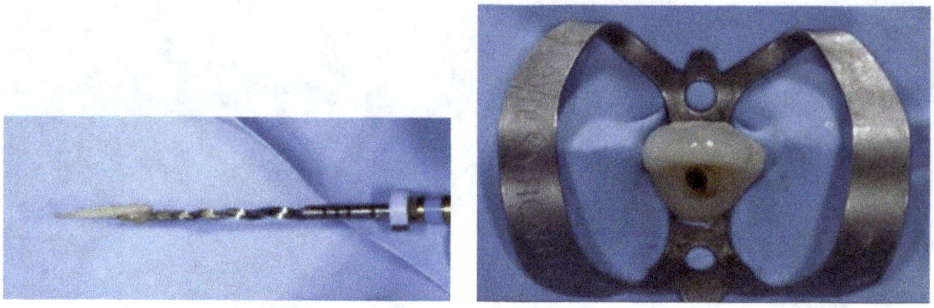

(a) (b)

Figure 5: (a) Necrotic pulp tissue and (b) rubber dam isolation.

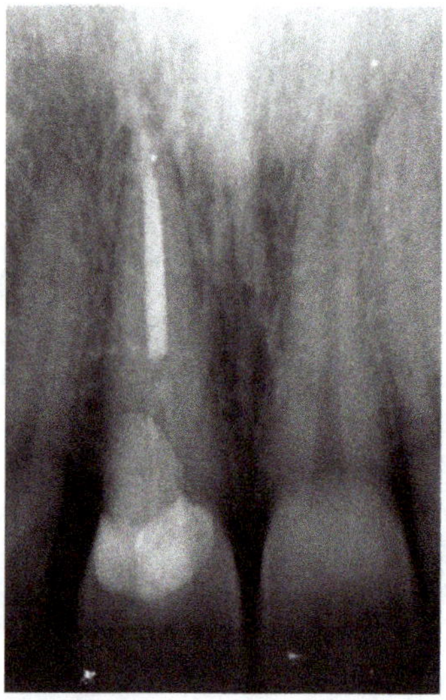

Figure 6: Postoperative X-ray of root canal treatment.

isolation was placed with No. 9 clamp on tooth 1.1 and No. 0 clamp on tooth 2.5 (Figure 7(a)).

The old resin restoration was removed, and total acid etching was performed for 20 seconds (Figure 7(b)). Then, a two-step bonding system (Scotchbond Universal Adhesive, 3M Company) was applied to the cavity (Figure 7(c)). The cavity was filled with resin composite (Filtek Z500, 3M Company), and finally, the restoration was polished and finished (Figure 7(d)).

Subsequently, the patient received monitoring visits during which clinical examination, and radiographs were performed; follow-up has been carried out, respectively, after 1, 2, and 3 year, and at each appointment, a periapical radiograph was taken (Figure 8).

Six years later, the patient was checked again, and the 6-year follow-up confirmed the treatment success; indeed, as is apparent in Figure 9, it showed that the absence of sign of gingival inflammation, no bleeding on probing, the absence of periodontal pocket, complete remission of symptoms, and the X-ray examination indicated that no bone loss occurred.

3. Discussion

Diagnosis is a key step when facing an insidious lesion, such as EICR; clinician may initially be disorientated, since a radiolucent image on the X-ray could be misdiagnosed as a subgingival caries. However, there are some distinctive features that allow the clinician to establish a differential diagnosis: a carious lesion in a healthy periodontium does not usually present bleeding on probing, which is usually observed instead in the case of EICR due to the high vascularization of the granulation tissue [6]; moreover, there is a typical pinkish discoloration (pathognomonic clinical sign) of the crown in the cervical region of the affected tooth, and in addition, the resorbed area produces a scraping sound on probing giving the feeling of hard tissue, quite different from the one that characterizes the softened dentine [7].

The introduction of CBCT imaging in dentistry, especially in endodontics, plays an important role in the diagnosis and management of pathologies, such as EICR; however, considering that the patient's radiation exposure should be kept "as low as reasonably achievable," the use of CBCT imaging should be limited to the cases in which the information gathered by conventional imaging systems is not enough.

At present, CBCT imaging has been recommended for the planning of endodontic surgery treatment [13–15]; indeed only with a 3D imaging, the clinician can assess the exact location and extension of the lesion, and therefore its real restorability. Furthermore, the increased precision of the CBCT imaging can also result in early detection of EICR and, in these cases, is of great importance [16, 17].

As previously reported, in the present case report, the treatment of a Heithersay class II lesion was performed. The Heithersay classification was the first developed, in which EICR lesions were classified into four classes according to the size and extension of the defect into dentine: from a small resorptive lesion in the cervical area (Class I) to an extensive resorptive defect beyond the coronal third of the root (Class IV) [3].

Depending on the severity and type of injury, the treatment plan will radically change from an external approach to an internal approach, up to orthodontic extrusion or, in some cases, even tooth extraction. Today, there are no clear treatment guidelines for EICR, and for this reason, clinical classifications, such as the Heithersay class I, are so useful. However, this classification was developed on two-dimensional images, which could offer an underestimated representation of the real situation. To overcome this

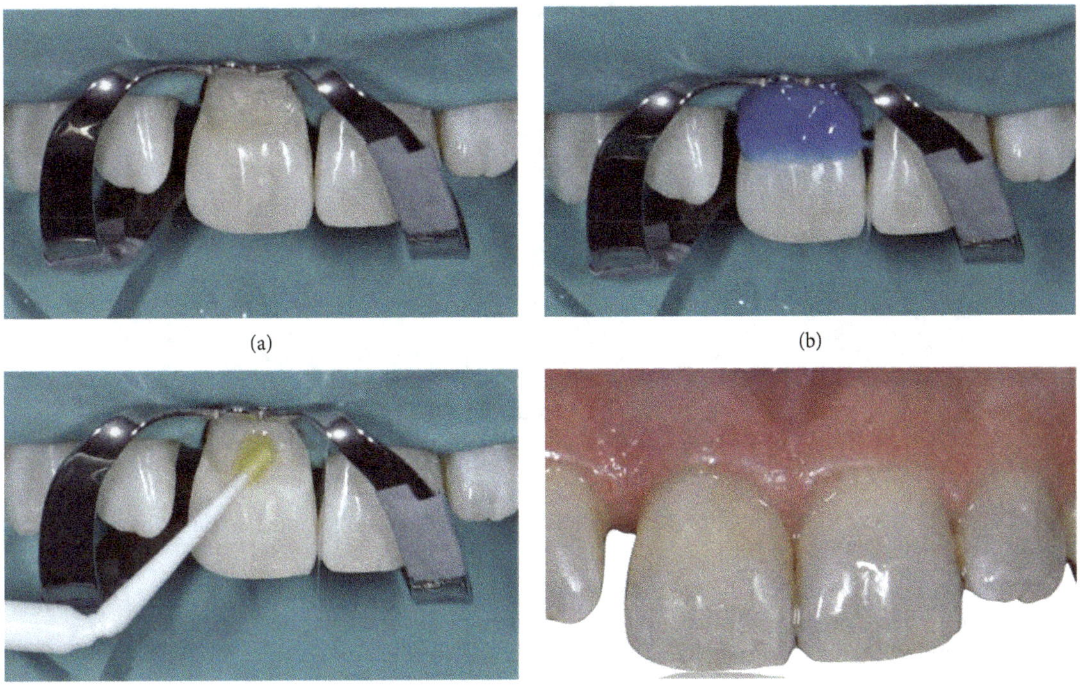

(a) (b) (c) (d)

FIGURE 7: Phases of class V restoration: (a) rubber dam isolation, (b) enamel total acid etching, (c) bonding agent application, and (d) final restoration results.

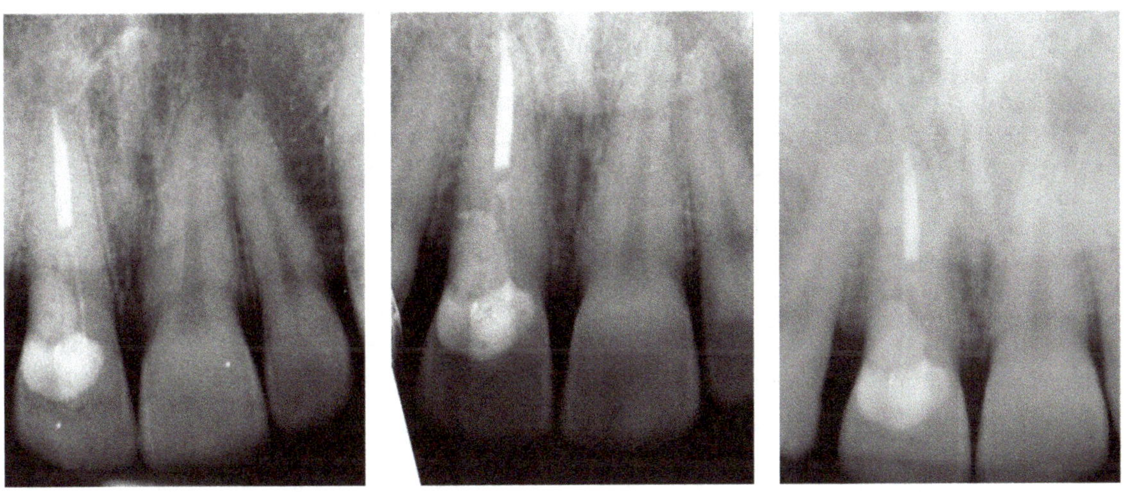

(a) (b) (c)

FIGURE 8: X-ray at (a) 1-year, (b) 2-year, and (c) 3-year follow-ups.

limitation, Patel et al. introduced a three-dimensional classification based on CBCT findings [8]. Three parameters were considered in this new classification: lesion height (1: at CEJ level or coronal to the bone crest (supracrestal), 2: extends into the coronal third of the root and apical to the bone crest (subcrestal), 3: extends into the middle third of the root, and 4: extends into the apical third of the root), circumferential spread (*A*: ≤90°, *B*: ≤180°, *C*: ≤270°, and *D*: >270°), and proximity to the root canal (d: lesion confined to dentine and p: probable pulpal involvement) [8]. Following these parameters, it is possible to classify EICR defects in three dimensions, thus improving communication between colleagues, prognostic, and treatment outcomes.

A careful removal of the resorptive tissue and thorough root canal cleaning [18] are absolutely necessary to guarantee a successful treatment outcome; regarding the restoration of the defect, as previously discussed, several materials have been proposed. Several studies have been conducted in recent years on the qualities and clinical performance of mineral trioxide aggregate "MTA" (Dentsply-Tulsa Dental); many favorable properties were described, among the most important being biocompatibility and optimal tissue response [10, 19].

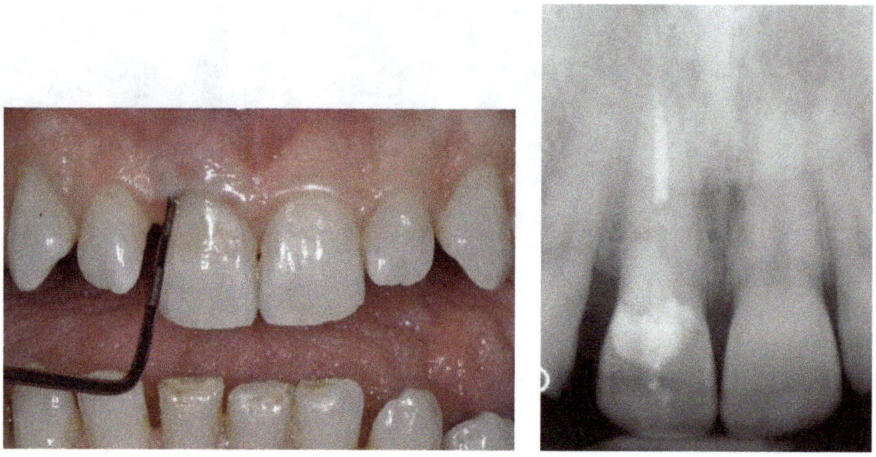

(a) (b)

Figure 9: (a) Probing and postoperative clinical condition and (b) X-ray at the 6-year follow-up.

Although several articles reported that Biodentine (Septodont), a calcium silicate-based product, has better physical properties (resistance and compressive strength) and handling properties than MTA, in fact, Biodentine was developed from MTA technology in order to improve some characteristics of these types of materials [11, 20].

Even if the efficacy of Biodentine and MTA is widely demonstrated, in this case report, composite resin (Filtek™ Universal Restorative, 3M Company) was preferred. Both the "white" and "pink" aesthetics of a smile are complex to imitate, especially if there is an impairment of the dental and periodontal tissues that entail the risk of losing a tooth in the aesthetic area [21]. However, modern composite resins offer a very satisfactory degree of integration when it is possible to restore the natural tooth. Adequate adhesive bond strength is ensured in root dentine by employing a proper self-etch adhesive system [12].

Additionally, composite resin has a faster setting time (20 seconds light-curing time) compared to the long setting time of the MTA. Moreover, the polishing of the restoration provides a smooth surface that prevents the accumulation of subgingival plaque, unlike the rough surface MTA. Although composite resins are not fully biologically acceptable for periodontal tissues, the "creeping attachment" described by Goldman and Cohen [22] develops, and coronal migration of gingival marginal tissue occurs [23]. In this case, the absence of gingival inflammation and the complete resolution of the symptoms support the clinical assessment of a new and healthy epithelial tissue gingival attachment.

4. Conclusions

Early detection of EICR lesion and an accurate endodontic and restorative treatment planning are paramount to achieve a favorable clinical outcome. This case report shows how accurate removal of resorption tissue followed by defect restoration with composite resins could be a good choice for EICR treatment in aesthetic zones. As reported, this treatment approach could result in a favorable periodontal tissue response. More research is needed to confirm the long-term outcome of this treatment modality.

References

[1] G. S. Heithersay, "External root resorption," *Annals of the Royal Australasian College of Dental Surgeons*, vol. 12, pp. 46–59, 1994.

[2] S. Patel, S. Kanagasingam, and F. T. Pitt, "External cervical resorption: a review," *Journal of Endodontia*, vol. 35, no. 5, pp. 616–625, 2009.

[3] G. Heithersay, "Invasive cervical resorption: an analysis of potential predisposing factors," *Quintessence International*, vol. 30, no. 2, pp. 83–95, 1999.

[4] O. Rotondi, P. K. S. Waldon, and S. G. Kim, "The disease process, diagnosis and treatment of invasive cervical resorption: a review," *Dental Journal*, vol. 8, no. 3, p. 64, 2020.

[5] H. M. Goldman, "Spontaneous intermittent resorption of teeth," *Journal of the American Dental Association*, vol. 49, no. 5, pp. 522–532, 1954.

[6] S. D. Kandalgaonkar, L. A. Gharat, S. D. Tupsakhare, and M. H. Gabhane, "Invasive cervical resorption: a review," *Journal of International Oral Health*, vol. 5, no. 6, pp. 124–130, 2013.

[7] G. Heithersay, "Invasive cervical resorption," *Endodontic Topics*, vol. 7, no. 1, pp. 73–92, 2004.

[8] S. Patel, F. Foschi, F. Mannocci, and K. Patel, "External cervical resorption: a three-dimensional classification," *International Endodontic Journal*, vol. 51, no. 2, pp. 206–214, 2018.

[9] G. Rabie, M. Trope, and L. Tronstad, "Treatment of a maxillary canine with external inflammatory root resorption," *Journal of Endodontia*, vol. 14, no. 2, pp. 101–105, 1988.

[10] C. J. White and N. Bryant, "Combined therapy of mineral trioxide aggregate and guided tissue regeneration in the treatment of external root resorption and an associated osseous defect," *Journal of Periodontology*, vol. 73, no. 12, pp. 1517–1521, 2002.

[11] Ö. Malkondu, M. K. Kazandağ, and E. Kazazoğlu, "A review on Biodentine, a contemporary dentine replacement and repair material," *BioMed Research International*, vol. 2014, p. 10, 2014.

[12] P. R. Pleffken, A. P. de Almeida Lourenço, C. R. Torres, and B. A. Bühler, "Influence of application methods of self-

etching adhesive systems on adhesive bond strength to dentin," *The Journal of Adhesive Dentistry*, vol. 13, no. 6, pp. 517–525, 2011.

[13] S. Patel, A. Dawood, T. P. Ford, and E. Whaites, "The potential applications of cone beam computed tomography in the management of endodontic problems," *International Endodontic Journal*, vol. 40, no. 10, pp. 818–830, 2007.

[14] S. Patel, "New dimensions in endodontic imaging: part 2. Cone beam computed tomography," *International Endodontic Journal*, vol. 42, no. 6, pp. 463–475, 2009.

[15] D. Vaz de Souza, E. Schirru, F. Mannocci, F. Foschi, and S. Patel, "External cervical resorption: a comparison of the diagnostic efficacy using 2 different cone-beam computed tomographic units and periapical radiographs," *Journal of Endodontia*, vol. 43, no. 1, pp. 121–125, 2017.

[16] T. Venskutonis, G. Plotino, G. Juodzbalys, and L. Mickevičiene, "The importance of cone-beam computed tomography in the management of endodontic problems: a review of the literature," *Journal of Endodontia*, vol. 40, no. 12, pp. 1895–1901, 2014.

[17] H. Ren, J. Chen, F. Deng, L. Zheng, X. Liu, and Y. Dong, "Comparison of cone-beam computed tomography and periapical radiography for detecting simulated apical root resorption," *The Angle Orthodontist*, vol. 83, no. 2, pp. 189–195, 2013.

[18] M. Dioguardi, V. Crincoli, D. Sovereto et al., "Effectiveness of vapor lock effect removal in endo training blocks: manual dynamic agitation versus passive ultrasonic irrigation," *Applied Sciences*, vol. 9, no. 24, p. 5411, 2019.

[19] M. Kuratate, K. Yoshiba, Y. Shigetani, N. Yoshiba, H. Ohshima, and T. Okiji, "Immunohistochemical analysis of nestin, osteopontin, and proliferating cells in the reparative process of exposed dental pulp capped with mineral trioxide aggregate," *Journal of Endodontia*, vol. 34, no. 8, pp. 970–974, 2008.

[20] L. Grech, B. Mallia, and J. Camilleri, "Investigation of the physical properties of tricalcium silicate cement-based root-end filling materials," *Dental Materials*, vol. 29, no. 2, pp. e20–e28, 2013.

[21] R. Crippa, R. Aiuto, M. Dioguardi, M. Peñarrocha-Diago, M. Peñarrocha-Diago, and F. Angiero, "Laser therapy for infected sites and immediate dental implants in the esthetic zone: a case report and review of literature," *Case Reports in Dentistry*, vol. 2020, 2020.

[22] H. M. Goldman and D. W. Cohen, *Periodontal Therapy*, Mosby, St. Louis, Mo, USA, 5th edition, 1973.

[23] L. A. Bell, T. A. Valluzzo, J. J. Garnick, and B. M. Pennel, "The presence of "creeping attachment" in human gingiva," *Journal of Periodontology*, vol. 49, no. 10, pp. 513–517, 1978.

24

Accidental Insertion of a Broken Needle into the Pterygoid Mandibular Space during Inferior Alveolar Nerve Block: A Case Report

Kazuhiro Terada,[1,2] Kenji Yamagata,[1] Fumihiko Uchida,[1] Satoshi Fukuzawa,[1] Naomi Ishibashi-Kanno,[1] and Hiroki Bukawa[1]

[1]*Department of Oral and Maxillofacial Surgery, Faculty of Medicine, University of Tsukuba, Tsukuba, Japan*
[2]*Department of Oral and Maxillofacial Surgery, Tsukuba Medical Center Hospital, Tsukuba, Japan*

Correspondence should be addressed to Kenji Yamagata; y-kenji@md.tsukuba.ac.jp

Academic Editor: Darko Macan

The incidence of needle breakage is estimated to be 0.000007%, and most needle breaks occur during inferior alveolar nerve block (IANB) administration and are localized to the pterygomandibular space. Although immediate surgical intervention is recommended for the removal of the fracture needles, intraoperative localization of a broken injection needle fragment can be challenging. Here, we present the case of a 36-year-old woman who underwent dental extraction of the left lower wisdom tooth under local anesthesia at a private office. At that time, a disposable 33G needle was broken and accidentally inserted into the pterygomandibular space during IANB. A broken injection needle was presented at the base of the left coronoid process of the mandible on computed tomography (CT). We successfully removed the broken injection needle using fluoroscopy and assisted endoscopy under general anesthesia.

1. Introduction

Local dental anesthesia via injection is a technique that is performed in daily dental practice. A very rare occurrence is a broken injection needle and accidental insertion. The incidence of needle breakage has been estimated to be 0.000007%, and most needle breaks (70%) occur during inferior alveolar nerve block (IANB) administration and are localized to the pterygomandibular space [1]. Needle fracturing is thought to be caused by manual bending of the needle, incorrect choice of needle diameter, or sudden patient movements [2]. One study reported a critical case in which the broken needle migrated toward the skull base into the carotid space and jugular foramen [3]. Although immediate surgical intervention is recommended for the removal of fractured needles, intraoperative localization of a broken needle fragment can be challenging. We report a case of successful removal of a broken injection needle inserted into the pterygomandibular space during IANB using fluoroscopy assisted by endoscopy, and discuss the possible cause, timing of removal, modern modalities of localization, techniques for removal, and preventive measures.

2. Case Report

A 36-year-old woman was referred to our department for removal of a broken injection needle from the site of a left mandibular third molar extraction. She underwent dental extraction of the left lower third molar under local anesthesia at the private office one month ago. At that time, a disposable 33G needle was broken and accidentally inserted into the pterygomandibular space during IANB. The patient had mild trismus, but no inferior alveolar nerve paralysis, and the extracted site was clearly cured. Mild tenderness was noted in the left submandibular and upper internal deep cervical lymph nodes (LNs). The mucosa on the medial side of the left mandible, which was accidentally inserted with a broken injection needle, was smooth and normal. Panoramic

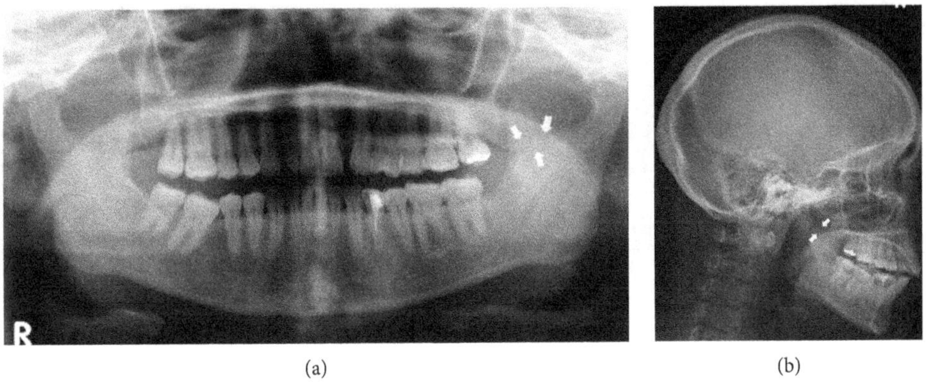

FIGURE 1: (a) Panoramic X-ray performed at the first visit. The broken injection needle can be seen at the base of the left coronoid process (arrows). (b) Lateral cephalometric X-ray. The broken injection needle can be seen at the base of the left coronoid process (arrows).

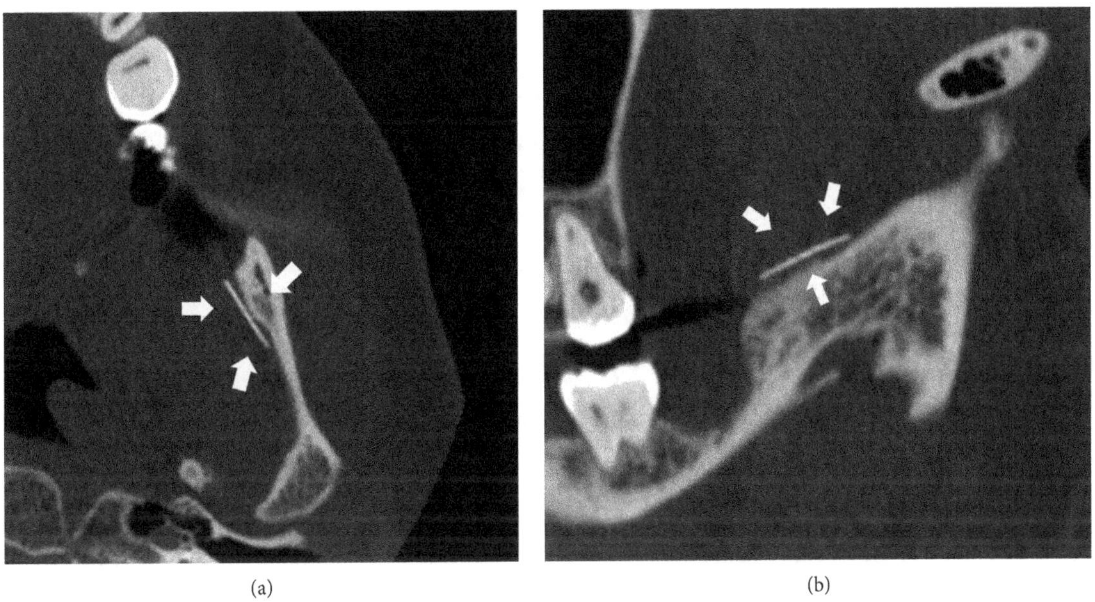

FIGURE 2: (a) Computed tomography (axial). The broken injection needle can be seen at the base of the left coronoid process (arrows). (b) Computed tomography (sagittal). The broken injection needle can be seen at the base of the left coronoid process (arrows).

and lateral radiographs revealed the broken injection needle at the base of the left coronoid process (Figure 1(a) and 1(b)). Computed tomography (CT) showed the broken injection needle along the bone surface inside the left coronoid process of the mandible (Figure 2(a) and 2(b)).

The plan was to remove the broken injection needle via an intraoral approach using fluoroscopy and endoscopy under general anesthesia. First, the position of the broken injection needle was examined using X-ray fluoroscopy (Figure 3(a)). An incision approximately 25 mm in length was made on the oblique line of the mandible. The broken injection needle pointing upward from the base of the coronoid process was confirmed in the medial pterygoid muscle by endoscopic examination (Figure 3(b) and 3(c)). The surgical time was 35 min, and there was a small amount of bleeding. The removed dental injection needle had broken at the base of the hub of the syringe adaptor (Figure 4). The postoperative course was uneventful, with no injury to the inferior alveolar or lingual nerves.

3. Discussion

In a meta-analysis, Ho et al. reviewed 78 articles of ocular and neurological adverse effects, allergies, hematomas, needle breakage, tissue necrosis, blanching, jaw ankylosis, osteomyelitis, and isolated atrial fibrillation during dental local anesthesia [4], and estimated that the incidence of needle breakage was around 0.000007%. Fifteen of 16 needle fractures occurred in connection with the IANB, and 13 involved a 30G needle [1]. Acham et al. reported that the diameters of the broken needles were 31G (2.5%), 30G (77.5%), and 27G (20%) [5]. In most cases, needle breakage is not due to a material defect but to preventable reasons such as inappropriate injection techniques or choosing the wrong type of needle [2]. Augello et al. stated that needle fracture is almost always preventable when all precautions are taken. To reduce the risk of needle fracture during dentistry, it is advisable to use a 35-mm-long, 25- or 27-gauge dental needle for administering an IANB [2]. When the

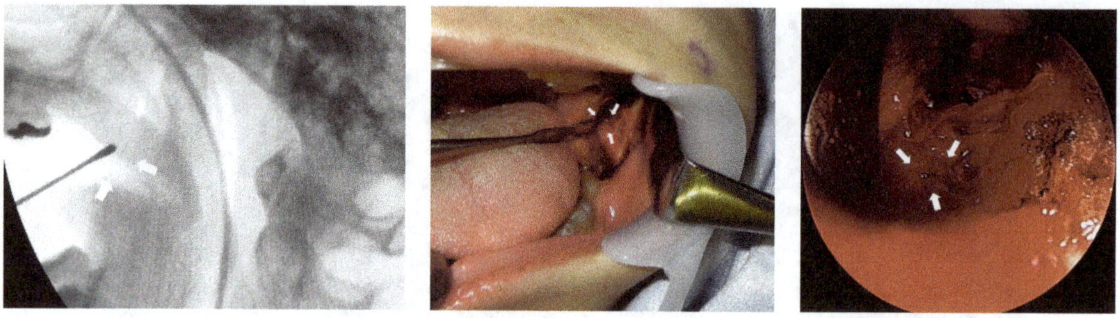

(a) (b) (c)

Figure 3: (a) Intraoperative X-ray transmission device images. The position of the broken injection needle was confirmed with a sonde using fluoroscopy. (b) Intraoperative photograph. (c) Endoscopic image taken intraoperatively. An incision approximately 25 mm in length was made on the oblique line of the mandible. A broken injection needle pointing upward from the base of the coronoid process was confirmed in the medial pterygoid muscle. Broken injection needles are shown by an arrow.

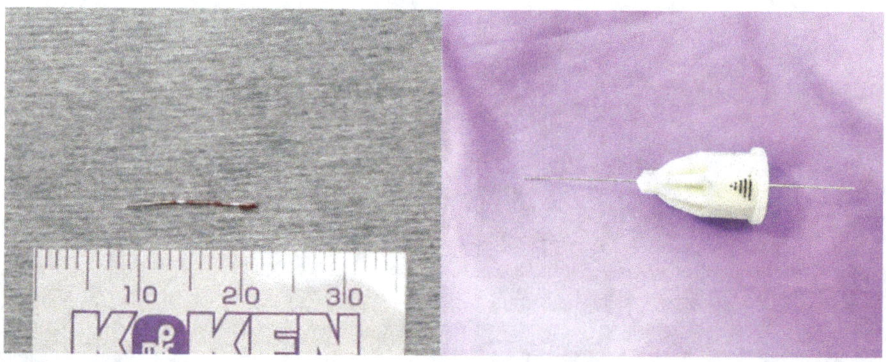

Figure 4: The removed disposable dental injection needle and unused disposable dental injection.

broken fragment is not fully buried in the tissues, it can be readily retrieved using a clamp. The patient should be well instructed to avoid sudden head movements before the injection [6]. Our patient was injected with a 33G needle, which is commonly used for pediatric injection. Choosing the wrong type of needle and the injection technique by inserting the base of the needle into the tissue were the reasons for needle breakage.

The timing of surgical removal of the needle fragment was reported to be 73% within 2 days after the incident [2]. In contrast, Acham et al. reported that 53.8% of needle fragments were removed immediately within 1 day after the event, 30.8% within 3 months, and 12.8% were delayed 3–12 months or later [5]. In the present study, the patient was referred to our hospital 1 month after the accident. Fortunately, there was no change in the position of the needle on imaging when she visited our department, and we were able to remove it. In the future, we believe that it will be necessary to inform dental practitioners to consult as soon as possible if a needle is accidentally broken. Brooks et al. reported a critical case of a broken dental anesthetic needle that migrated for several weeks toward the skull base into the carotid space and jugular foramen. They postulated that the broken needle migrated because of the cutting nature of the bevel as well as the musculature of the nasopharynx and oropharynx, specifically the contraction of the superior and middle pharyngeal constrictor muscles [3]. In another case, subcutaneous migration of a broken dental needle from the mandibular gingiva to the neck has been reported. The 33G thick needle migrated to the subcutaneous submandible for 11 months, and was retrieved using an extraoral approach [7]. Therefore, immediate surgical intervention is recommended for fractures of the dental anesthetic needles.

Although the success rate of removal is 95% [5], intraoperative localization of a broken dental needle fragment can be challenging. Conventional CT, intraoperative cone beam CT, sonography, intraoperative navigation, fluoroscopy, metal detectors, and simple plain radiography have all been reported to triangulate broken needles [3]. Recently, Lukas et al. reported successful needle removal using a three-dimensionally printed surgical guide [6]. Real-time intraoperative confirmation of a broken injection needle includes fluoroscopy, endoscopy, and ultrasonography, all of which aid successful removal. In our case, intraoperative fluoroscopy was used to confirm the setting of the incision line and the position of the needle during surgery. The endoscope confirmed the broken injection needle in a bright and magnified image.

Needle breakage prevention is based on three main principles: proper equipment, techniques, and patient care. Most broken needles occur during the administration of IANB. To avoid breakage, long needles, no smaller than 27G, should be used without bending the needle before insertion and without inserting into hub to the tissue. When working with anxious patients, clinicians should be cognizant of sudden or rapid movements [3].

References

[1] M. A. Pogrel, "Broken local anesthetic needles: a case series of 16 patients, with recommendations," *Journal of the American Dental Association*, vol. 140, no. 12, pp. 1517–1522, 2009.

[2] M. Augello, J. von Jackowski, K. W. Grätz, and C. Jacobsen, "Needle breakage during local anesthesia in the oral cavity-a retrospective of the last 50 years with guidelines for treatment and prevention," *Clinical Oral Investigations*, vol. 15, no. 1, pp. 3–8, 2011.

[3] J. Brooks and M. T. Murphy, "A novel case of a broken dental anesthetic needle transecting the right internal carotid artery," *Journal of the American Dental Association*, vol. 147, no. 9, pp. 739–742, 2016.

[4] J.-P. T. F. Ho, T. C. T. van Riet, Y. Afrian et al., "Adverse effects following dental local anesthesia: a literature review," *Journal of Dental Anesthesia and Pain Medicine*, vol. 21, no. 6, pp. 507–525, 2021.

[5] S. Acham, A. Truschnegg, P. Rugani, B. Kirnbauer, K. E. Reinbacher, W. Zemann et al., "Needle fracture as a complication of dental local anesthesia: recommendations for prevention and a comprehensive treatment algorithm based on literature from the past four decades," *Clinical Oral Investigations*, vol. 23, pp. 1109–1119, 2019.

[6] D. Lukas, M. Jan, P. Constantinus, and L. Paul, "Fractured needle removal with a 3-dimensionally printed surgical guide: a case report and literature review," *Journal of Oral and Maxillofacial Surgery*, vol. 79, pp. 1019–1024, 2021.

[7] K. Karakida, M. Takahashi, H. Sakamoto, Y. Nakanishi, and M. Tamura, "Subcutaneous migration of a broken dental needle from the mandibular gingiva to the neck: a case report," *Tokai Journal of Experimental and Clinical Medicine*, vol. 45, pp. 108–112, 2020.

25

The Importance of Histopathological Examination to the Final Diagnosis of Peripheral Odontogenic Tumors: A Case Report of a Peripheral Odontoma

Marcio Augusto de Oliveira,[1] Bruna Reis,[2] Debora Pallos,[2] Yeon Jung Kim,[2] Paulo Henrique Braz-Silva,[1,3] and Fabiana Martins[2]

[1] *Department of Stomatology, School of Dentistry, University of São Paulo, Av Prof. Lineu Prestes 2227, 05508-000 São Paulo, Brazil*
[2] *Dental School, University of Santo Amaro, R. Prof. Eneas de Siqueia Neto 340, 04829-300 São Paulo, Brazil*
[3] *Laboratory of Virology, Institute of Tropical Medicine of São Paulo, University of São Paulo, v. Dr. Enéas Carvalho de Aguiar 470, 05403-000 São Paulo, Brazil*

Correspondence should be addressed to Fabiana Martins; fmoliveira@prof.unisa.br

Academic Editor: Rui Amaral Mendes

A 30-year-old Caucasian man presented with an 18-month history of an asymptomatic calcified mass, located on the buccal side of the alveolar ridge. Medical records did not present any underlying conditions. On intraoral examination, the lesion was located on the right side of the maxilla, showing mucosal fenestration with mineralized tissue measuring approximately 1 cm in diameter. Radiographic examination showed multiple radiopaque masses. Incisional biopsy was performed, and histological analysis revealed a presence of enamel matrix, dentin, and cementum, resembling tooth-like structures. Surgical removal was offered after the diagnostic confirmation of peripheral odontoma, but the patient refused because of the asymptomatic nature of the lesion.

1. Introduction

Odontomas are the most common type of odontogenic tumors, being considered hamartomas when associated with dental development failure [1]. Two types of odontomas can be recognized: complex and compound odontomas, with the former being characterized by a mineralized mass and the latter by multiple small calcifications [2, 3]. Clinically, odontomas can be intraosseous or extraosseous. The intraosseous type can eventually erupt into the oral cavity, whereas the peripheral odontoma (PO) occurs in the soft tissues and is considered rare, with a higher tendency to exfoliate [4].

PO is extremely uncommon, with less than 25 cases reported in the literature [4, 5]. PO arises in young individuals and children, rarely reported in adults. Histologically, both complex and compound types can be seen in more than 50% of the cases affecting the anterior region of the maxilla [4].

The purpose of this article is to present a new case of erupted peripheral odontoma of the maxilla in a 30-year-old patient and to review and discuss the characteristics of the cases of PO in the craniofacial region described in the literature.

2. Case Report

A 30-year-old male patient was referred with a diagnosis of an asymptomatic calcified mass located on the right side of the anterior maxilla, lasting 18 months. On the intraoral examination, a mucosal cutaneous fenestration with a mineralized tissue measuring approximately 1 cm in diameter was observed (Figure 1(a)). A periapical radiograph revealed an image exhibiting discrete radiopacity in the region of upper premolars (Figure 1(b)). The diagnostic hypothesis was maxillary exostosis.

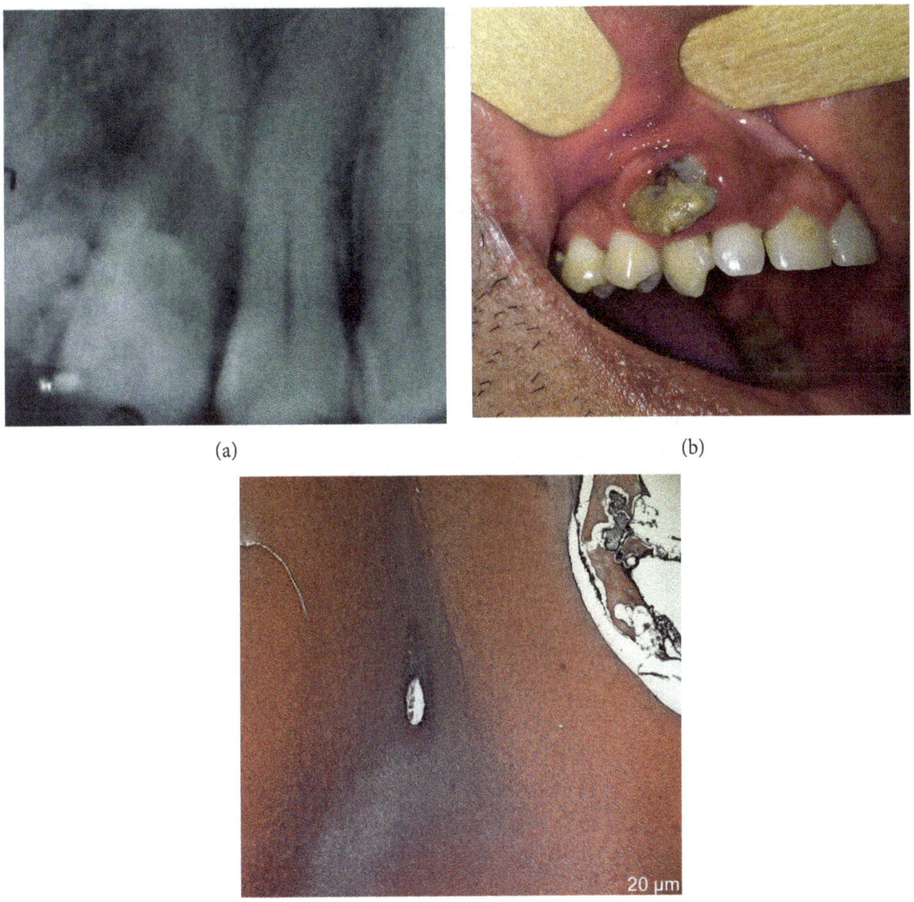

(a) (b) (c)

Figure 1: Radiographic examination showing multiple radiopaque masses (a). Fenestration of the mucosa with a display of mineralized tissue (b). Histological analysis revealed the presence of enamel matrix, dentin, and cementum, resembling tooth-like structures (c).

Incisional biopsy was performed for the removal of the fragment, which then was placed in 10% neutral-buffered formalin and sent for histopathological analysis. The gross examination of the calcified specimen revealed a yellowish tumor with $4 \times 4 \times 5$ mm.

The histopathological analysis revealed structures composed of enamel, dentin, pulp chamber, and cement in the same order of arrangement as that of a normal tooth. A mature tubular dentin and an enamel matrix were also observed (Figure 1(c)).

After the diagnostic confirmation of erupted peripheral odontoma, surgical removal was performed to reduce the lesion. The patient was free of symptoms after the procedure, and no complications were recorded.

3. Discussion

Odontomas, by definition, refer to any tumor of odontogenic origin, although these entities are truly considered hamartomas [2]. Odontomas occur at any age but are most commonly seen in the first two decades of life [2], which is not coincident with the present case of a 30-year-old adult, denoting the rarity of this lesion. Table 1 demonstrates a review of peripheral odontomas in adults and children, reported in English literature (Table 1 [3, 4, 6–15]). Among the cases described, only 5 [2, 9, 11, 13, 15] were histologically confirmed cases of erupted peripheral compound odontoma in adults, and among these, the present case and three additional cases were not associated with an impacted tooth [9, 13, 15–22].

PO is usually asymptomatic and detected during routine radiographic examinations or once there is a delay in tooth eruption [Rajendran et al., 2012]. The differential diagnosis of OP includes other tumors of odontogenic origin, exostoses, and osteomas [6], with the latter being considered our first diagnostic hypothesis.

The histogenesis of odontomas is primarily associated with remnants of soft tissues of the odontogenic epithelium, such as the gingival rests of Serres, which could lead to the production of mineralized structures similar to teeth as a result of odontoblastic hyperactivity and changes in the genetic component responsible for controlling dental development, including a reduction of epithelial-mesenchymal interactions [2].

This condition can also be attributed to some pathological conditions, such as local trauma, inflammatory process, and infectious and genetic anomalies [4, 5].

Some of the peripheral odontomas reported in the literature might be erupted odontomas because of intraosseous lesions, often related to unerupted or spontaneously erupted

Table 1: Review of peripheral odontoma cases described in the literature.

Author	Age*	Gender	Location	Erupted PO	Histopathologic diagnosis
Present case	30	Male	Anterior maxillary region	Yes	Compound odontoma
Custódio et al.	11	Female	Anterior maxillary region	No	Complex odontoma
Sfakianou et al.	7 Mo**	Male	Posterior mandible region	No	Peripheral developing odontoma
Ahmed	24	Male	Posterior mandible region	Yes	Complex odontoma
Bagewadi et al.	22	Male	Posterior mandible region	Yes	Complex odontoma
Bereket et al.	19	Male	Posterior maxillary region	Yes	Compound odontoma
Kudva et al.	23	Male	Posterior mandible region	Yes	Complex odontoma
Raval et al.	22	Male	Anterior maxillary region	Yes	Compound odontoma
Ohtawa et al.	10	Female	Posterior maxillary region	Yes	Complex odontoma
Arunkumar et al.	22	Male	Posterior maxillary region	Yes	Complex odontoma
Tejasvi and Babu	22	Female	Anterior mandible region	Yes	Compound odontoma
Friedrich et al.	3	Male	Posterior maxillary region	No	Peripheral developing odontoma
Serra-Serra et al.	11	Male	Posterior maxillary region	Yes	Complex odontoma
	27	Male	Anterior mandible region	Yes	Compound odontoma
Shekar et al.	15	Female	Posterior mandible region	Yes	Compound odontoma
Silva et al.	5 Mo	Male	Anterior maxillary region	No	Peripheral developing odontoma
	8 Mo	Male	Anterior maxillary region	No	Peripheral developing odontoma
Ilief-Ala et al.	2	Female	Posterior maxillary region	Yes	Complex odontoma
Vengal et al.	23	Male	Posterior mandible region	Yes	Complex odontoma
Junquera et al.	23	Female	Posterior maxillary region	Yes	Complex odontoma
Ide et al.	39	Male	Anterior maxillary region	No	Complex odontoma
Ledesma-Montes et al.	3	Female	Posterior mandible region	No	Compound odontoma
Giunta et al.	21	Male	Posterior mandible region	No	Compound odontoma

*Patient's age at the time of the oral examination. **Months

teeth [2]. However, it can be postulated that the eruptive force of nonerupted teeth plays an important role in the eruption of odontoma. In the absence of unerupted teeth, some authors assume that the odontoma eruption is caused by local bone resorption, which may involve both the bone remodeling of the jaws and the increase in the size of the tumor over time, since movement forces are not linked to fibroblast contractility, unlike teeth [7]. Another hypothesis described in the literature is that PO is an erupted form of an extraosseous mesiodens [1].

In the present case, the patient was referred to an evaluation due to exposure of the mineralized tissue in the oral cavity, suggesting a growth of the lesion and the presence of mild discomfort in the adjacent periodontal area. The type of force that may have led to mucosal fenestration was probably caused by physiological bone resorption, since there was no report of delayed dental eruption.

Histologically, PO resembles intraosseous odontomas, which can be classified as compound and complex. However, the absence of bone tissue is a finding also observed in the present case. This fact occurs due to the absence of bone erosion under the tumor, supporting the hypothesis of the development of this odontoma in the gingival tissue [6, 8].

Clinically, some authors have described odontomas that erupted in older patients and whose lesions were histologically characterized as complex odontomas associated with noneruption of posterior teeth [6]. Conversely, the lesion described was located in gingival tissues and was not associated with an impacted tooth, being histologically described as a compound odontoma.

Peripheral odontoma is a rare benign odontogenic lesion that can be treated by local excision with good results. Both young and adult patients can present these alterations. A comprehensive evaluation with radiographic and histological examinations is important to establish the differential diagnosis and prevent unnecessary extensive resections.

Acknowledgments

This work was supported by São Paulo Research Foundation (FAPESP) [2015/07727-9 and 2018/02568-8].

References

[1] J. A. C. Hanemann, D. T. Oliveira, N. G. Garcia, M. R. G. Santos, and A. A. C. Pereira, "Peripheral compound odontoma erupting in the gingiva," *Head & Face Medicine*, vol. 9, no. 1, pp. 1–4, 2013.

[2] S. E. Shekar, R. S. Rao, B. Gunasheela, and N. Supriya, "Erupted compound odontome," *Journal of Oral and Maxillo Facial Pathology*, vol. 13, no. 1, pp. 47–50, 2009.

[3] G. Serra-Serra, L. Berini-Aytés, and C. Gay-Escoda, "Erupted odontomas: a report of three cases and review of the litera-

ture," *Medicina Oral, Patología Oral y Cirugía Bucal*, vol. 14, no. 6, pp. 299–303, 2009.

[4] M. Vengal, H. Arora, S. Ghosh, and K. M. Pai, "Large erupting complex odontoma: a case report," *Journal of the Canadian Dental Association*, vol. 73, no. 2, pp. 169–173, 2007.

[5] C. Seckinger, S. Wang, and D. Anastasio, "Extraosseous odontoma in the mouth floor: report of a case and literature review," *Medecine Buccale Chirurgie Buccale*, vol. 21, pp. 253–256, 2015.

[6] L. Junquera, J. C. Vicente, P. Roig, S. Olay, and O. Rodríguez-Recio, "Intraosseus odontoma erupted into the oral cavity: an unusual pathology," *Medicina Oral, Patología Oral y Cirugía Bucal*, vol. 10, no. 3, pp. 248–251, 2005.

[7] K. A. Ahmed, "Large eruption complex odontome in a Saudi patient," *Saudi Medical Journal*, vol. 36, no. 2, pp. 228–232, 2015.

[8] S. B. Bagewadi, R. Kukreja, G. N. Suma, B. Yadav, and H. Sharma, "Unusually large erupted complex odontoma: a rare case report," *Imaging Science in Dentistry*, vol. 45, no. 1, pp. 49–54, 2015.

[9] C. Bereket, N. Çakır-Özkan, İ. Şener, E. Bulut, and M. Tek, "Complex and compound odontomas: analysis of 69 cases and a rare case of erupted compound odontoma," *Nigerian Journal of Clinical Practice*, vol. 18, no. 6, pp. 726–730, 2015.

[10] A. Kudva, A. Chithra, N. N. Rao, and K. M. Cariappa, "An erupted silent tumour," *Journal of Maxillofacial and Oral Surgery*, vol. 15, no. S2, pp. 320–324, 2016.

[11] N. Raval, D. Mehta, K. Vachhrajani, and A. Nimavat, "Erupted odontoma: a case report," *Journal of Clinical and Diagnostic Research*, vol. 8, no. 7, pp. 10-11, 2014.

[12] K. V. Arunkumar, Vijaykumar, and N. Garg, "Surgical management of an erupted complex odontoma occupying maxillary sinus," *Annals of Maxillofacial Surgery*, vol. 2, no. 1, pp. 86–89, 2012.

[13] M. L. Tejasvi and B. B. Babu, "Erupted compound odontomas: a case report," *Journal of Dental Research, Dental Clinics, Dental Prospects*, vol. 5, no. 1, pp. 33–36, 2011.

[14] F. Ide, T. Shimoyama, and N. Horie, "Gingival peripheral odontoma in an adult: case report," *Journal of Periodontology*, vol. 71, no. 5, pp. 830–832, 2000.

[15] J. L. Giunta and M. A. Kaplan, "Peripheral, soft tissue odontomas: two case reports," *Oral Surgery, Oral Medicine, and Oral Pathology*, vol. 69, no. 3, pp. 406–411, 1990.

[16] C. Ledesma-Montes, A. Perez-Bache, and M. Garcés-Ortíz, "Gingival compound odontoma," *International Journal of Oral and Maxillofacial Surgery*, vol. 25, no. 4, pp. 296-297, 1996.

[17] M. A. Ilief-Ala, E. Eisenberg, and G. J. Mathieu, "Peripheral complex odontoma in a pediatric dental patient: a case report," *Journal of the Massachusetts Dental Society*, vol. 56, no. 4, pp. 24–26, 2008.

[18] A. R. Silva, R. Carlos-Bregni, P. A. Vargas, O. P. de Almeida, and M. A. Lopes, "Peripheral developing odontoma in newborn. Report of two cases and literature review," *Medicina Oral, Patología Oral y Cirugía Bucal*, vol. 14, no. 11, pp. 612–615, 2009.

[19] R. E. Friedrich, A. Fuhrmann, H. A. Scheuer, and J. Zustin, "Small peripheral developing odontoma of the maxilla in a 3-year-old patient depicted on cone-beam tomograms," *In Vivo*, vol. 24, no. 6, pp. 895–898, 2010.

[20] Y. Ohtawa, S. Ichinohe, E. Kimura, and S. Hashimoto, "Erupted complex odontoma delayed eruption of permanent molar," *The Bulletin of Tokyo Dental College*, vol. 54, no. 4, pp. 251–257, 2013.

[21] A. Sfakianou, D. E. Emmanouil, K. I. Tosios, and A. Sklavounou, "Peripheral tumor with osteodentin and cementum-like material in an infant: odontogenic hamartoma or odontoma?," *Journal of Dentistry for Children (Chicago, Ill.)*, vol. 83, no. 1, pp. 38–41, 2016.

[22] M. Custódio, J. P. Araujo, C. B. Gallo, and M. Trierveiler, "Gingival complex odontoma: a rare case report with a review of the literature," *Autopsy & Case Reports*, vol. 8, no. 1, article e2018009, 2018.

26

Diagnosis and Management of a Unilateral Posterior Open Bite using a Temporary Anchorage Device (TAD): Case Report and Review of the Literature

Bandar Alyami

Department of Preventive Dentistry, Faculty of Dentistry, Najran University, Najran, Saudi Arabia

Correspondence should be addressed to Bandar Alyami; bsalyami@nu.edu.sa

Academic Editor: Daniel Torres-Lagares

This report describes the diagnosis and successful treatment of a unilateral posterior open bite (POB) in a 15-year-old Caucasian boy. Simple mechanics were used to rule out ankylosis of left posterior teeth as the etiological factor of the POB. Thereafter, the same mechanics were continued to expand the unilateral constricted maxilla, to create a space, and to close POB. Sectional biomechanics were applied to avoid undesirable tooth movements. Then, continuous arch wires were employed to coordinate arches and to achieve treatment objectives.

1. Introduction

A posterior open bite (POB) is defined as failure of a number of teeth in either or both opposing buccal segments to reach occlusion while there is an incisal contact [1]. Two scenarios have been described in POB: the first one is when only the anterior teeth are touching with no single posterior teeth touching and the second one is when the anterior teeth and some of the posterior teeth are touching. Generally, an open bite is present in about 25%-38% of patients treated orthodontically [2], and the etiology is multifactorial from interaction between genetic and environmental factors [1]. POB is a rare condition and can be attributed to conditions like interpositional tongue habit, digit habit (sucking or chewing), mouth breathing, adenoid hypertrophy, syndromes, and partial eruption of the first premolars [3]. Other causes of open bite include obstacles in the path of eruption such as supernumerary teeth and nonresorbing deciduous roots [3–5].

Patients with POB can have functional and psychological problems [1]. The functional problems include defective speech, mastication challenges, and problems with deglutition resulting in child's impaired development [1]. Treatment of POB and the retention of the posterior teeth in occlusion can be two of the most difficult problems an orthodontist can face. When this condition occurs unilaterally, it requires complex management strategies [6]. Several treatment options have been reported for the management of POB. These methods include habit breakers, myofunctional appliances in the growing child, orthodontic removable appliances, fixed orthodontic appliances including temporary anchorage device (TAD), and orthognathic surgery for a skeletal open bite [7–12]. In this case report, the TAD was used to confirm if the unilateral POB was a result of ankylosis and thereafter used to successfully treat the condition. A literature search has not highlighted this concept in the management of POB.

2. Case Report

A 15-year-old Caucasian male presented with the complaints "I cannot bite properly on left side." His medical, dental, familial, and social history was not contributory. He has no abnormal oral habit. On examination, he has an asymmetrical dolichofacial face (Figure 1(a)), competent lips, an obtuse nasolabial angle, and an orthognathic slightly convex profile. His upper lip was 9 mm behind the E-line, and his lower lip was 4 mm behind the E-line. His maxillary midline was

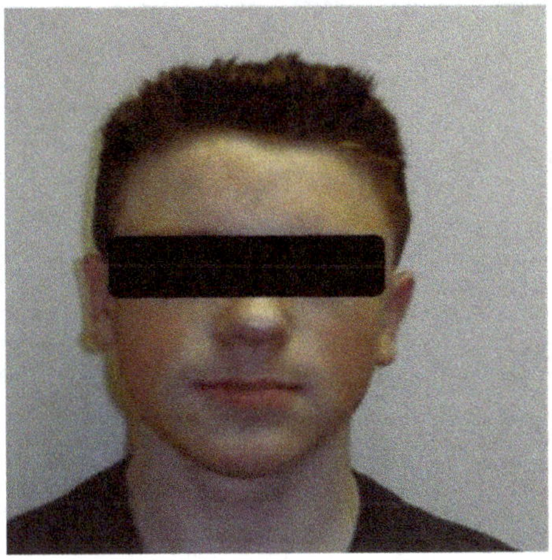

(a)

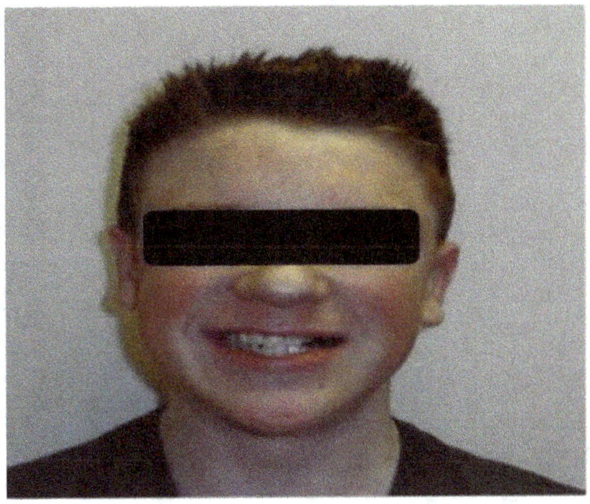

(b)

FIGURE 1: (a) Pretreatment frontal view of the patient. (b) Pretreatment frontal smile view of the patient.

TABLE 1: Cephalometric evaluation: normal, pretreatment, and posttreatment.

	Normal values	Pretreatment	Posttreatment
SNA	81 ± 2	84	85.1
SNB	80 ± 2	83.4	83.4
ANB	4 ± 2	1.4	1.7
Convexity	6.8	0.9	1.1
SN-Go Gn	32.9	29.3	28
UFH:LFH, lower (ANS-Gn/N-Gn)	55	62.8	63.3
U1-SN (°)	103.1	106.3	109.3
L1-NB (°)	25.3	25.9	23
Mandibular length (Co-Gn) (mm)	122.1	179.5	181.6
Maxillary length (Co-A) (mm)	90.0	121.5	121.3

1 mm to the left of the facial midline, and his mandibular midline is 2 mm to the left of the chin (Figure 1(b)).

Cephalometric analyses (Table 1) revealed a normodivergent profile. Figure 2(a) shows a skeletal class I pattern with an increase in the length of the mandible and maxilla and increased lower facial height. Panoramic X-ray showed that all teeth were present with no pathology seen (Figure 2(b)). He has a dentally class III molar and canine relationship on the right while the left molar and canine relationships cannot be determined (Figures 3(a) and 3(b)). In addition, there were 6.71 mm and 4 mm of crowding in the upper and lower arches, respectively. He also has an edge-to-edge incisor relationship (Figure 3(c)), a posterior open bite on the left side, and a curve of Spee of 3.5 mm. Figures 4(a)–4(c) show pretreatment cast views of the patient.

3. Problem List

The problem list included a unilateral posterior open bite and constricted maxilla on the left side, severe maxillary crowding (blocked out upper left canine) and moderate mandibular crowding, edge-to-edge incisal relationship, deep curve of Spee, class III molar and canine relationship, maxillary midline shift of about 1 mm to the left, and mandibular left midline shift of about 2 mm.

4. Treatment Objectives

The objectives of the treatment were to initially find out if etiology of the POB was due to ankylosis (if not, treatment will proceed with the closing of the left posterior open bite), to alleviate crowding and bring the upper left canine to normal position, to improve overbite and overjet, to level the curve of Spee, to achieve a class I molar and canine relationship, and to correct midline shifts in the maxillary and mandibular arches.

5. Treatment Plan

The treatment plan included bonding of the upper left first premolar, upper left second premolar, and upper left first molar and placement of a palatal button, a TAD between the lower left second premolar and lower left first molar buccally, a sectional arch wire in the upper left side, and rubber bands from the palatal button to the TAD; use of an advanced arch wire 2 × 4 to correct edge-to-edge

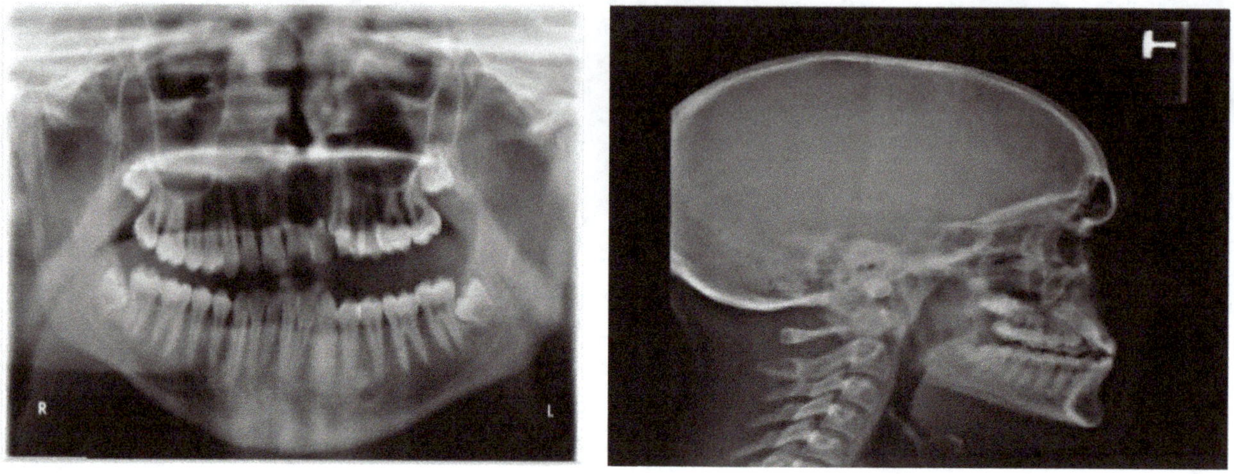

(a) (b)

Figure 2: (a) Pretreatment panoramic X-ray showing all teeth present without any pathology and unlevelled upper and lower left posterior segments. (b) Pretreatment cephalometric X-ray of the patient's skeletal class I pattern with an increase in the length of the mandible and maxilla and increased lower facial height.

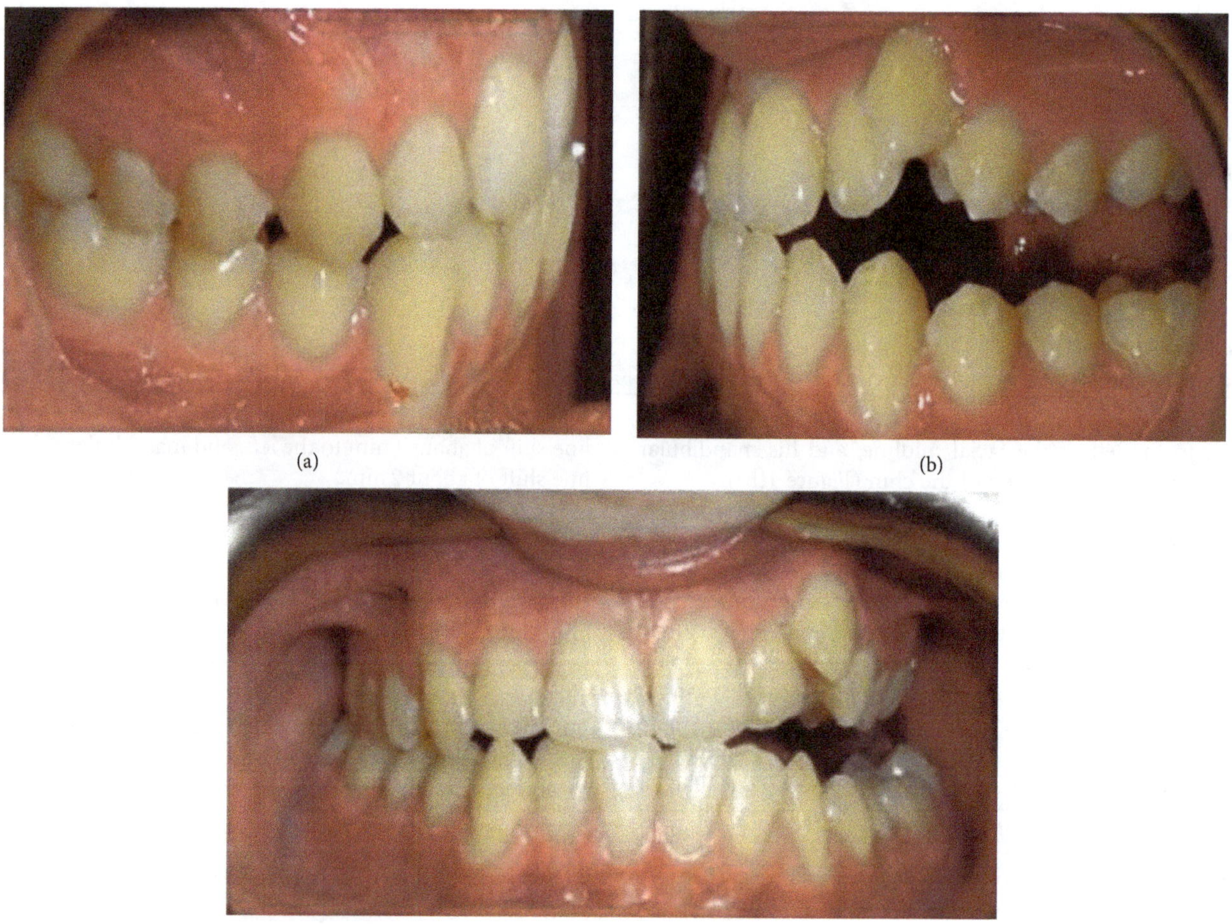

(a) (b) (c)

Figure 3: (a) Intraoral lateral view showing the right class III molar and canine relationships. (b) Intraoral lateral view showing the left POB and undetermined molar and canine relationships. (c) Intraoral view showing maxillary crowding with the blocked out upper left canine.

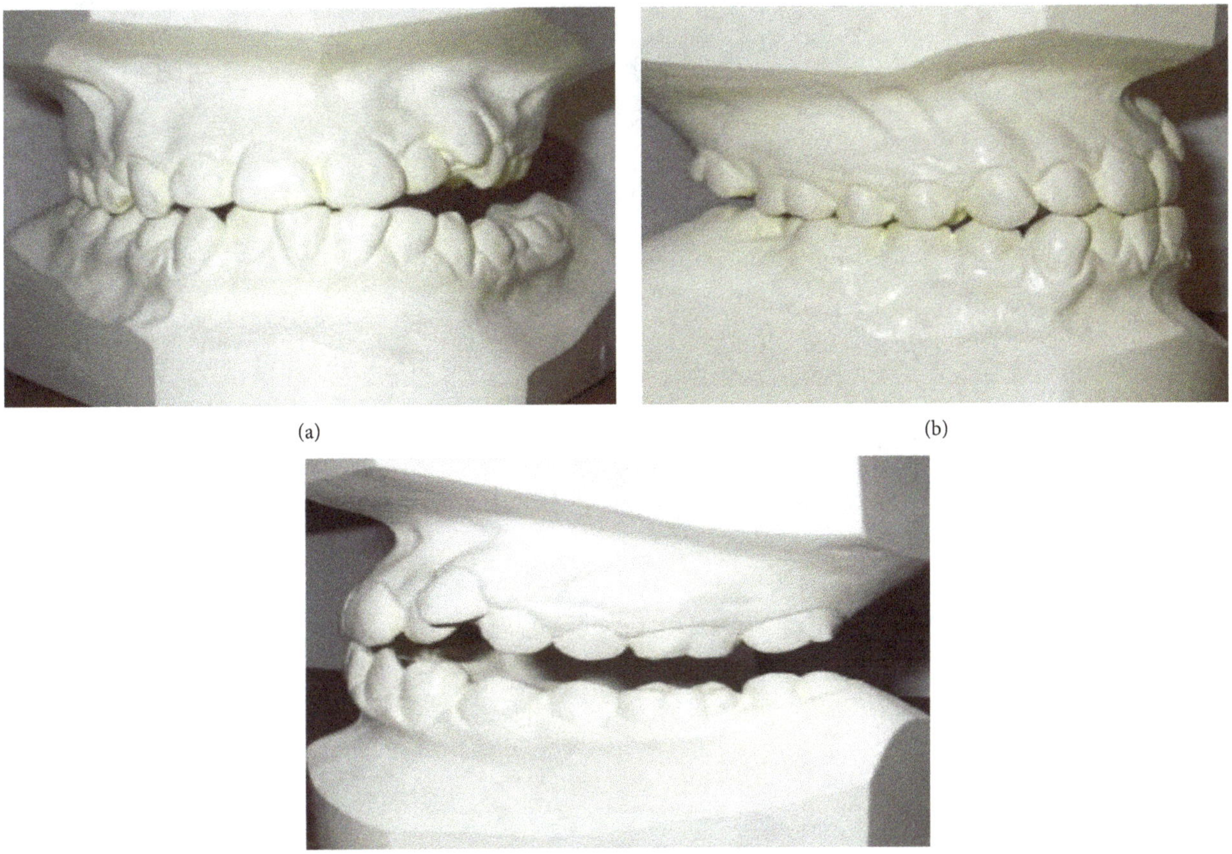

(a) (b) (c)

FIGURE 4: (a) Pretreatment frontal view of the patient's cast. (b) Pretreatment right lateral view of the patient's cast. (c) Pretreatment left lateral view of the patient's cast.

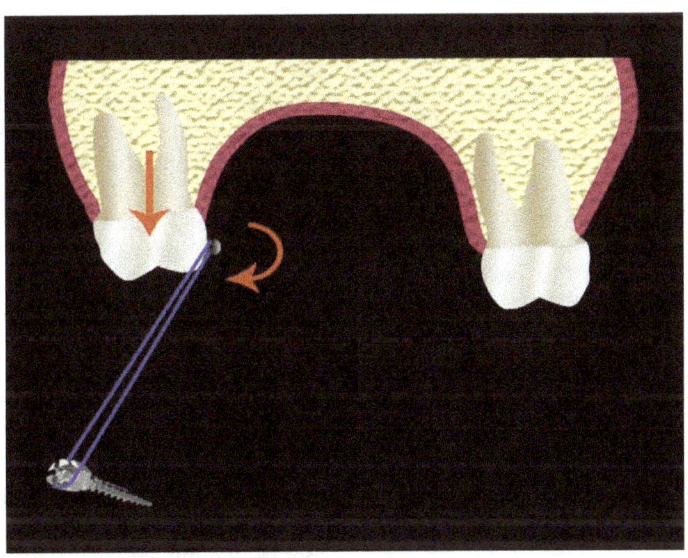

FIGURE 5: Schematic diagram showing the mechanotherapy principle employed.

anterior bite and bonding of lower arches from the right second molar to the left second molar; and then placement of a sectional arch wire, leveling and aligning of upper and lower arches, interproximal reduction (IPR) of upper and lower teeth, coordination of arches, finishing, detailing, and finally retention.

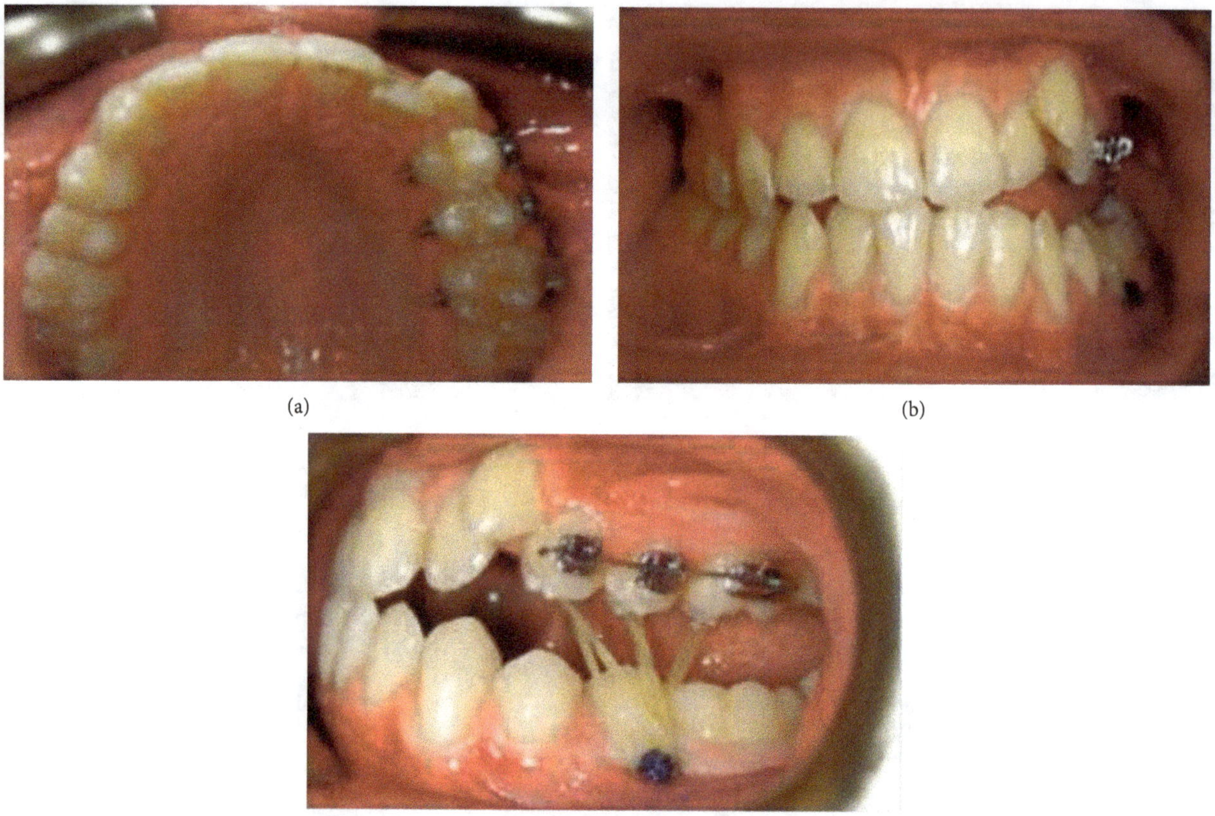

(a) (b) (c)

Figure 6: (a) Intraoral radiograph showing palatal buttons. (b) Intraoral radiograph showing TAD between the second premolar and first molar. (c) Intraoral radiograph showing elastics 5/16 4 oz placed from the palatal buttons to the TAD.

6. Mechanotherapy

The challenge in this case was what kind of mechanics can correct the constricted maxilla, create a space, and extrude teeth to close the POB without any side effect on other teeth that are in a proper position.

The patient was asked to wear the elastic from the palatal button of the upper teeth to the TAD on the lower arch (Figure 5). The force applied from the palatal button was passing away from the center of resistance of the segment which creates a moment leading to buccal tipping and downward movement of the segment. The use of these mechanics allowed us to diagnose any possible presence of ankylosed teeth with no effect on adjacent and/or opposing teeth. After extruding the posterior segment to the same level of adjacent teeth, an advanced arch wire was used to correct the edge-to-edge bite. Then, continuous arch wires were used to coordinate arches.

7. Treatment Progress

After taking initial records, the upper left first premolar, upper left second premolar, and upper left first molar were bonded at the same level to allow the insertion of a 0.018 × 0.025 TMA wire (Figure 6(a)). Thereafter, palatal buttons were bonded and TAD was placed between the lower left second premolar and lower left first molar. The patient was asked to wear elastics size 5/16 4 oz from the palatal buttons to the TAD (Figures 6(b) and 6(c)). After 2 months of treatment, the use of elastics was stopped and the lower left canine, lower left first premolar, lower left second premolar, and lower left first molar were bonded to commence levelling and alignment. The patient was lost to follow-up for 4 months.

Following 5 months of leveling and alignment, the TAD was removed and the upper right central incisor, upper right lateral incisor, upper right first molar, upper left central incisor, and upper left lateral incisor were bonded, and an advancement arch wire size 0.018 SS was placed to correct the overjet.

A lower sectional arch wire was then upgraded from sectional 0.016 NITI to sectional 0.016 × 0.022 NITI. After one month of treatment, the overjet improved and thereafter the posterior left side elastic was placed from the upper lingual button to the lower buccal brackets. In the following month, the lingual button was placed on the lower left first premolar, lower left second premolar, and lower left first molar and 3/16 4 oz elastics were placed. These mechanics were maintained for another 2 months. The remaining upper teeth were bonded for levelling and alignment. IPR was done for the lower right central incisor, lower right lateral incisor, and lower left central incisor and from the upper right second

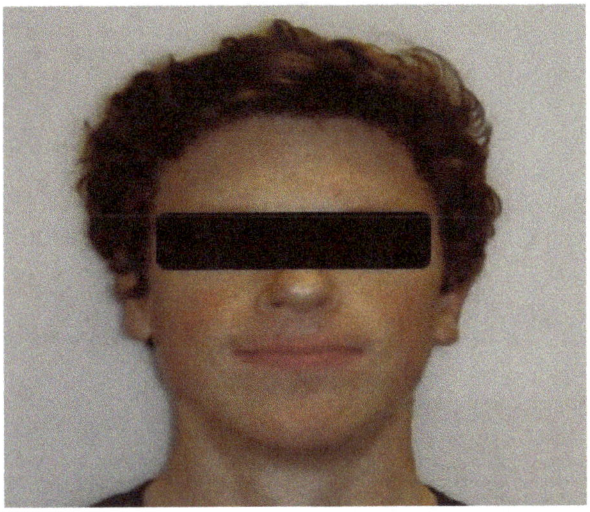

(a)

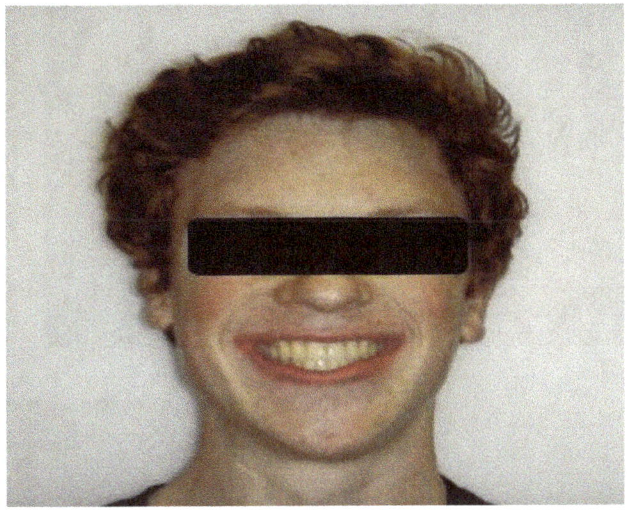

(b)

FIGURE 7: (a) Posttreatment frontal view of the patient. (b) Posttreatment frontal smile view of the patient.

premolar to the upper left second premolar. The upper arch wire was then upgraded to 0.018 × 0.025SS and lower arch wire upgraded to 0.020 SS for another 6 months.

8. Result

After 18 months of active treatment, the overjet and overbite were within a normal value and the left unilateral open bite and midline shift were corrected (Figures 7(a) and 7(b)). In addition, there were satisfactory leveling and alignment, and alleviation of crowding and a class I molar and canine relationship were achieved (Figures 8(a)–8(c)). Cephalometric X-ray (Figure 9(a)) showed minor skeletal changes posttreatment (Table 1). Panoramic X-ray (Figure 9(b)) showed levelling of the upper and lower left posterior segments posttreatment. Figure 10 shows cephalometric superimpositions. Figures 11(a)–11(c) show posttreatment casts.

9. Retention

Because of the strong cheek muscle observed in this patient which might have been the etiological factor of the POB, modified Hawley's retainer with acrylic part on the buccal side was fabricated to hold the cheek away from the occlusion thereby allowing maximum intercuspation of the posterior segment during the retention period.

10. Discussion

Management of open bites is often challenging because of high relapse rate, and patients' cooperation is highly important. When such open bites are skeletal and the patient declines surgery, then an orthodontic option for treatment is opted for which needs more time and patient cooperation [13]. Studies have recommended TADs for the provision of anchorage in the extrusion and intrusion of posterior teeth [7, 10, 14, 15]. This mechanism had been shown to close POB and reduce facial height without any form of surgical intervention [10, 16]. Etiologies of POB are countless, and diagnosis of a particular cause can be challenging. In this report, the TAD was used as both diagnostic and therapeutic devices. Clinically, it is important to differentiate whether the failure of eruption was due to disruption of the eruption mechanism or primary failure [16]. In this case, the patient did not give any history of habit therefore making decision on the mode of intervention difficult. To unravel this impasse, it was decided to place the TAD to see if there will be any form of tooth movement. When movement was observed, the device then proceeded to the treatment phase. If the POB was due to ankylosis, then no tooth movement will be observed and the device should be terminated immediately to prevent complications. In the current report, tooth movement was observed thereby eliminating ankylosis as the etiological factor. A literature search did not report this novel option of the diagnostic effect of TAD.

During the initial active treatment phase, a sectional biomechanics principle was employed to avoid undesirable tooth movement and to directly target the problem site. Undesirable tooth movement during the active treatment phase will result in a side effect of which the solution requests additional treatment time. It may also result in increased biological damage to the dentition and possible root resorption [17]. Sectional biomechanics were introduced by Dr. Charles Burstone in 1962 and consist of a sequence of orthodontic procedures based on the mechanical principles of mechanics [18]. In this case, the dental arch was divided into three major segments, one anterior (incisors and canines) and two posterior (premolars to molars) [19]. The rationale behind this division was to have a better controlled tooth movement than arch wire-guided tooth movement [19]. In the present case report, the left posterior upper and lower segments were focused

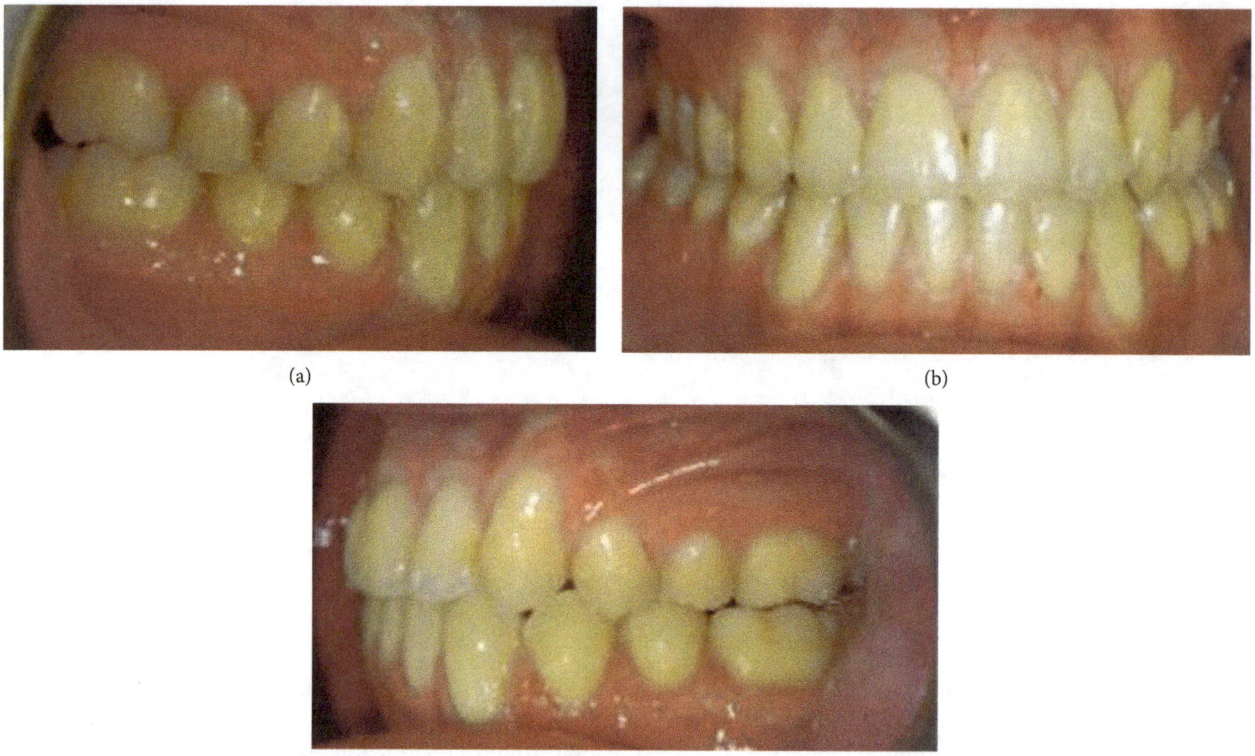

(a) (b) (c)

Figure 8: (a) Posttreatment intraoral lateral photograph showing the right class I molar and canine relationship. (b) Posttreatment intraoral photograph showing the corrected midline. (c) Posttreatment intraoral photograph showing the left class I molar and canine relationship and correction of the left POB.

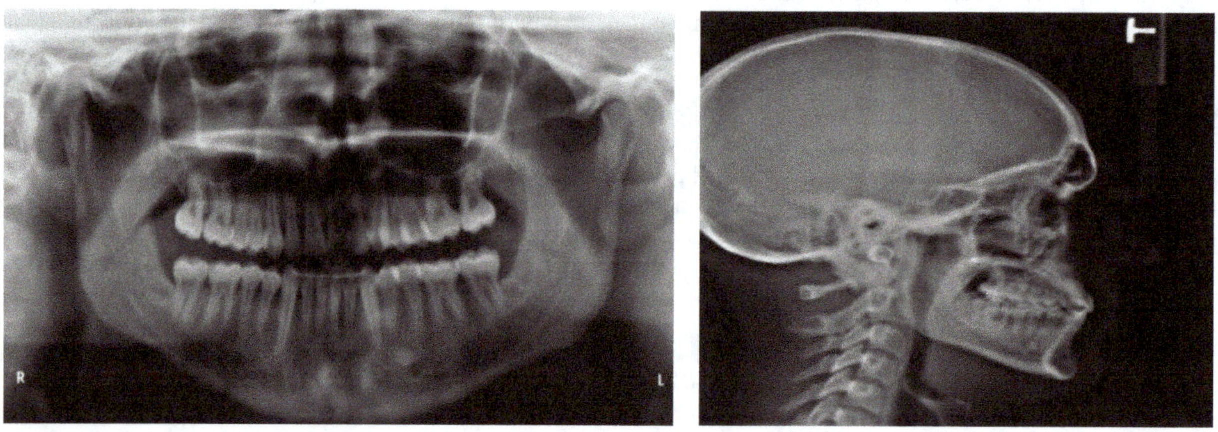

(a) (b)

Figure 9: (a) Posttreatment panorama showing levelling of the upper and lower left posterior segments. (b) Posttreatment cephalometric X-ray showing minor skeletal changes with slight changes in the upper and lower incisor inclination.

on the principle of sectional biomechanics. Following the extrusion of the teeth in the upper left and lower left segments, the sectional biomechanics were changed to a continuous arch wire mechanism for levelling and alignment.

In order to correct the edge-to-edge bite, a two-by-four sectional appliance was applied after the correction of the unilateral POB. This fixed orthodontic appliance comprises four brackets bonded onto the four erupted maxillary permanent incisors and two bands cemented or two tubes bonded on the first permanent molars with a continuous arch wire to provide and maintain a good arch form [20]. This fixed appliance allows swift correction of many emerging malocclusions in a distinct short phase of fixed appliance therapy during the early mixed dentition stage [21]. In addition, a two-by-four appliance may also lessen the complexity and interval of any future treatment.

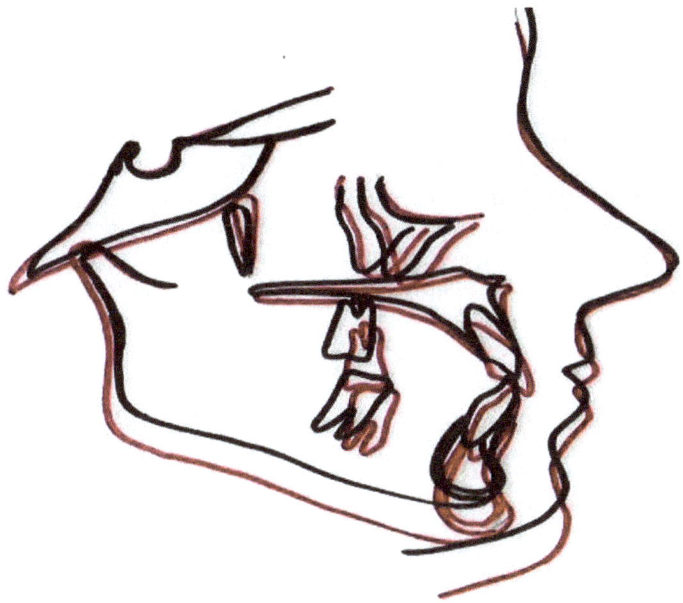

Figure 10: Cephalometric superimpositions showing skeletal changes (black is pretreatment and red is posttreatment).

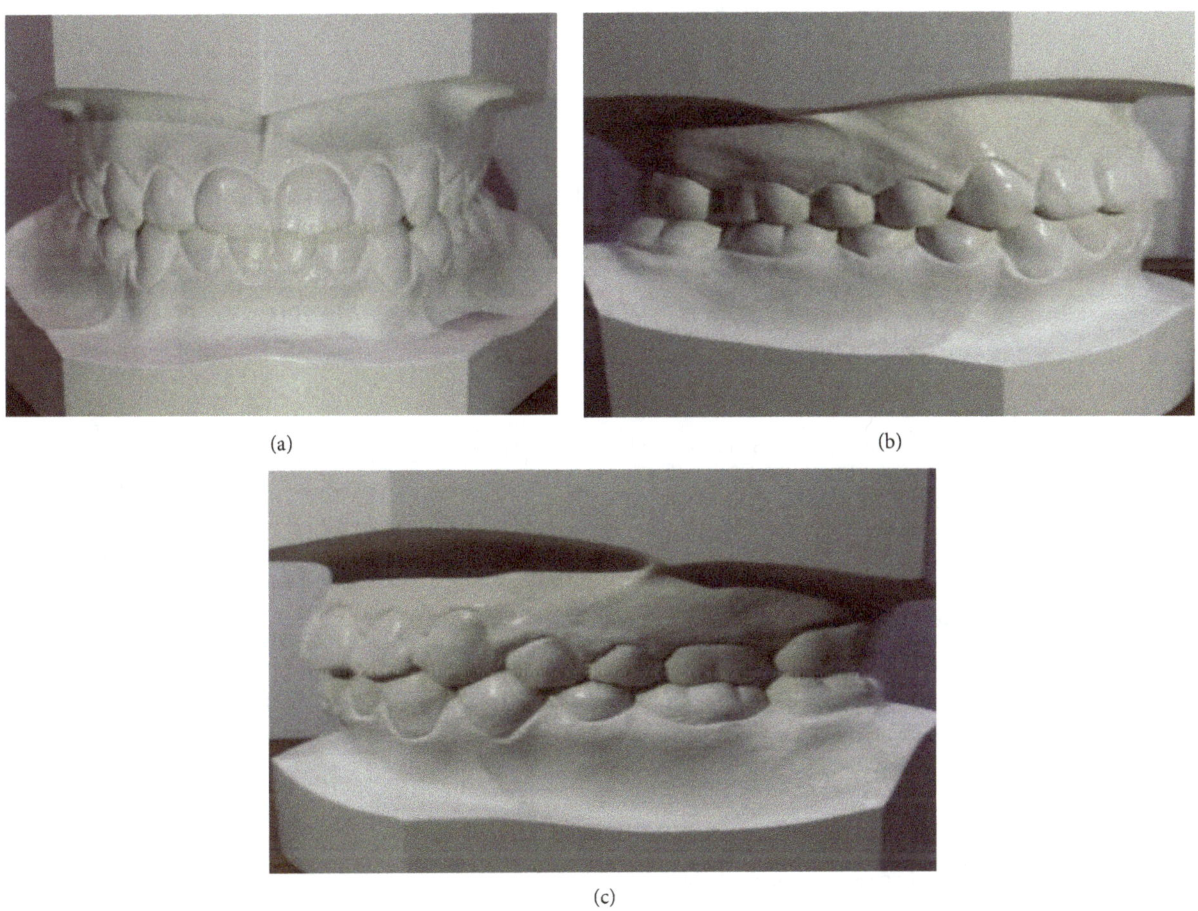

Figure 11: (a) Posttreatment frontal view of the patient's cast. (b) Posttreatment right lateral view of the patient's cast. (c) Posttreatment left lateral view of the patient's cast.

11. Conclusion

Diagnosing the etiological factors and treatment of posterior open bite malocclusion is often challenging. Treatment modalities include myofunctional appliances in growing children and surgeries in adults. Minor cases can be managed by fixed orthodontics especially with TADs alongside with some habit-breaking appliances if any form of it was identified. Additional care should be taken while diagnosing and planning treatment for such cases as any mistake in identifying the etiological factor may lead to a poor end result.

Acknowledgments

The author acknowledged the technical input of Dr. Ramat Braimah of the Department of Oral and Maxillofacial Surgery, Najran Specialty Dental Center, Najran, Kingdom of Saudi Arabia.

References

[1] M. A. Wajid, P. Chandra, R. Kulshrestha, K. Singh, R. Rastogi, and V. Umale, "Open bite malocclusion: an overview," *Journal of Oral Health and Craniofacial Science*, vol. 3, pp. 11–20, 2018.

[2] L. Espeland, P. A. Dowling, K. A. Mobarak, and A. Stenvik, "Three-year stability of open-bite correction by 1-piece maxillary osteotomy," *American Journal of Orthodontics and Dentofacial Orthopedics*, vol. 134, no. 1, pp. 60–66, 2008.

[3] M. A. N. Matsumoto, F. L. Romano, J. T. L. Ferreira, and R. A. Valerio, "Open bite: diagnosis, treatment and stability," *Brazilian Dental Journal*, vol. 23, no. 6, pp. 768–778, 2012.

[4] T. E. Southard, S. D. Marshall, and L. L. Bonner, "Posterior Open Bites," in *Orthodontics in the vertical dimension: a case-based review*, pp. 457–571, John Wiley & Sons, Inc., New Jersey, USA, 2015.

[5] M. Atobe, T. Sekiya, K. Tamura, Y. Hamada, and Y. Nakamura, "Severe lateral open bite caused by multiple ankylosed teeth: a case report," *Oral Surgery, Oral Medicine, Oral Pathology, Oral Radiology, and Endodontology*, vol. 107, no. 4, pp. e14–e20, 2009.

[6] J. M. Cafferty, E. A. Awadi, and A. C. O'Connell, "Management of severe posterior open bite due to primary failure of eruption," *European Archives of Paediatric Dentistry*, vol. 11, no. 3, pp. 158–158, 2010.

[7] Y. H. Kim, U. K. Han, D. D. Lim, and M. L. Serraon, "Stability of anterior openbite correction with multiloop edgewise archwire therapy: a cephalometric follow up study," *American Journal of Orthodontics and Dentofacial Orthopedics*, vol. 118, no. 1, pp. 43–54, 2000.

[8] J. Sugawara, U. B. Baik, M. Umemori et al., "Treatment and posttreatment dentoalveolar changes following intrusion of mandibular molars with application of a skeletal anchorage system (SAS) for open bite correction," *The International Journal of Adult Orthodontics and Orthognathic Surgery*, vol. 17, no. 4, pp. 243–253, 2002.

[9] B. Melsen, J. A. McNamara Jr., and D. C. Hoenie, "The effect of bite-blocks with and without repelling magnets studied histomorphometrically in the rhesus monkey (Macaca mulatta)," *American Journal of Orthodontics and Dentofacial Orthopedics*, vol. 108, no. 5, pp. 500–509, 1995.

[10] Y. C. Park, H. A. Lee, N. C. Choi, and D. H. Kim, "Open bite correction by intrusion of posterior teeth with miniscrews," *The Angle Orthodontist*, vol. 78, no. 4, pp. 699–710, 2008.

[11] M. de Castro Cabrera, C. A. G. Cabrera, K. M. S. de Freitas, G. Janson, and M. R. de Freitas, "Lateral open bite: treatment and stability," *American Journal of Orthodontics and Dentofacial Orthopedics*, vol. 137, no. 5, pp. 701–711, 2010.

[12] H.-W. Ahn, K.-R. Chung, S.-M. Kang, L. Lin, G. Nelson, and S.-H. Kim, "Correction of dental class III with posterior open bite by simple biomechanics using an anterior C-tube miniplate," *The Korean Journal of Orthodontics*, vol. 42, no. 5, pp. 270–278, 2012.

[13] M. B. S. Stuani, A. S. Stuani, and A. S. Stuani, "Modified Thurow appliance: A clinical alternative for correcting skeletal open bite," *American Journal of Orthodontics and Dentofacial Orthopedics*, vol. 128, no. 1, pp. 118–125, 2005.

[14] C. H. Moon, J. S. Lee, H. S. Lee, and J. H. Choi, "Non-surgical treatment and retention of open bite in adult patients with orthodontic mini-implants," *The Korean Journal of Orthodontics*, vol. 39, no. 6, pp. 402–419, 2009.

[15] M.-J. Kim, S.-H. Park, H.-S. Kim et al., "Effects of orthodontic mini-implant position in the dragon helix appliance on tooth displacement and stress distribution: a three-dimensional finite element analysis," *The Korean Journal of Orthodontics*, vol. 41, no. 3, pp. 191–199, 2011.

[16] T. Deguchi, H. Kurosaka, H. Oikawa et al., "Comparison of orthodontic treatment outcomes in adults with skeletal open bite between conventional edgewise treatment and implant-anchored orthodontics," *American Journal of Orthodontics and Dentofacial Orthopedics*, vol. 139, no. 4, pp. S60–S68, 2011.

[17] S. G. F. R. Caldas, A. A. Ribeiro, H. Simplício, and A. W. Machado, "Segmented arch or continuous arch technique? A rational approach," *Dental Press Journal of Orthodontics*, vol. 19, no. 2, pp. 126–141, 2014.

[18] C. J. Burstone, "Rationale of the segmented arch," *American Journal of Orthodontics*, vol. 48, no. 11, pp. 805–822, 1962.

[19] T. El-Bialy, "Segmented and sectional orthodontic technique: review and case report," *Journal of Health Specialties*, vol. 1, no. 2, pp. 90–96, 2013.

[20] V. Quinzi, R. Ferro, F. A. Rizzo et al., "The two by four appliance: a nationwide cross-sectional survey," *European Journal of Paediatric Dentistry*, vol. 19, no. 2, pp. 145–150, 2018.

[21] H. F. McKeown and J. Sandlerd, "The two by four appliance: a versatile appliance," *Dental Update*, vol. 28, no. 10, pp. 496–500, 2001.

Management of OSAS: The ELIBA® Device Can Help the Patient?

Eleonora Ortu,[1] Davide Pietropaoli,[1] Alessandra Mummolo,[1] IAPNOR,[2] Mario Giannoni,[1] and Annalisa Monaco[1]

[1]*MeSVA Department, Division of Dentistry, University of L'Aquila, P.le Salvatore Tommasi, 67100 L'Aquila, Italy*
[2]*I. A.P.N.O.R.–International Academy of Posture and Neuromyofascial Occlusion Research, Viale Gino Moretti 37, 63074 San Benedetto del Tronto, AP, Italy*

Correspondence should be addressed to Eleonora Ortu; eleortu@gmail.com

Academic Editor: Asja Celebic

Obstructive sleep apnea syndrome (OSAS) is one of the most challenging diseases to treat in medicine. Here, the authors describe a case of OSAS treated with a lingual elevator of Balercia (ELIBA®). The patient, a forty-five-year-old Caucasian male, had a chief complaint of numerous episodes of nocturnal apnea. After several visits with specialists, a polysomnographic examination was performed, in which the patient's apnea hypopnea index (AHI) was 30.4, and a lingual elevator was prescribed. The lingual elevator helped to keep the patient's tongue in the correct position and prevented the tongue from reverting back to the soft tissue spaces in the mouth. After six months of treatment with the lingual elevator and dietary adjustments, the patient's AHI decreased to 11.6. This simple yet customizable approach is a comfortable and easy option for patients to reduce night apnea episodes.

1. Introduction

OSAS is characterized by repeated episodes of complete, partial, and/or prolonged obstruction of the upper airway during sleep, normally associated with a reduction in blood oxygen saturation. It occurs in all ages and it is certainly more common in males [1]. Patients present a high number of apneas during the night and complain of excessive sleepiness during the day. Other common symptoms are headache upon waking up, snoring reported by the partner as intermittent (because interrupted by apnea), reduced memory capacity, reduced ability to concentrate, hypertension, and dry mouth upon waking up [2, 3]. The airways can be blocked in several ways. For example, a large tongue, associated with normal muscle relaxation and consequent soft tissue collapse that occurs during sleep, may be one of the causes of apnea [3–5]. Further, overweight or obese people have a predisposition for apnea; symptom severity often increases with increased body weight. Another major risk factor for apnea is nasopharyngeal abnormalities that reduce the upper airway diameter. Though generalized narrowing is common in adults and in children, anatomopathological anomalies such as adenotonsillar hypertrophy can increase the risk of apnea, and deviations of the nasal septum are often observed [6]. A fundamental premise for the treatment of OSAS is an accurate and multidisciplinary diagnosis: the reference centers for sleep medicine usually have a team that includes, in addition to the sleep doctor (specialist in pneumology or neurology) who coordinates activities, other specialists (maxillofacial specialist, orthodontist, otolaryngologist, and nutritionist) who each deal with their own skills to best treat this disease [3, 7]. To reach a correct diagnosis, the clinical work-up requires the association of comprehensive clinical evaluation (anamnesis, physical examination) and nocturnal polysomnography [8]. The last one uses a simultaneous recording of several physiological parameters during the night, using a polysomnograph. Normally, during the test, two or more electroencephalography channels, various electromyographic channels, chest and abdomen movements, oronasal flow, and oxygen saturation in the blood are recorded [9]. There is a variety of

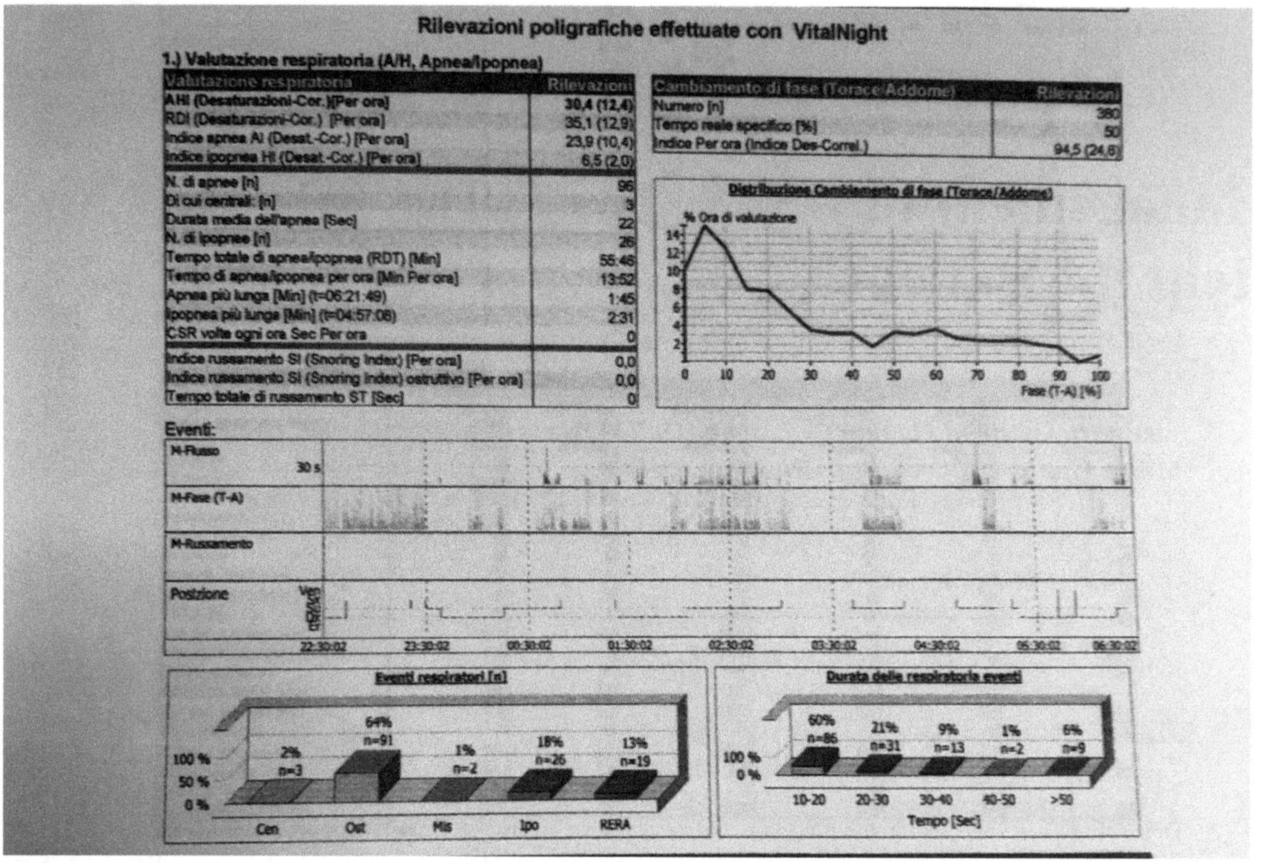

Figure 1: Polysomnographic report before treatment with the ELIBA® device. The apnea hypopnea index (AHI) was 30.4.

treatments for obstructive sleep apnea syndrome, which depends on the medical history of the individual, the severity of the disorder and, mainly, the specific cause of the obstruction. Although there are various oral devices to treat OSAS, many of these devices are cumbersome for patients to use at night because they act to advance the position of the jaw [10–12].

2. Case Report

A forty-five-year-old male Caucasian patient had a chief complaint of numerous episodes of nocturnal apnea and daytime sleepiness. The patient had no history of diabetes and asthma. The dental history was insignificant. The patient's body mass index was 29 (overweight), and he was being treated by a nutritionist to improve alimentation and lose weight [13]. The patient's arterial blood pressure was 120/80 mmHg, his pulse was 95 beats/min, and his respiratory rate was 20 breaths/min. The results of the laboratory (i.e., complete blood count, hematocrit, mean corpuscular value, erythrocyte sedimentation rate, and lipid panel) examinations were normal. Chest X-ray, respiratory function tests, and bronchoscopic test results were also normal. The upper airway appeared normal in ear-nose-throat and laryngoscopy examinations. The patient's neck and tongue muscles were enlarged. Written consent was obtained from the patient.

Upon polysomnographic examination, the subject was diagnosed with positional preference obstructive sleep apnea syndrome (OSAS), with 70% of episodes occurring while the patient was in the supine position (Figure 1). During the test, he had 96 apneas, 3 of which were central. The patient's apnea hypopnea index (AHI) was 30.4, a value that meets the criterion for severe sleep apnea [14, 15]. Treatment options for reduction of the OSAS, including a lingual elevator by Balercia (ELIBA® device that properly spaces the orolingual space for better breathing) and continuous positive airway pressure (CPAP) therapy, were discussed with the patient. Because the patient refused CPAP therapy due to discomfort, the patient was prescribed an ELIBA®, which is a small, comfortable to wear device that does not change the position of the jaw.

Briefly, dental stone models of the dental arches and Myoprint impressions of the physiological free orolingual space were made using Bosworth Sapphire acrylic resin (custom acrylic material; Bosworth Company) under ultra-low-frequency-transcutaneous nervous stimulation (ULF-TENS) [16–20]. The low-frequency neurostimulator (J5 Myomonitor® TENS Unit, Myotronics-Noromed Inc., Tukwila, WA) generated a repetitive, synchronous, and bilateral stimulus through pulsed currents delivered at 1.5 s intervals and a frequency of 0.66 Hz. The two TENS electrodes (Myotrode SG Electrodes®, Myotronics-Noromed Inc., Tukwila, WA) were then placed bilaterally over the cutaneous projection of the fifth pair of cranial nerves notch,

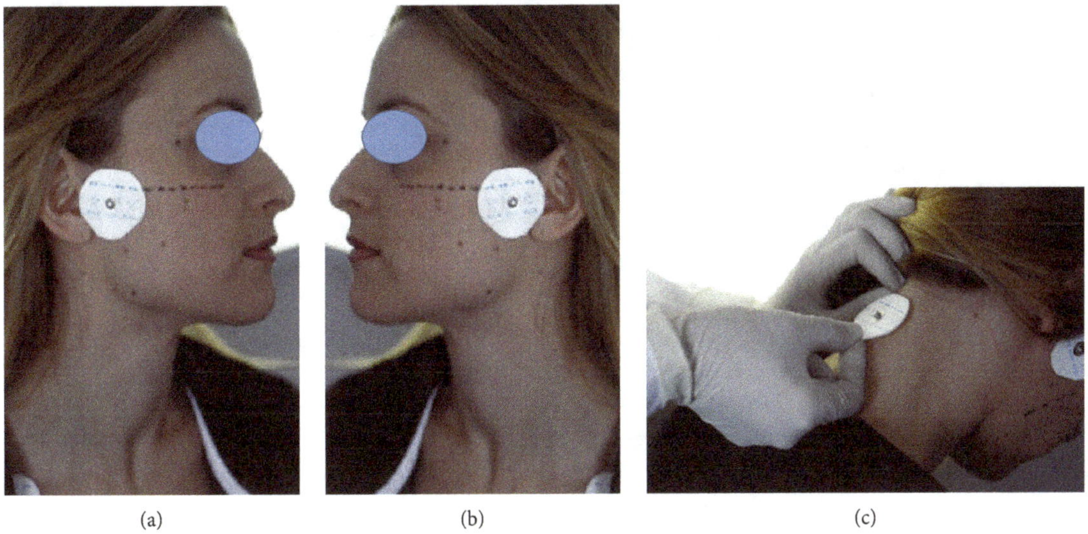

FIGURE 2: Application of TENS electrodes. (a, b) The two TENS electrodes are placed bilaterally over the cutaneous projection of the fifth pair of cranial nerves notch, which is located between the coronoid and condylar processes. (c) A third grounding electrode is placed in the center of the back of the neck.

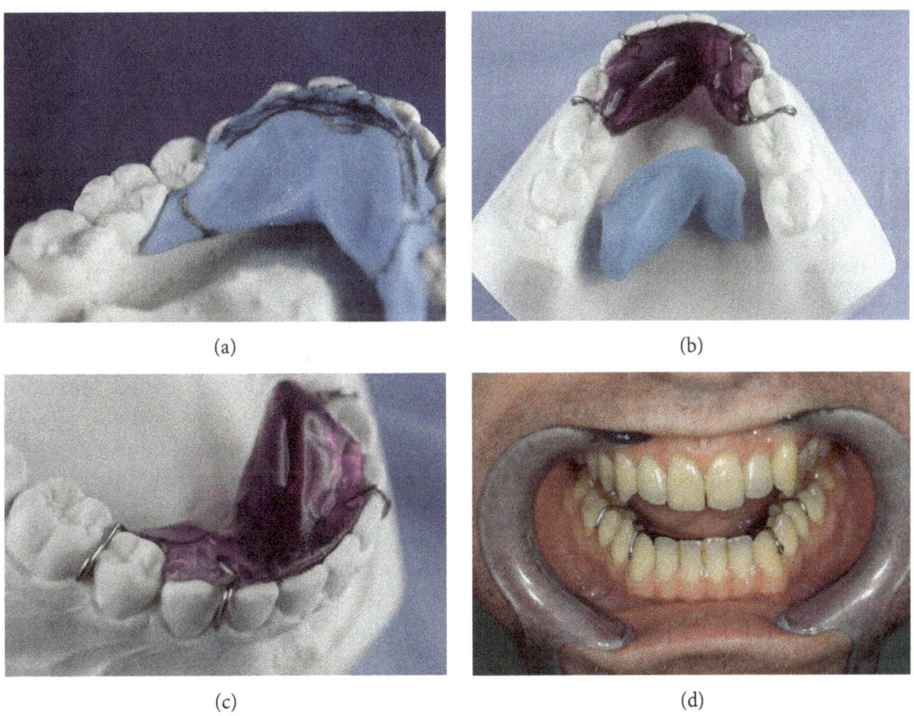

FIGURE 3: ELIBA® construction phases and oral aspect of the device. (a) Marking of the lateral/distal borders of the ELIBA® device, as specified by the clinician. (b) The ELIBA® appliance on the plastic cast and impression of the ELIBA® device. (c) Enlargement of the device ELIBA® applied on the plastic cast with hooks in front area in cobalt chrome. (d) Intraoral views of the ELIBA® appliance fitted to the oral cavity of the patient.

which was located between the coronoid and condylar processes. This location was determined by manual palpation of the zone anterior to the tragus (Figures 2(a) and 2(b)). A third grounding electrode was placed in the center of the back of the neck [21, 22] (Figure 2(c)). Central nervous system stimulation was produced by sensory stimulation of cranial nerves V and VII with low-frequency TENS [18]. Typically, low-frequency ULF-TENS is applied to bring the mandible in a neutral position that can obviate the need for occlusal adjustments [19]. Once the threshold of sensory stimulus is identified, identified by the sensation of tingling at the level of the electrodes, the stimulus is administered

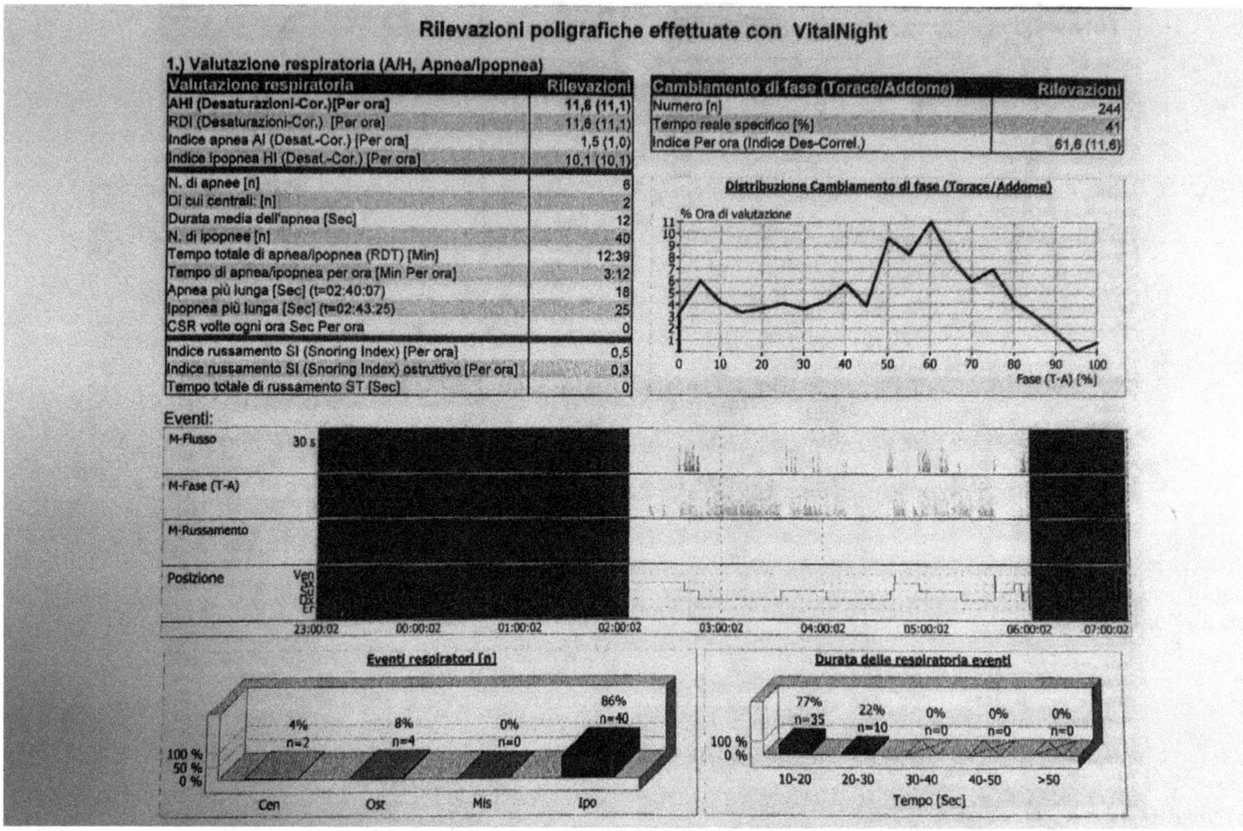

FIGURE 4: Polysomnographic report after treatment with the ELIBA® device. The apnea hypopnea index (AHI) decreased to 11.6.

with the ULF-TENS. The patient is asked to rest the apex of the tongue against the back incisive papilla and keep it relaxed in this position for the duration of the procedure. When the resin reached a solid but elastic consistency, before complete hardening, it was extracted from the oral cavity and inserted into the master model to complete its hardening. The clinician indicated to the dental laboratory (enabled to manufacture) the distal lateral limits for the construction of the artifact and the most suitable retentive devices for the stabilization of ELIBA®. ELIBA® must be totally passive and must not touch the oral mucosa [4–9, 19, 23–27] (Figures 3(a)–3(d)).

After six months of using the ELIBA® device, the patient's apnea improved, and the second polysomnographic examination revealed only six apnea episodes, two of which were central. The patient's AHI decreased to 11.6 after implementation of the ELIBA® device (Figure 4). Moreover, the patient's overall health improved owing to dietary adjustments. He lost ten kilograms, and his body mass index decreased to 25. The patient appeared satisfied with the results of the ELIBA® and dietary adjustments.

3. Discussion

The patient described in this case was treated with an ELIBA® device, in strict accordance with the principles of neuromyofascial occlusal dynamics. The ELIBA®, which was designed to treat atypical swallowing and yields better patient compliance than those prescribed CPAP, modifies the position of the tongue by acting on the inner component of the trigeminal system and partly on the autonomic nervous system. ELIBA® seizes the patient's physiological free orolingual space, defined anteriorly and laterally by the lower jaw, inferiorly by the tongue floor, and superiorly by the ventral surface of the tongue. The Medium Longitudinal File, which allows a direct connection between the various cranial nerves, can provide a way to link the upper spinal cord to the mesencephalus. The ELIBA® works by way of proprioception and interception, in which it stimulates the trigeminal system and, consequently, activates the oculomotor system to help maintain appropriate tongue position and movement [28]. Contact of the tongue apex with its designated spot during the night together with perioral muscle-generated centripetal force is indicative of functional improvement. The tongue and neck muscles are related by way of proprioception via a common trunk from the ansa cervicalis through the hypoglossal nerve [29]. Currently, tongue position studies have suggested that it may not be possible to improve OSAS, at least not without difficult-to-use devices, because it is related to a subcortical abnormality, specifically in the ventral part of the rostral brainstem [30, 31].

The ELIBA® is a simple, customizable device that is comfortable for patients to wear and does not have any contraindications in children or adults. In the current case study, ELIBA® implementation combined with dietary changes improved the patient's sleep quality while maintaining patient comfort [32]. The patient was satisfied with the outcome of the ELIBA®. The authors hope to treat further patients with this approach to understand more about its advantages and possible limitations.

References

[1] D. M. Toraldo, D. Passali, A. Sanna, F. De Nuccio, L. Conte, and M. De Benedetto, "Cost-effectiveness strategies in OSAS management: a short review," *Acta Otorhinolaryngologica Italica*, vol. 37, no. 6, pp. 447–453, 2017, Strategie e costi/benefici nella gestione dell'OSAS.

[2] D. Manzanares, M. E. Monzon, R. C. Savani, and M. Salathe, "Apical oxidative hyaluronan degradation stimulates airway ciliary beating via RHAMM and RON," *American Journal of Respiratory Cell and Molecular Biology*, vol. 37, no. 2, pp. 160–168, 2007.

[3] S. M. Caples, A. S. Gami, and V. K. Somers, "Obstructive sleep apnea," *Annals of Internal Medicine*, vol. 142, no. 3, pp. 187–197, 2005.

[4] R. Del Pinto and C. Ferri, "Inflammation-accelerated senescence and the cardiovascular system: mechanisms and perspectives," *International Journal of Molecular Sciences*, vol. 19, no. 12, p. 3701, 2018.

[5] R. Del Pinto and C. Ferri, "Hypertension management at older age: an update," *High Blood Pressure & Cardiovascular Prevention*, vol. 26, no. 1, pp. 27–36, 2019.

[6] I. Helena, E. Margareta, L. Eva, and Å. Pernilla, "Tailored behavioral medicine intervention for enhanced physical activity and healthy eating in patients with obstructive sleep apnea syndrome and overweight," *Sleep and Breathing*, vol. 18, no. 3, pp. 655–668, 2014.

[7] D. Pietropaoli, E. Ortu, M. Severino, I. Ciarrocchi, R. Gatto, and A. Monaco, "Glycation and oxidative stress in the failure of dental implants: a case series," *BMC Research Notes*, vol. 6, no. 1, 2013.

[8] S. Baiardi and F. Cirignotta, "The clinical diagnosis of obstructive sleep apnea syndrome (OSAS)," *La Medicina del lavoro*, vol. 108, no. 4, pp. 267–275, 2017, La diagnosi clinic-strumentale della Sindrome delle Apnee Ostrutiive nel Sonno (OSAS).

[9] V. Ibanez, J. Silva, and O. Cauli, "A survey on sleep assessment methods," *PeerJ*, vol. 6, article e4849, 2018.

[10] R. Marco Pitarch, M. Selva García, J. Puertas Cuesta, J. Marco Algarra, E. Fernández Julian, and A. Fons Font, "Effectiveness of a mandibular advancement device in obstructive sleep apnea patients: a prospective clinical trial," *European Archives of Oto-Rhino-Laryngology*, vol. 275, no. 7, pp. 1903–1911, 2018.

[11] E. Ortu, M. Giannoni, M. Ortu, R. Gatto, and A. Monaco, "Oropharyngeal airway changes after rapid maxillary expansion: the state of the art," *International Journal of Clinical and Experimental Medicine*, vol. 7, no. 7, pp. 1632–1638, 2014.

[12] E. Ortu, D. Pietropaoli, M. Ortu, M. Giannoni, and A. Monaco, "Evaluation of cervical posture following rapid maxillary expansion: a review of literature," *The Open Dentistry Journal*, vol. 8, no. 1, pp. 20–27, 2014.

[13] K. M. Flegal, M. D. Carroll, B. K. Kit, and C. L. Ogden, "Prevalence of obesity and trends in the distribution of body mass index among US adults, 1999-2010," *JAMA*, vol. 307, no. 5, pp. 491–497, 2012.

[14] W. R. Ruehland, P. D. Rochford, F. J. O'Donoghue, R. J. Pierce, P. Singh, and A. T. Thornton, "The new AASM criteria for scoring hypopneas: impact on the apnea hypopnea index," *Sleep*, vol. 32, no. 2, pp. 150–157, 2009.

[15] D. Passali, M. C. Spinosi, and F. M. Passali, "Ear nose and throat (ENT) aspects of obstructive sleep apnea syndrome (OSAS) diagnosis and therapy," *La Medicina del lavoro*, vol. 108, no. 4, pp. 288–292, 2017, Sindrome delle Apnee Ostruttive nel Sonno (OSAS): aspetti diagnostici e terapeutici otorinolaringoiatrici.

[16] A. Monaco, R. Cattaneo, M. C. Marci, D. Pietropaoli, and E. Ortu, "Central sensitization-based classification for temporomandibular disorders: a pathogenetic hypothesis," *Pain Research & Management*, vol. 2017, article 5957076, pp. 1–13, 2017.

[17] G. Aprile, E. Ortu, R. Cattaneo, C. Pietropaoli, M. Giannoni, and A. Monaco, "Orthodontic management by functional activator treatment: a case report," *Journal of Medical Case Reports*, vol. 11, no. 1, 2017.

[18] A. Monaco, R. Cattaneo, E. Ortu, M. V. Constantinescu, and D. Pietropaoli, "Sensory trigeminal ULF-TENS stimulation reduces HRV response to experimentally induced arithmetic stress: a randomized clinical trial," *Physiology & Behavior*, vol. 173, pp. 209–215, 2017.

[19] E. Ortu, D. Pietropaoli, G. Mazzei, R. Cattaneo, M. Giannoni, and A. Monaco, "TENS effects on salivary stress markers: a pilot study," *International Journal of Immunopathology and Pharmacology*, vol. 28, no. 1, pp. 114–118, 2015.

[20] V. Parlati, E. Ortu, R. Cattaneo, A. Mummolo, D. Pietropaoli, and A. Monaco, "Electric activity of stomatognatic muscles and opening of the lower jaw [Attività elettrica dei muscoli del sistema stomatognatico e apertura della mandibola]," *Dental Cadmos*, vol. 87, no. 7, pp. 422–442, 2019.

[21] R. Cattaneo and A. Monaco, *La TENS per uso odontoiatrico*, Futura publishing Society, 2016.

[22] L. Guerrini, A. Monaco, D. Pietropaoli, E. Ortu, M. Giannoni, and M. C. Marci, "Antibiotics in dentistry: a narrative review of literature and guidelines considering antibiotic resistance," *The Open Dentistry Journal*, vol. 13, pp. 383–398, 2019.

[23] T. Castroflorio, D. Farina, A. Bottin et al., "Non-invasive assessment of motor unit anatomy in jaw-elevator muscles," *Journal of Oral Rehabilitation*, vol. 32, no. 10, pp. 708–713, 2005.

[24] D. Falla, P. Dall'Alba, A. Rainoldi, R. Merletti, and G. Jull, "Location of innervation zones of sternocleidomastoid and scalene muscles–a basis for clinical and research electromyography applications," *Clinical Neurophysiology*, vol. 113, no. 1, pp. 57–63, 2002.

[25] A. Monaco, R. Cattaneo, A. Spadaro, and G. Marzo, "Neuromuscular diagnosis in orthodontics: effects of TENS on the sagittal maxillo-mandibular relationship," *European Journal of Paediatric*, vol. 9, no. 4, pp. 163–169, 2008.

[26] E. Ortu, M. Lacarbonara, R. Cattaneo, G. Marzo, R. Gatto, and A. Monaco, "Electromyographic evaluation of a patient treated with extraoral traction: a case report," *European Journal of Paediatric Dentistry*, vol. 17, no. 2, pp. 123–128, 2016.

[27] E. Ortu, D. Pietropaoli, F. Adib, C. Masci, M. Giannoni, and A. Monaco, "Electromyographic evaluation in children

orthodontically treated for skeletal class II malocclusion: comparison of two treatment techniques," *CRANIO®*, vol. 37, no. 2, pp. 129–135, 2019.

[28] N. Marchili, E. Ortu, D. Pietropaoli, R. Cattaneo, and A. Monaco, "Dental occlusion and ophthalmology: a literature review," *The Open Dentistry Journal*, vol. 10, no. 1, pp. 460–468, 2016.

[29] I. J. Edwards, V. K. Lall, J. F. Paton et al., "Neck muscle afferents influence oromotor and cardiorespiratory brainstem neural circuits," *Brain Structure & Function*, vol. 220, no. 3, pp. 1421–1436, 2015.

[30] A. Monaco, R. Cattaneo, C. Masci, A. Spadaro, and G. Marzo, "Effect of ill-fitting dentures on the swallowing duration in patients using polygraphy," *Gerodontology*, vol. 29, no. 2, pp. e637–e644, 2012.

[31] F. Sista, V. Abruzzese, M. Schietroma, E. M. Cecilia, A. Mattei, and G. Amicucci, "New harmonic scalpel versus conventional hemostasis in right colon surgery: a prospective randomized controlled clinical trial," *Digestive Surgery*, vol. 30, no. 4-6, pp. 355–361, 2013.

[32] E. Ortu, D. Pietropaoli, R. Cattaneo, M. Giannoni, and A. Monaco, "Overjet reduction with the use of the ELIBA device: a case report," *Journal of Clinical and Diagnostic Research*, vol. 12, no. 12, pp. 8–10, 2018.

28

Oral Management of a Haematopoietic Stem Cell Transplant Recipient with Chédiak–Higashi Syndrome

Kasumi Shimizu, Miho Hayashi, Nozomi Ito, Kokoro Hamada, Gaku Koizumi, Kazuto Kurohara, and Naoya Arai

Department of Oral and Maxillofacial Surgery, Department of Clinical Sciences, Medical Life Science, Mie University Graduate School of Medicine, Tsu, Mie 514-8507, Japan

Correspondence should be addressed to Kasumi Shimizu; skasumi@clin.medic.mie-u.ac.jp

Academic Editor: Giuseppe Colella

Chédiak–Higashi syndrome (CHS), a rare autosomal recessive disorder associated with leukocyte dysfunction, is characterised by partial skin and hair albinism, immunodeficiency, and abnormal bleeding. Furthermore, it may be associated with cognitive and neurological impairments. The long-term prognosis of patients is generally poor, and haematopoietic stem cell transplantation is a radical immunodeficiency treatment. Here, we report a case of successful oral management of an 18-year-old woman with CHS accompanied by aggressive periodontitis who underwent haematopoietic stem cell transplantation.

1. Introduction

Chédiak–Higashi syndrome (CHS) is a rare congenital recessive disorder caused by mutations in the lysosomal trafficking regulator gene (*LYST*) [1]. A murine model of CHS suggested that *LYST* encodes a cytoplasmic protein and is involved in granule transport and fusion; however, the exact cellular function of this protein is unclear. Histologically, mutations of *LYST* result in large intracellular granules that are characteristic of CHS. The encapsulation of giant melanosomes and large amounts of lysosomes can be observed in melanocytes and leukocytes, respectively, and are associated with hypopigmentation and impaired cellular immunity. Defective organelle transport also markedly reduces the number of dense granules present in platelets [2].

Only approximately 500 cases of CHS have been reported worldwide. CHS has multiple clinical features, including hypopigmentation of the skin and hair, reduced platelet and leukocyte counts, abnormal organelles in circulating granulated cells, and neurological dysfunction. Patients often exhibit a severe phenotype and die in the first decade of life; however, in approximately 10%–15% of patients, the disease has a relatively milder clinical course.

Even patients with comparatively mild CHS reportedly experience severe periodontitis due to immunodeficiency. Thumbigere Math et al. [3] reported that *LYST* mutations in patients with CHS can affect the expression and function of Toll-like receptor 2 and Toll-like receptor 4, leading to dysregulation of immune reactions and affecting the status of periodontitis.

Therefore, oral management is of utmost importance in patients undergoing haematopoietic stem cell transplantation. However, few reports have discussed oral management in patients with CHS undergoing haematopoietic stem cell transplantation.

In this study, we describe the oral management for a patient with CHS who had severe periodontitis before undergoing haematopoietic stem cell transplantation.

2. Case Presentation

An 18-year-old woman was referred to our department in a wheelchair for oral management before undergoing bone marrow transplant. She was diagnosed with atypical CHS 3 years prior by LYST RNA analysis and based on her clinical course. Because of repeated infections, she was scheduled to

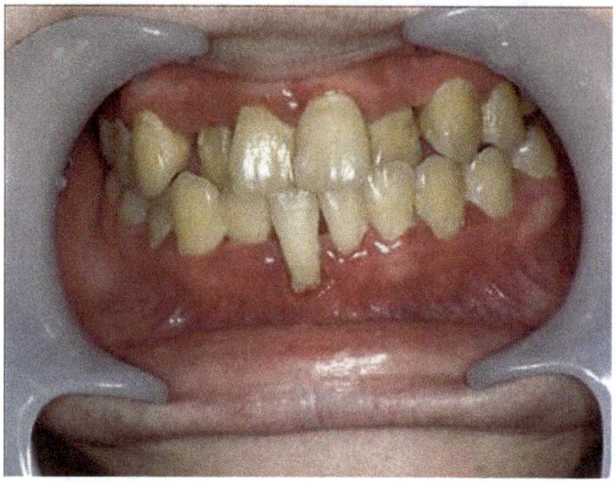

FIGURE 1: Intraoral view at the initial visit. Gingival swelling and redness were present throughout the oral cavity, and gingival retraction of the right lower central incisor was evident.

TABLE 1: Periodontal examination chart 7 weeks before the transplantation.

Grade of mobility	—	1	1	1	1	1	1	1	1	1	1	1	1	1	1	—
Probing depth	—	5	5	5	5	5	6	6	6	5	6	5	5	5	5	—
Tooth	8	7	6	5	4	3	2	1	1	2	3	4	5	6	7	8
Tooth	8	7	6	5	4	3	2	1	1	2	3	4	5	6	7	8
Probing depth	—	5	5	5	5	5	5	5	5	5	5	5	5	5	5	—
Grade of mobility	—	1	1	1	1	1	1	1	1	1	1	1	1	1	1	—

Plaque control record (O'Leary) 80%.

undergo haematopoietic stem cell transplantation in our paediatrics department after the completion of treatment for her limb pain, which is one of the neurological symptoms of CHS. At her first visit, the general findings included hyperpigmentation on the facial skin, which is often seen in Asian CHS. Her intraoral examination revealed extensive gingival swelling and redness and gingival retraction in the right lower central incisor (Figure 1). The gingival pocket depth was 5–6 mm, the degree of movement was grade 1, and the O'Leary plaque control record (PCR) value was 80% (Table 1).

We initiated professional oral care and self-administered oral care education 7 weeks before transplantation (Table 2). Her intelligence quotient was 75, and she feared using the ultrasonic scaler, so we made an effort to eliminate her fear. We performed professional mechanical tooth cleaning and cleaned the periodontal pockets. The O'Leary PCR value was very high on her first visit. However, it decreased following the educational sessions, and it was 58% at the final session before bone marrow transplantation. Approximately 2 weeks before transplantation, she entered the cleaning room. Etoposide, busulfan, and cyclophosphamide were administered, and grade 1 mucositis was observed as a side effect on the day before transplantation. The Common Terminology Criteria for Adverse Events version 4.0 was used to evaluate mucositis. From the day after transplantation, redness was observed on her oral mucosa as a side effect of methotrexate, and she experienced pain that rendered brushing impossible (Table 3). A gargle containing lidocaine (Xylocaine®) was effective. The use of Episil® oral liquid was also attempted, but she used it only once for irritation. Six days after transplantation, she developed grade 3 mucositis and underwent nutritional management via infusion. From 2 weeks after transplantation, her oral condition improved slightly (Figure 2). At 20 days after transplantation, the mucositis gradually improved, and brushing became possible. At 27 days after transplantation, the mucositis disappeared. The gingival swelling became mild, redness improved, and no gingival bleeding was detected during brushing (Figure 3). She was discharged 84 days after transplantation. Although there was no change in the degree of tooth movement, the gingival pocket depth and gingival swelling in the lower anterior region improved, and the O'Leary PCR value was 24.1%, which was lower than that before transplantation (Table 4).

3. Discussion

CHS is characterised by severe periodontitis from childhood due to its adverse effects on immunity; however, its management is rarely reported due to its low incidence. Shibutani et al. [4] conducted long-term follow-up observations in a patient with CHS and reported that periodontal treatment resulted in a limited response. Our patient appeared to have atypical CHS as she had not been diagnosed even until the age of 16 years. Irrespective of age, her periodontitis was moderate, with a periodontal pocket depth of 5–6 mm and tooth mobility. She often experienced fever and salivary gland inflammation, possibly caused by oral bacterial infection.

The treatment for CHS is bone marrow transplantation; its success depends on professional oral health care and self-administered oral care. CHS can be associated with cognitive and neurological impairments [5]. Certain et al. [6] described patients with CHS with low intellectual capacity, mental retardation, and poor school performance. Our patient was borderline in this respect as she has an intelligence quotient of 75. Despite being aged 18 years, she was initially scared of using the ultrasonic scaler and it was difficult for her to brush her teeth independently. The interventions were initiated 7 weeks before bone marrow transplantation, and subsequently, she has become accustomed to dental instruments and dental hygienists. In addition, we provided professional oral health care and self-care guidance to the patient and her parents. Kashiwazaki et al. [7] reported that professional oral health care reduces the incidence of oral mucositis and febrile neutropenia after bone marrow transplantation. Yoneyama et al. [8] reported that control of dental plaque by professional brushing combined with frequent tooth cleaning and self-administered oral care could reduce microbial counts.

In the present case, the chemo-induced oral mucositis progressed to grade 3 and required tube feeding, but there was no febrile neutropenia. Oral mucositis was alleviated using a mouthwash containing lidocaine. Episil® has recently been used to control pain in oral mucositis. It protects the oral mucosa and controls and alleviates oral pain caused by

Table 2: Treatment schedule and oral condition before the transplantation.

Week	−7	−6	−5	−4	−3	−2	−1	0 (transplantation)
Pretransplant treatment							VP-16, BU, CY	
O'Leary PCR (%)	80.0	74.1	64.3	54.5	53.0	58.0		
Stomatitis (grade)							1	
Treatment for stomatitis								

Table 3: Treatment schedule and oral condition after the transplantation.

Day	0	1	2	3	4	5	6	7	8	9	13	14	15	16	20	84
Immuno-suppressive therapy			MTX													
O'Leary PCR(%)		2														24.1
Stomatitis(grade)							3				2				1	
Treatment for stomatitis		Mouthwash containing lidcaine					episil® →									

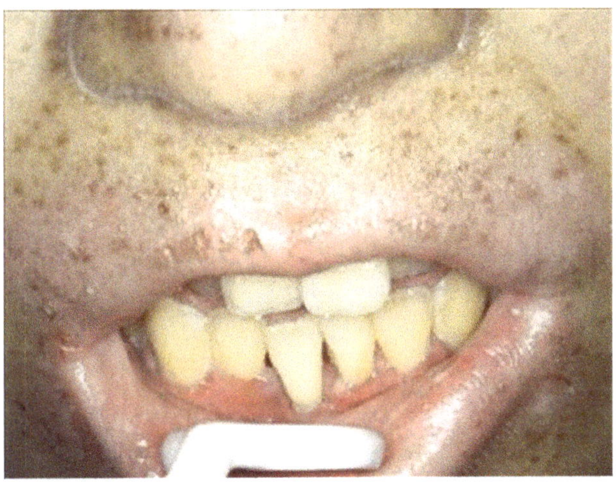

Figure 2: Oral condition 2 weeks after stem cell transplantation. Oral mucositis improved slightly. Hyperpigmentation was noted around the lips, but this was also present at the first visit.

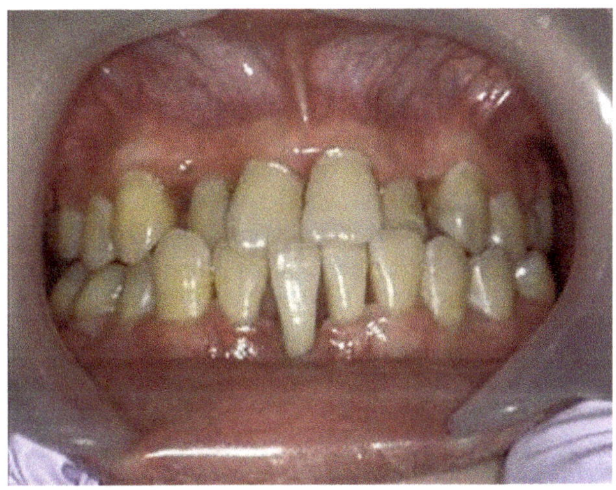

Figure 3: Oral condition 7 weeks after stem cell transplantation. Mild gingival swelling was evident, and the redness had improved. Bleeding was absent during scaling or brushing.

stomatitis associated with chemotherapy and radiotherapy through a physical mode of action. It became commercially available in Japan in 2018. It protects the surfaces of ulcers and erosions and relieves pain by forming a bioadhesive film. Hadjieva et al. [9] reported that the use of Episil® in patients who underwent radiotherapy for head and neck cancer provided significant pain relief.

Because Episil® is a spray, our patient could not use it because it caused painful irritation during spraying. We determined that as the mucositis had progressed to grade 3, the spray should have been used earlier. Eventually, her mucositis and oral hygiene improved, and she was successfully discharged.

This is the first report of the oral management of a patient with CHS undergoing haematopoietic stem cell transplantation to the best of our knowledge. We performed oral care in this patient with CHS accompanied by periodontitis, and it contributed to successful haematopoietic stem cell transplantation and improved her periodontitis. Periodontitis tends to become severe in patients with CHS; however, early management is important as stem cell transplantation is performed for the treatment.

Table 4: Periodontal examination chart 12 weeks after the transplantation.

Grade of mobility	—	1	1	1	1	1	1	1	1	1	1	1	1	1	1	—
Probing depth	—	3	3	3	2	2	3	3	2	2	2	2	3	3	3	—
Tooth	8	7	6	5	4	3	2	1	1	2	3	4	5	6	7	8
Tooth	8	7	6	5	4	3	2	1	1	2	3	4	5	6	7	8
Probing depth	—	3	2	2	2	3	3	2	2	2	2	2	3	4	3	—
Grade of mobility	—	1	1	1	1	1	1	1	1	1	1	1	1	1	1	—

Plaque control record (O'Leary) 24.1%.

References

[1] J. Kaplan, I. de Domenico, and D. M. Ward, "Chediak-Higashi syndrome," *Current Opinion in Hematology*, vol. 15, no. 1, pp. 22–29, 2008.

[2] J. Masliah-Planchon, L. Darnige, and S. Bellucci, "Molecular determinants of platelet delta storage pool deficiencies: an update," *British Journal of Haematology*, vol. 160, no. 1, pp. 5–11, 2013.

[3] V. Thumbigere Math, P. Rebouças, P. A. Giovani et al., "Periodontitis in Chédiak-Higashi syndrome: an altered immunoinflammatory response," *JDR clinical & translational research*, vol. 3, no. 1, pp. 35–46, 2018.

[4] T. Shibutani, K. Gen, M. Shibata, Y. Horiguchi, N. Kondo, and Y. Iwayama, "Long-term follow-up of periodontitis in a patient with Chédiak-Higashi syndrome. A case report," *Journal of Periodontology*, vol. 71, no. 6, pp. 1024-1028, 2000.

[5] T. N. Shirazi, J. Snow, L. Ham et al., "The neuropsychological phenotype of Chediak-Higashi disease," *Orphanet Journal of Rare Diseases*, vol. 14, no. 1, p. 101, 2019.

[6] S. Certain, F. Barrat, E. Pastural et al., "Protein truncation test of LYST reveals heterogenous mutations in patients with Chediak-Higashi syndrome," *Blood*, vol. 95, no. 3, pp. 979–983, 2000.

[7] H. Kashiwazaki, T. Matsushita, J. Sugita et al., "Professional oral health care reduces oral mucositis and febrile neutropenia in patients treated with allogeneic bone marrow transplantation," *Supportive Care in Cancer*, vol. 20, no. 2, pp. 367–373, 2012.

[8] T. Yoneyama, M. Yoshida, T. Matsui, and H. Sasaki, "Oral care and pneumonia," *The Lancet*, vol. 354, p. 515, 1999.

[9] T. Hadjieva, E. Cavallin-Ståhl, M. Linden, and F. Tiberg, "Treatment of oral mucositis pain following radiation therapy for head-and-neck cancer using a bioadhesive barrier-forming lipid solution," *Supportive Care in Cancer*, vol. 22, no. 6, pp. 1557–1562, 2014.

29

Clinical, Imaging and Histopathology of Angioleiomyoma of the Buccal Cheek

Mohammad Jafarian,[1] Fatemeh Mashhadi Abbas,[2] Mitra Ghazizadeh Ahsaie,[3] and Homeira Saebnoori[2]

[1]Department of Oral and Maxillofacial Surgery, School of Dentistry, Shahid Beheshti University of Medical Sciences, Tehran, Iran
[2]Department of Oral and Maxillofacial Pathology, School of Dentistry, Shahid Beheshti University of Medical Sciences, Tehran, Iran
[3]Department of Oral and Maxillofacial Radiology, School of Dentistry, Shahid Beheshti University of Medical Sciences, Tehran, Iran

Correspondence should be addressed to Mitra Ghazizadeh Ahsaie; mitraghazizadeh@gmail.com

Academic Editor: Giovanni Mergoni

Angioleiomyoma is a benign neoplasia originating from vascular smooth muscle and very uncommon in the oral cavity. In this report, we present a rare case of angioleiomyoma in oral cavity in a 46-year-old female buccal cheek and discuss the clinical, histological, and immunohistochemical characteristics. As the treatment of choice is the complete excision, the lesion was excised under local anesthesia with no further complications. In addition, a brief update on other reported cases of angiomyoma in the oral cavity is further discussed.

1. Introduction

Angiomyoma or angioleiomyoma (also known as vascular leiomyoma) are benign neoplasms originating from vascular smooth muscle [1, 2]. Histologically, there are subgroups in three categories: solid, venous, and cavernous [3]. They commonly occur in the extremities and female genital tract and rarely in the oral cavity [4, 5]. The most common site in the oral cavity is in the lips [1]. Other reported sites were the palate, tongue, cheek, gingiva, retromolar area, and submandibular triangle [2, 6–10]. Although the etiology is still unclear, previous studies report trauma or spontaneous development as the causes of origin in oral cavity [10, 11]. The lesion is most often detected in adults of 30 to 50 years old [3]. Clinically, it usually presents as a slow growing, painless nodule or mass of variable size; however, pain has also been reported [12]. The final treatment and diagnosis is based on surgical excision and hematoxylin and eosin (H&E) staining and immune-histochemical (IHC) assessments [1]. In this report, a rare case of angioleiomyoma in the cheek along with a complete imaging assessment including color Doppler ultrasonography, computed tomography (CT), and magnetic resonance imaging (MRI) with an update on the literature is presented.

2. Case Report

A 46-year-old female was referred to a private clinic of an Oral and Maxillofacial Surgeon with complaint of a painless swelling in the right side of her cheek since 6 years ago. The swelling was initially small in size and slowly enlarged, although the patients faced no tenderness in the area. The patient had diabetes mellitus and anemia. In addition, no history of previous trauma to the area was present. Extraoral examination showed no asymmetry or marked expansion on the right cheek. On intraoral examination, no clinically visible lesion was detected. The mucosa was intact with no color change. When the area was palpated, a firm, compressible solid mass was detected with moderate attachment to the adjacent tissues. The estimated size of the lesion was $1.5 * 1$ cm, and the approximate diameter was 1.5 cm. No pulsation or bruit was present. The patient had previously visited and had prior imaging including Doppler ultrasonography, multidetector computed tomography (MDCT), and MRI. The

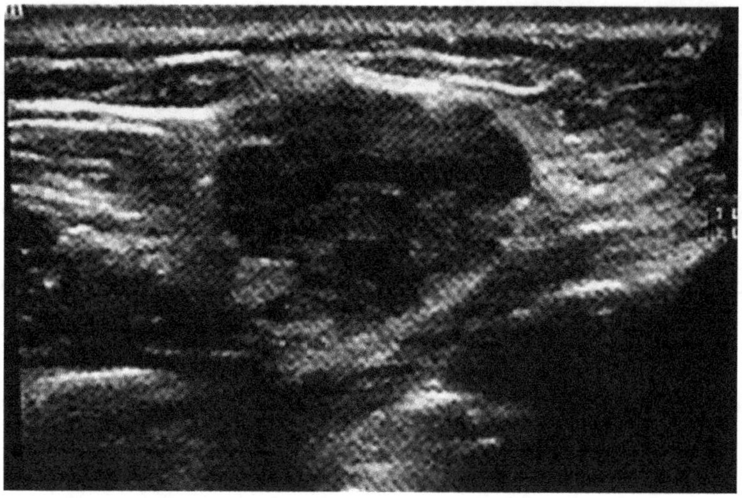

FIGURE 1: Ultrasonography shows a well-defined hypoechoic heterogenous mass lying between the skin and buccinator muscle.

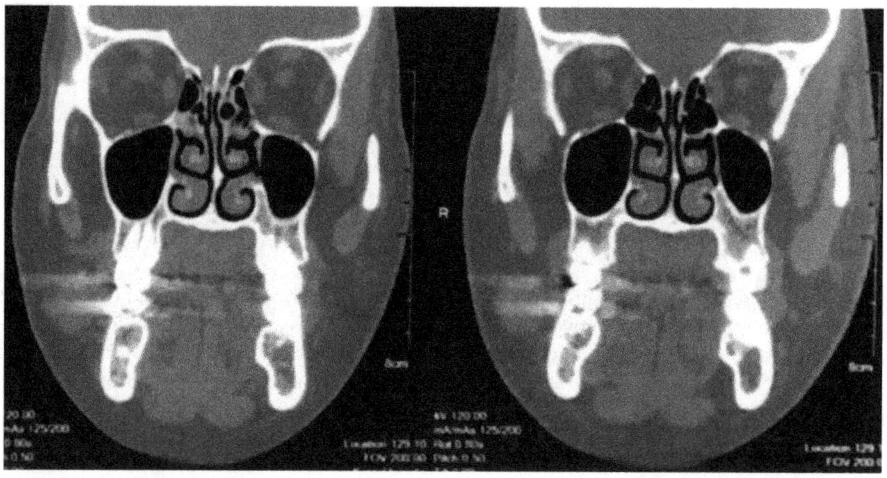

FIGURE 2: Coronal MDCT image shows a circular well-defined homogenous mass in the right buccal area.

results of ultrasonography indicated a well-defined hypoechoic heterogeneous mass lying beneath the skin measuring 13 * 18 mm (Figure 1). The lesion had moderate vascular flow. MDCT showed a circular well-defined homogenous mass over the buccinator muscle (Figure 2). The MRI T1 sequence showed a well-defined low signal mass between the buccinator muscle and buccal fat (Figure 3(a)). The MRI T2 sequence showed that the mass is homogenous and high signal (Figure 3(b)). A soft tissue mass was suspected, and an intraoral surgical excisional biopsy was planned. Upon obtaining consent, an excisional biopsy was performed under local anesthesia and incision was made on the buccal mucosa just over the palpated mass (Figure 4). The lesion was completely excised (Figure 5). H&E staining histopathological examination demonstrated an encapsulated mass composed of fully developed cavernous angioma in a fibrous stroma and occasionally myxomatous change. The thin-wall blood vessels showed papillary projections to the lumen which some had become irregular, large in size, and even sinusoid in some areas (Figure 6(a)). The stroma contains immature spindle-shaped fibroblasts with a paralleling fascicle pattern next to the blood vessels (Figure 6(b)). The mixed inflammatory infiltration and hyalinized area intermixed with adipose tissue were also found. In the IHC staining analysis, the specimen was positive for both SMA (smooth muscle actin) (Figures 7(a) and 7(b)) and desmin (Figures 7(c) and 7(d)); however, the microscopic features in combination with IHC findings were consistent with angioleiomyoma diagnosis. A postoperative follow-up of the patient was uneventful. The area had healed with no complication, and no signs of recurrence were detected.

3. Discussion

Angioleiomyoma is a rare benign soft tissue neoplasm of oral cavity [7]. Although hormonal changes, trauma, and venous stasis are suggested as possible causes, the etiology is still unknown [5]. On our latest review of literature from year 2000 to 2020 using the PubMed Central search engine, 25 articles (32 cases) were retrieved (Table 1). The most common sites of oral angiomyomas were the lip [2, 4, 12–15], cheek or buccal mucosa [5, 8, 14, 16–18], palate [7, 19–21],

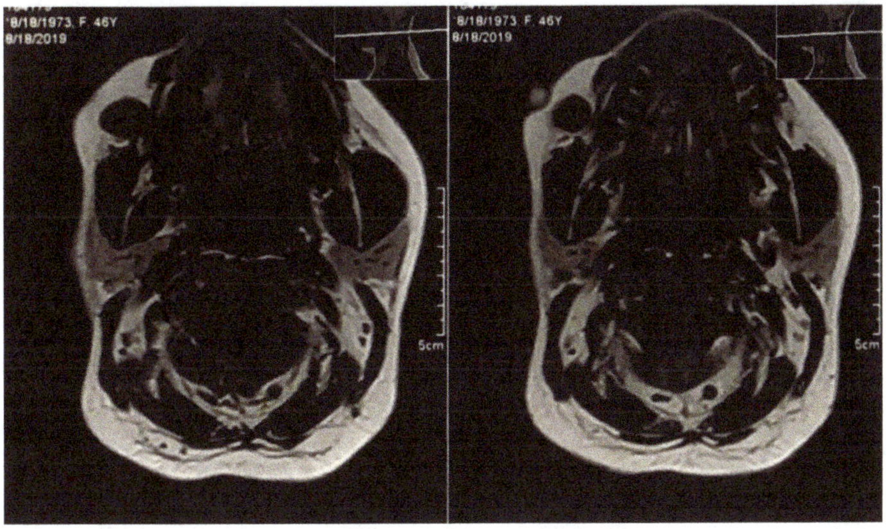

(a)

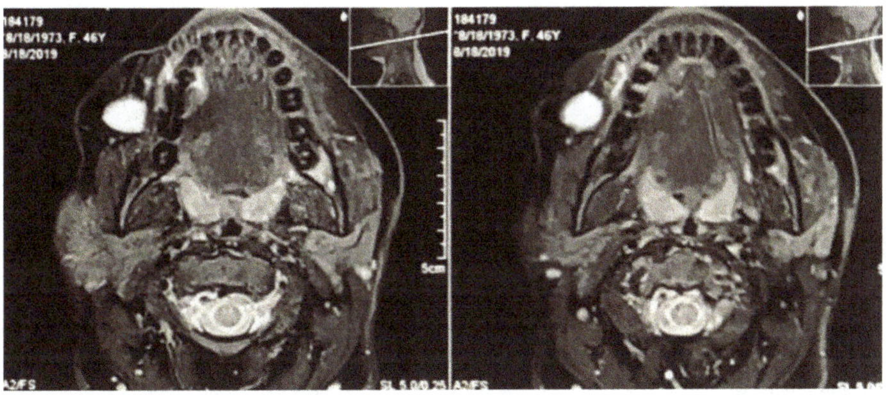

(b)

FIGURE 3: (a) Axial T1 MRI shows a low signal homogenous mass in the right lying over the buccinator muscle and under the skin. (b) Axial T2 MRI shows the lesion as high signal and homogenous.

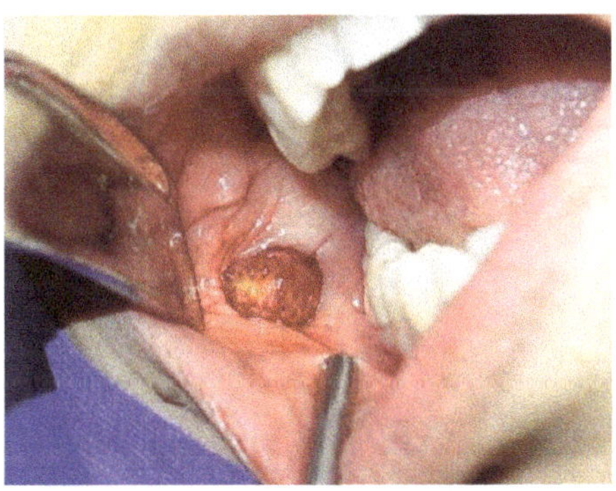

FIGURE 4: Intraoral incision on the buccal mucosa revealed a spherical lesion just underneath the buccinator muscle.

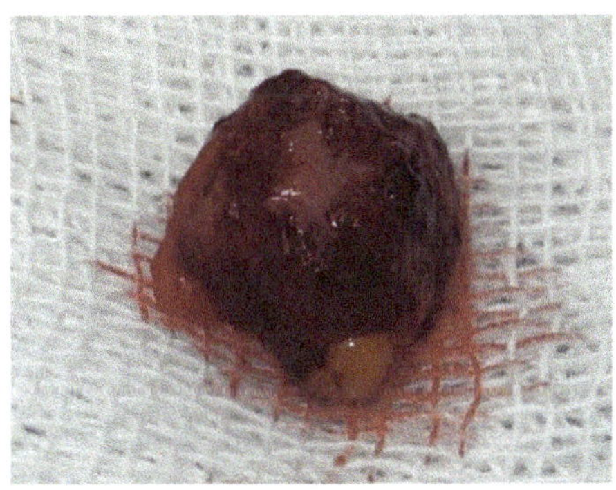

FIGURE 5: Image shows gross specimen, a spherical brown-gray firm tissue, measuring 1 cm in diameter.

tongue [6, 22, 23], and submandibular area [9, 11, 24]. The gingiva [10], mandible [2], retromolar area [2], and anterior maxillary labial fold [17] were each reported once among the studies. 73% of patients were male, and 27% were females, which is consistent with previous studies [25, 26]. The mean age was 43 ± 16.57 years old (range 2 to 79). Only one study reported a congenital angiomyoma in the tongue [3]. In all reviewed studies, the patient faced a painless swelling. Only three cases reported pain associated with the lesion [7, 21, 24].

Preoperative radiologic assessments varied among the studies, from no radiographic assessments and plain radiography to ultrasound, MRI, and CT evaluations. To our knowledge, this is the first case report of angioleiomyoma

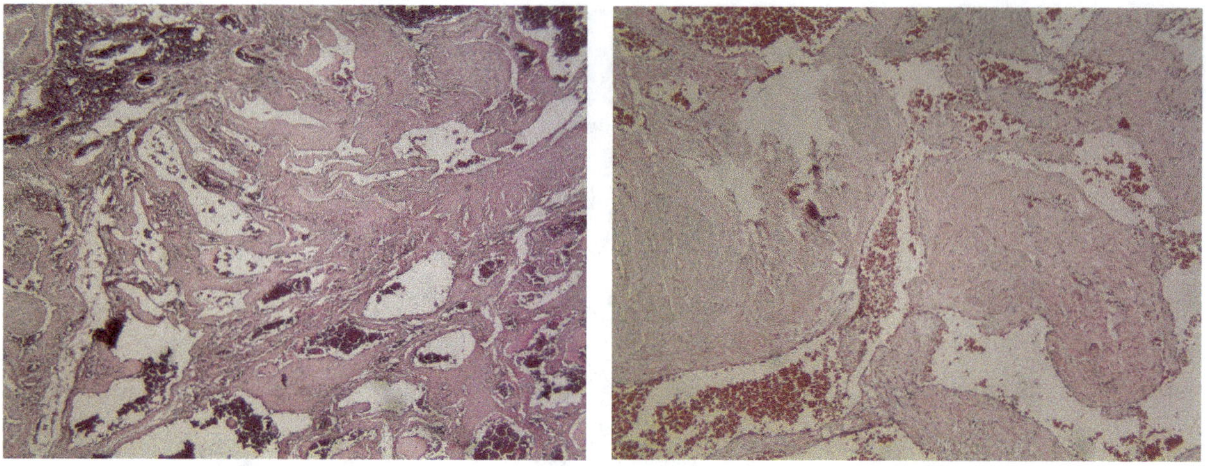

(a) (b)

FIGURE 6: (a) Thin blood vessels with papillary projections in the fibrous stroma (×40). (b) Paralleling pattern of fascicle and glomus cells around the blood vessels (×100).

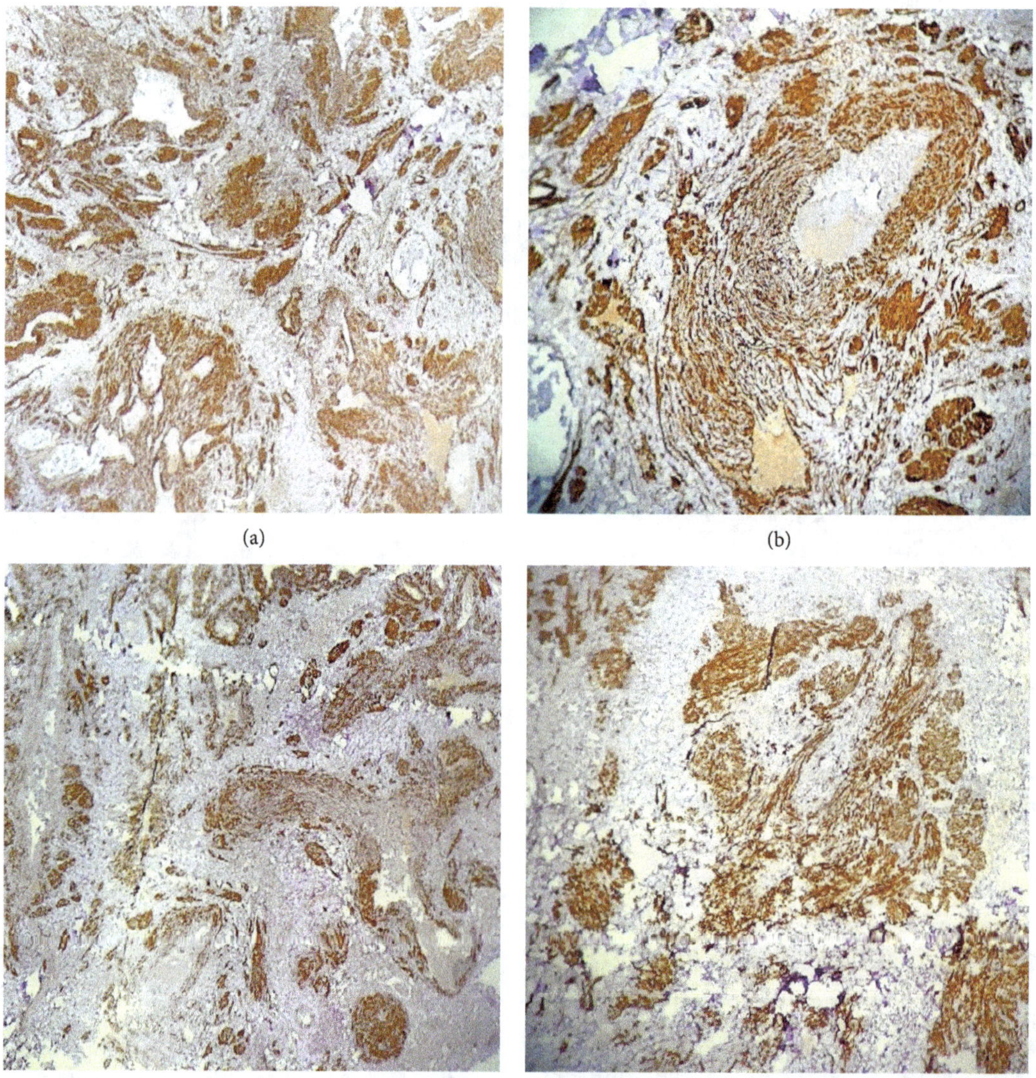

(a) (b) (c) (d)

FIGURE 7: (a) ×40 and (b) ×100 positive IHC staining for SMA. (c) ×40 and (d) ×100 positive for desmin.

Table 1: Review of various studies on angioleiomyoma of head and neck. cm: centimeter; CT: computed tomography; D: day; F: female; H&E: hematoxylin and eosin; IHC: immunohistochemistry; M: male; Mo: month; mm: millimeter; MRI: magnetic resonance imaging; SMA: smooth muscle actin; Y: year; YO: years old.

No	Author & year	Age & sex	Location	Size	Sign & symptoms	Radiologic assessments	Treatment plan	Anesthesia	Histologic assessments	Follow-up
1	Mehta et al., 2020 [15]	57 YO, M	Lower lip	1 × 1 cm	Exophytic nodular swelling	—	Surgical excision	Local	H&E: Large vascular channels of varying caliber, surrounded by thick walls of irregularly arranged spindle-shaped cells. Whorled bundles of muscle fibers were seen fused with the vessel walls IHC: SMA+	3 Mo, no recurrence
2	Giudice et al., 2019 [32]	17 YO, F	Cheek	1.5 × 1.0 cm	Swelling	—	Surgical excision	Local	H&E: Uniform spindle smooth muscle cells with pale eosinophilic cytoplasm, low amount of fibrous connective tissue, and distributed around numerous small tortuous "slit-like" vessels IHC: SMA+ CD34+ Desmin+ Vimentin+	1 week, 4 weeks, 6 months No recurrence
3	Pandya et al., 2019 [23]	46 YO, F	Palate	1.5 × 1.5 × 0.5 cm	Exophytic growth, pain	Occlusal plain film	Surgical excision	Local	H&E: Numerous thick-walled blood vessels in the connective tissue formed of hyperplastic smooth muscle fibers IHC: SMA+	6 Mo, no recurrence
4	Perić et al., 2019 [4]	36 YO, M	Lip	5 × 3 mm	Painless swelling	—	Surgical excision	Local	H&E: Numerous thick-walled vessel IHC: CD34+ SMA+	7 D, normal healing

Table 1: Continued.

No	Author & year	Age & sex	Location	Size	Sign & symptoms	Radiologic assessments	Treatment plan	Anesthesia	Histologic assessments	Follow-up
5	Ribeiro et al., 2019 [18]	60 YO, M	Anterior maxillary labial fold	—	Swelling	—	Surgical excision	—	H&E: Multiple vessels, thickened muscular layer IHC: CD34+ SMA+	2 Y, no recurrence
6	Ribeiro et al., 2019 [18]	33 YO, M	Buccal mucosa		Submucosal nodule	Color Doppler ultrasonography: well-limited hyperechoic area between cutaneous and muscular layers, no change in blood flow	Surgical excision		H&E: Multiple vascular spaces of various sizes and calibers, sometimes congested and interconnected IHC: CD34- SMA+	
7	S.Y. Rawal and Y.B. Rawal, 2018 [22]	70 YO, M	Hard palate	2.0 × 1.5 cm	Painless mass	—	Surgical excision	—	H&E: Brightly eosinophilic, spindle-shaped cells IHC: SMA+	—
8	Hassona et al., 2017 [14]	52 YO, F	Upper lip	—	Painless mass	—	Surgical excision	Local	H&E: Vascular channels surrounded by fascicles of concentrically arranged spindle cells with eosinophilic cytoplasm IHC: SMA+	12 Mo, no recurrence
9	Osano et al., 2015 [5]	45 YO, M	Cheek	22 × 15 × 11 mm	Painless mass	MRI: T1+contrast: homogeneously enhanced mass and a vessel leading to the tumor T2: Uniform signal and hyperintense signal	Surgical excision	General	H&E: Proliferation of vessels with a smooth muscle wall and vessels surrounded by smooth muscle cells IHC: SMA+ Desmin+ Vimentin+	18 Mo, no recurrence

Table 1: Continued.

No	Author & year	Age & sex	Location	Size	Sign & symptoms	Radiologic assessments	Treatment plan	Anesthesia	Histologic assessments	Follow-up
10	Ishikawa et al., 2014 [6]	51 YO, M	Tongue	11 mm	Nodular mass	—	Surgical excision	—	H&E: Brightly eosinophilic, spindle-shaped cells IHC: SMA+ HHF-35 actin+ Vimentin+ Desmin+ S100- CD34-	8 Mo, no recurrence
11	Tsuji et al., 2014 [7]	79 YO, M	Hard palate	1.5 × 1.5 cm	Painless swelling	Panoramic: No source of odontogenic infection CT: Well-circumscribed mass, no evidence of surrounding bone resorption	Surgical removal and curettage	Local	H&E: Vascular spaces and redundant smooth muscle IHC: Desmin+ SMA+	6 Mo, no recurrence
12	Eley et al., 2012 [21]	39 YO, M	Hard palate	2 cm	Painless swelling	MRI: T1: Slightly higher than the surrounding soft tissue T2: Marked hyper intensity	Surgical excision	General	H&E: Vascular channels surrounded by fascicles of spindle cells IHC: Desmin+ SMA+	3 Mo, no recurrence
13	Minni et al., 2012 [11]	54 YO, F	Submandibular space	3 × 3 cm	Painless swelling	MRI: Displacement of submandibular gland, tongue, and oropharynx airway Compressing the right tonsil Ultrasound-guided FNA: Blood-stained aspirate	Complete surgical removal	General	H&E: Smooth muscle tissue punctuated with thick-walled vessels, capillary, and venous-type vessels IHC: SMA+	6 Mo, no recurrence
14	Menditti et al., 2012 [10]	14 YO, M	Gingiva	1-2 cm	Painless swelling	—	Radical excision with 2 mm free margins	Local	H&E: Vascular spaces and redundant smooth muscle IHC: SMA+	1 Y, no recurrence
15	Gueiros et al., 2011 [16]	-54 YO, M -66 YO, M -53 YO, M	Lower lip Upper lip Upper lip	−1 × 1 cm −0.8 × 0.5 × 0.5 cm	Painless nodule	—	Surgical excision	Local	H&E: Spindle-shaped cells and blood vessels IHC: MSA+	-2 Y -1 Y -6 Mo, no recurrence

Table 1: Continued.

No	Author & year	Age & sex	Location	Size	Sign & symptoms	Radiologic assessments	Treatment plan	Anesthesia	Histologic assessments	Follow-up
16	Vidaković et al., 2011 [8]	58 YO, M	Cheek	2 × 1.5 cm	Painless swelling	—	Surgical excision	Local	H&E: Thick-walled vessels with partially patent and smooth muscle fibres	7 D, normal healing of wound
17	Kim et al., 2010 [3]	2 YO, M	Tongue	2.5 × 2 cm	Soft tissue mass	MRI: Elevated mass on the base of the tongue T1: Isointense signal to muscle T2: Slightly hyperintense signal with hyperintense rim	Surgical removal	General	H&E: Prominent and thickened vessel walls consisting of benign and mature smooth muscle cells IHC: Desmin+ SMA+	26 Mo, no recurrence
18	Nonaka et al., 2010 [25]	38 YO, M	Tongue	2 cm	Painless exophytic mass	—	Surgical excision	—	H&E: Proliferation of spindle-shaped nucleus cells, numerous blood vessels IHC: SMA+	1 Y, no recurrence
19	Keerthi et al., 2009 [17]	32 YO, M	Cheek	4.5 × 4 cm	Painless swelling	CT: Large nonhomogenously enhancing mixed density lesion in the infratemporal fossa and the buccal space, moderately enhancing soft tissue component superolaterally, with no calcification or necrosis	Surgical removal	General	H&E: Multiple blood vessels with proliferation of smooth muscle	6 Y, no recurrence
20	Keerthi et al., 2009 [17]	32 YO, M	Cheek	3 × 3 cm	Painless swelling	Plain film radiograph: No bony changes Ultrasound: Hypoechoic lesion more in favor of soft tissue swelling	Surgical removal	General	H&E: Spindle-shaped fascicles and many blood vessels IHC: Masson trichrome stain (+)	1 Y, no occurrence
21	McParland et al., 2009 [19]	42 YO, M	Buccal mucosal	3 × 3 cm	Painless swelling	—	Surgical excision	Local	H&E: Smooth muscle bands are surrounded by slit-like vascular spaces	6 Mo, no recurrence

Table 1: Continued.

No	Author & year	Age & sex	Location	Size	Sign & symptoms	Radiologic assessments	Treatment plan	Anesthesia	Histologic assessments	Follow-up
22	Cepeda et al., 2008 [2]	39 YO, F 27 YO, F 43 YO, F 36 YO, M 48 YO, M	Retromolar area Mandibular region Lower lip Upper lip Upper lip	0.9 × 0.6 × 1 cm 1.4 × 1.3 × 1 cm 0.7 × 0.5 × 0.4 cm 1.5 × 1.0 × 1.0 cm 1.7 × 1.0 × 1.0 cm	Painless mass	Routine radiographic inspection: A unilocular radiolucency located in a mandibular region (in case 2)	Surgical excision	—	H&E: Several blood vessels lined by a thin layer of endothelial cells were observed intercalated in the fascicules IHC: SMA+ Vimentin+ Desmin+ CD34-	
23	Manor et al., 2007 [20]	39 YO, M	Buccal vestibule	8	Asymptomatic mass	CT: Hypervascular soft tissue mass, with no invasion of the periosteum or bone	Surgical excision	—	H&E: Bands of smooth muscle cells surrounding multiple vascular spaces of varying size IHC: SMA+	12 Mo, no recurrence
24	Ide et al., 2003 [26]	40 YO, F	Submandibular gland	2.0 × 1.8 × 1.5 cm	Painful swelling	—	Surgical excision		H&E: Tortuous thick-walled vessels in varying sizes, proliferation of smooth muscle IHC: SMA+ CD31– CD34– S-100-	
25	Toida et al., 2000 [12]	10 YO, M	Lower lip	2 × 1.5 cm	Painful mass	—	Surgical excision	Local	H&E: Spindle cells surrounded by numerous slit-like vessels IHC: SMA+ S-100-	3 Y, no recurrence
26	Simon et al., 2000 [9]	59 YO, F	Submandibular triangle	15 × 13 mm	Nontender mass	Color Doppler ultrasound: Well-circumscribed, homogeneous solid mass attached to the posterior surface of the submandibular gland, vascularity within the mass	Surgical excision	General	H&E: Smooth muscle punctuated with thick-walled venous vascular channels	—

with a thorough imaging assessment including color Doppler sonography, MDCT, and MRI. The lesion was slightly heterogeneous hypoechoic mass with slight vascular flow in the color Doppler sonography; in addition, the T1-weighted and T2-weighted sequences were low and high, respectively. The high T2-weighted sequence may be seen in cysts, benign or low-grade minor salivary gland tumors, and rare hemangiomatous lesions [27]. In this case, differential diagnosis such as benign lesions of salivary gland origin was suggested in lower possibility because the lesion was located between the buccinator muscle and skin. Cystic lesions were also excluded as the sonography of the cyst is homogenous and unechoic [28]. Differential diagnosis may suggest other benign mesenchymal tumors such as fibroma, lipoma, and neurofibroma and vascular lesions including arteriovenous malformation, lymphangioma, and hemangioma. However, these lesions may have different radiographic and imaging characteristics. According to previous studies, the intraosseous angioleiomyomas are radiographically unilocular or multilocular radiolucent lesions. They can have either an ill-defined or a well-defined sclerotic border [2, 11].

In this case, H&E histologic examination showed a tumor consisting of thin- and thick-walled blood vessels in a background of smooth muscle proliferation. Having numerous blood vessels may pretend other benign vascular tumors such as hemangioma, hemangiopericytoma, hemangioendothelioma, vascular malformation, and other neurovascular hamartomas [29], but a definite examination could rule out these lesions because of the smooth muscle background. Immunohistochemically markers like SMA and MSA (muscle-specific actin) can be useful in identification of smooth muscle nature of the cellular stroma [15, 30, 31]. In the present study, IHC staining was positive for both desmin and SMA. Various IHC stainings were carried out among studies (Table 1) although SMA and desmin were the most frequent. Depending on the apparent features of the blood vessels, IHC staining of endothelial cell markers such as CD34 and CD31 was not recommended. Other differential diagnosis histopathologically is leiomyosarcoma if there were more cellular pleomorphism and mitosis figures. In addition to well circumscribing of this tumor, lacking of anaplasia and bizarre cells, fewer than 5 mitoses per 20 high-power fields could rule out sarcoma.

In all evaluated cases, the lesion was resected with an excisional biopsy under local or general anesthesia. There are no recurrences after resection.

4. Conclusion

In conclusion, we have reported a case of angioleiomyoma of the buccal cheek that resulted in a good outcome. Among various studies, the most common sites of oral angiomyomas were the lip [2, 4, 12–15, 32], cheek or buccal mucosa [5, 8, 14, 16–18], palate [7, 19–21], tongue [6, 22, 23], and submandibular area [9, 11, 24]. Other areas such as the gingiva, mandible, retromolar area, and anterior maxillary labial fold were only reported once among studies [2, 10, 17]. Due to the benign nature of this lesion, the treatment is excisional biopsy and there have been no recurrences or complications reported so far [32].

References

[1] J. Aitken-Saavedra, K.-D. da Silva, A.-C. Ana-Paula-Neutzling Gomes, U. Vasconcelos, A. Etges, and T.-G. Nóbrega, "Clinicopathologic and immunohistochemical characterization of 14 cases of angioleiomyomas in oral cavity," *Medicina Oral, Patologia Oral y Cirugia Bucal*, vol. 23, no. 5, p. e564, 2018.

[2] L. G. Cepeda, D. Q. Rivera, F. T. Rocha, E. Huerta, and E. Sanchez, "Vascular leiomyoma of the oral cavity. Clinical, histopathological and immunohistochemical characteristics. Presentation of five cases and review of the literature," *Medicina Oral, Patología Oral y Cirugía Bucal*, vol. 13, no. 8, pp. e483–e488, 2008.

[3] Y. Kim, Y. Jang, H. Pai, and S. Kim, "Congenital angiomyoma of the tongue: case report," *Dentomaxillofacial Radiology*, vol. 39, no. 7, pp. 446–448, 2010.

[4] B. Perić, B. Vidaković, N. Grgić, S. Manojlović, and H. Čavka, "Angiomyoma of the upper lip–case report and review of the literature," *Acta Clinica Croatica*, vol. 58, no. 1, pp. 183–186, 2019.

[5] H. Osano, Y. Ioka, R. Okamoto et al., "Angioleiomyoma of the cheek: a case report," *Journal of Oral Science*, vol. 57, no. 1, pp. 63–66, 2015.

[6] S. Ishikawa, S. Fuyama, T. Kobayashi, Y. Taira, A. Sugano, and M. Iino, "Angioleiomyoma of the tongue: a case report and review of the literature," *Odontology*, vol. 104, no. 1, pp. 119–122, 2016.

[7] T. Tsuji, K. Satoh, H. Nakano, and M. Kogo, "Clinical characteristics of angioleiomyoma of the hard palate: report of a case and an analysis of the reported cases," *Journal of Oral and Maxillofacial Surgery*, vol. 72, no. 5, pp. 920–926, 2014.

[8] B. Vidaković, A. Kotarac Knežević, S. Manojlović, and G. Knežević, "Angiomyoma–angioleiomyoma of the cheek," *Collegium Antropologicum*, vol. 35, no. 1, pp. 207–209, 2011.

[9] K.-H. W. Simon, A. Ahuja, J. Chow, and W.-K. K. Walter, "Angioleiomyoma in the submandibular region: an unusual tumor in an unusual site," *Otolaryngology—Head and Neck Surgery*, vol. 122, no. 1, pp. 144-145, 2000.

[10] D. Menditti, L. Laino, L. Nastri, U. Caruso, and P. Fiore, "Oral angioleiomyoma: a rare pathological entity," *In Vivo*, vol. 26, no. 1, pp. 161–163, 2012.

[11] A. Minni, A. De Carlo, R. Roukos, G. Illuminati, and B. Cerbelli, "Angioleiomyoma of the oral cavity extended to submandibular space; an unusual tumor in an unusual deep-seated space: a case report," *European Review for Medical and Pharmacological Sciences*, vol. 16, no. 4, pp. 134–137, 2012.

[12] M. Toida, H. Koizumi, and K. Shimokawa, "Painful angiomyoma of the oral cavity: report of a case and review of the literature," *Journal of Oral and Maxillofacial Surgery*, vol. 58, no. 4, pp. 450–453, 2000.

[13] P. Ramesh, S. Annapureddy, F. Khan, and P. Sutaria, "Angioleiomyoma: a clinical, pathological and radiological review," *International Journal of Clinical Practice*, vol. 58, no. 6, pp. 587–591, 2004.

[14] Y. Hassona, F. Sawair, and C. Scully, "Angioleiomyoma of the upper lip," *Case Reports*, vol. 2017, p. bcr-2016-219172., 2017.

[15] P. D. Mehta, N. Desai, K. Makwana, and Y. Patel, "Angioleiomyoma of the lower lip," *Annals of Maxillofacial Surgery*, vol. 10, no. 1, pp. 251–253, 2020.

[16] L.-A. Gueiros, M.-J. Romañach, A.-M. Pires-Soubhia, F.-R. Pires, O. Paes-de-Almeida, and P.-A. Vargas, "Angioleiomyoma affecting the lips: report of 3 cases and review of the literature," *Medicina Oral, Patología Oral y Cirugía Bucal*, vol. 16, no. 4, pp. e482–e487, 2011.

[17] R. Keerthi, M. Nanjappa, S. S. Deora, and S. Kumaraswamy, "Angioleiomyoma of cheek: report of two cases," *Journal of Maxillofacial and Oral Surgery*, vol. 8, no. 3, pp. 298–300, 2009.

[18] J.-L. Ribeiro, F.-H. Costa, E. K. Ana-Sueli-Rodrigues Cavalcante, Y.-R. Carvalho, and A.-L. Anbinder, "Vascular leiomyoma in the oral cavity–report of two cases," *Journal of Clinical and Experimental Dentistry*, vol. 11, no. 6, article e582, 2019.

[19] H. McParland, S. Warnakulasuriya, and R. J. Cook, "Angioleiomyoma: an unusual diagnosis for a lump in the cheek," *British Journal of Oral and Maxillofacial Surgery*, vol. 47, no. 8, pp. 641-642, 2009.

[20] E. Manor, N. Sion-Vardy, M. Nash, and L. Bodner, "Angiomyoma of buccal vestibule: a rare case with a normal karyotype," *The Journal of Laryngology & Otology*, vol. 121, no. 12, pp. 1210–1212, 2007.

[21] K. A. Eley, S. Alroyayamina, S. J. Golding, R. N. Tiam, and S. R. Watt-Smith, "Angioleiomyoma of the hard palate: report of a case and review of the literature and magnetic resonance imaging findings of this rare entity," *Oral Surgery, Oral Medicine, Oral Pathology and Oral Radiology*, vol. 114, no. 2, pp. e45–e49, 2012.

[22] S. Y. Rawal and Y. B. Rawal, "Angioleiomyoma (vascular leiomyoma) of the oral cavity," *Head and Neck Pathology*, vol. 12, no. 1, pp. 123–126, 2018.

[23] M. Pandya, D. S. Rao, G. Mamatha, and R. G. Annigeri, "Angiomyoma–a requisite in differential diagnosis of palatal growths," *International Journal of Health Sciences*, vol. 13, no. 6, p. 47, 2019.

[24] H.-Y. Kim, S.-N. Jung, H. Kwon, W.-I. Sohn, and S.-H. Moon, "Angiomyoma in the buccal space," *Journal of Craniofacial Surgery*, vol. 21, no. 5, pp. 1634-1635, 2010.

[25] C. F. W. Nonaka, K. M. A. Pereira, and M. C. D. C. Miguel, "Oral vascular leiomyoma with extensive calcification areas," *Brazilian Journal of Otorhinolaryngology*, vol. 76, no. 4, p. 539, 2010.

[26] F. Ide, K. Mishima, and I. Saito, "Angiomyoma in the submandibular gland: a rare location for a ubiquitous tumour," *The Journal of Laryngology & Otology*, vol. 117, no. 12, pp. 1001-1002, 2003.

[27] T. M. Yoon, H. C. Yang, Y.-D. Choi, D. H. Lee, J. K. Lee, and S. C. Lim, "Vascular leiomyoma in the head and neck region: 11 years experience in one institution," *Clinical and Experimental Otorhinolaryngology*, vol. 6, no. 3, pp. 171–175, 2013.

[28] P. M. Som and H. D. Curtin, *Head and Neck Imaging E-Book*, Elsevier Health Sciences, 2011.

[29] C. Whittle, A. Retamal, D. Kramer, and C. Silva, "Sonographic diagnosis of periorbital dermoid cyst," *Ultrasound Quarterly*, vol. 33, no. 1, pp. 37–40, 2017.

[30] G. E. Anastassov and P. A. van Damme, "Angioleiomyoma of the upper lip: report of a case," *International Journal of Oral and Maxillofacial Surgery*, vol. 24, pp. 301-302, 1995.

[31] J. K. Brooks, N. G. Nikitakis, N. J. Goodman, and B. A. Levy, "Clinicopathologic characterization of oral angioleiomyomas," *Oral Surgery, Oral Medicine, Oral Pathology, Oral Radiology, and Endodontology*, vol. 94, no. 2, pp. 221–227, 2002.

[32] A. Giudice, F. Bennardo, C. Buffone, Y. Brancaccio, F. M. Plutino, and L. Fortunato, "Clinical and immunohistochemical features of oral angioleiomyoma: a comprehensive review of the literature and report of a case in a young patient," *Case Reports in Dentistry*, vol. 2019, Article ID 2498353, 9 pages, 2019.

30

Silane Heat Treatment Could Eliminate the Hydrofluoric Acid Etching of Lithium Disilicate Overlays: A Four-Year Follow-Up

Spartak Spasov Yanakiev[1] **and Mirela Borislavova Marinova-Takorova**[2]

[1]*Medical College, Medical University of Sofia, Yordanka Filaretova Str. No. 3, Sofia, Bulgaria*
[2]*Department of Conservative Dentistry, Faculty of Dental Medicine, Medical University of Sofia, Georgi Sofiiski 3 Str., Sofia, Bulgaria*

Correspondence should be addressed to Spartak Spasov Yanakiev; s.yanakiev@mc.mu-sofia.bg

Academic Editor: Konstantinos Michalakis

A four-year follow-up of a novel silane heat treatment method for bonding lithium disilicate overlays to tooth structures without hydrofluoric acid etching of the ceramic surface is presented in this case report. Silane heat treatment modifies the silane layer and thus enhances resin ceramic bond strength without hydrofluoric acid etching. The standard ceramic preparation technique prior to bonding silicate ceramics to tooth structure is hydrofluoric acid etching and applying a silane coupling agent, followed by dental adhesive. In this case, the micromechanical roughening of the ceramic surface was performed by air abrasion with Al_2O_3. Silane heat treatment with constant 120°C airflow, applied for 60 sec, followed by dental adhesive application enhanced the resin-ceramic bond strength. After a four-year follow-up, the restorations' clinical appearance could be defined as excellent/very good according to the FDI clinical criteria for the evaluation of direct and indirect restorations. This clinical result supports many in vitro studies regarding the resin-ceramic bond strength and durability obtained through postsilanization heat treatment.

1. Introduction

Lithium disilicate (LiS_2) is one of the most widely applied metal-free materials due to its high aesthetics, adequate mechanical properties, and favorable bonding strength, ensuring functional durability and high short- and medium-term survival rates [1–4]. It can be used for both tooth- and implant-supported restorations, including single crowns, bridges, anterior veneers, posterior inlays, onlays, and overlays [5]. In cases when single restorations like inlays, onlays, and partial crowns are needed, they present advantages such as high fracture resistance, low wear and abrasive potential, biocompatibility, adhesive bonding, and strength which make them preferable in cases with significant loss of tooth structure and abrasion or when occlusal correction is needed [5]. Bonded restorations with full occlusal coverage preserve tooth structure compared to full-coverage crowns and increase the fracture resistance of endodontically treated teeth compared to direct MOD restorations [6]. LiS_2 has shown promising clinical results for posterior endodontically treated teeth with or without fiber posts [7]. These restorations' success depends on many factors—tooth preparation, presence of enamel, bonding procedures, and material selection [8, 9].

The adequate adhesive bonding procedure for glass-ceramics needs proper preparation of the inner surface of the restoration. The significant adhesive strength is due to both micromechanical and chemical bonding mechanisms. The surface microirregularities for the micromechanical interlocking between the ceramic and the cement could be made by acid etching, sandblasting, or diamond bur grinding [5]. The application of a silane coupling agent ensures chemical interaction between the ceramics and the adhesive resin [10].

Hydrofluoric acid (HF) etching of glass-ceramics proved very efficient since it creates a large bonding surface [11, 12]. On the other hand, if it comes in contact with skin, eyes, or mucosa, HF could be harmful to both the patient and the clinician [13, 14] and is acknowledged as a highly hazardous chemical in dentistry [15, 16]. That is why some authors exert efforts on improving the chemical bond between dental ceramics and composite resin provided by the silane coupling

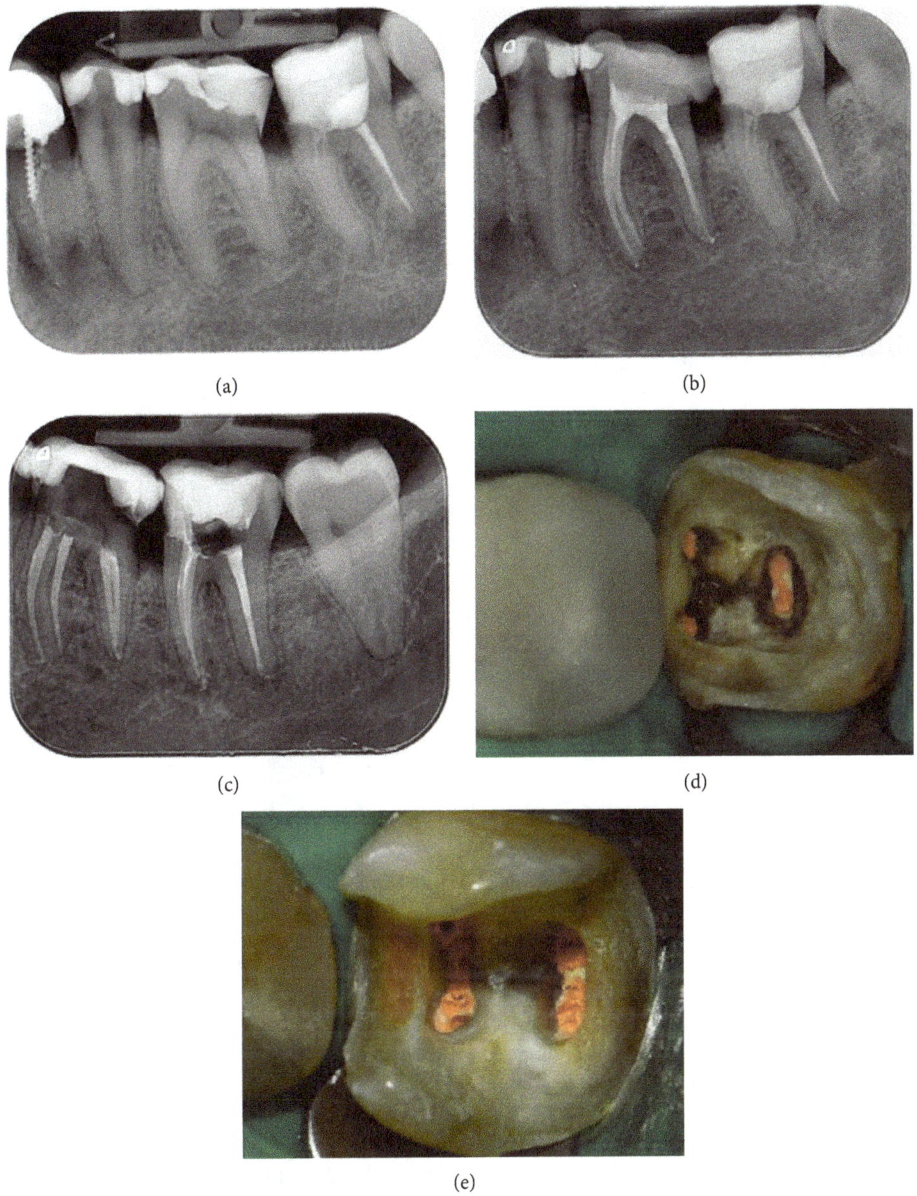

FIGURE 1: Preoperative images: radiograph images of tooth 36 (a) and 37 (b) prior to endodontic treatment and postendodontic treatment (c) and clinical view of tooth 37 (d) and 36 (e).

agents, thus trying to eliminate the use of HF acid. Silane treatment with heated airflow or in an oven is one of the most frequently used methods [17–20]. The proposed heating temperatures vary from 38 to 100°C. In a recent study, a 120°C heating temperature of the silane was presented [21]. This temperature was the most efficient treatment method, providing the highest bond strength among all heating temperatures. According to some studies, HF's effect in the bonding procedure could be compensated by micromechanical roughening of the ceramic restoration and silane heat treatment to obtain high bond strength [17, 18]. Despite the large number of in vitro studies in the literature, there is still a lack of clinical evidence of these methods' effectiveness in vivo.

This clinical case report describes two ceramic overlays' bonding procedures made from LiS_2 without HF etching and a 4-year follow-up.

2. Case Description

The patient is a 34 year old male, a smoker with good oral hygiene, who presented into our office for a routine examination. There was secondary caries around a composite resin restoration on tooth 36. The X-ray image of the tooth verified secondary caries on tooth 36 and revealed poor marginal adaptation of the restoration and an inadequate root canal treatment of tooth 37. After discussing the clinical options, the patient signed informed consent—root canal treatment and ceramic overlay restorations of both teeth were planned.

The endodontic treatment of the teeth was performed under microscope Zumax OMS2350 (Zumax Medical Co., Ltd., Suzhou New District, China) in several visits one by one. Root canals were shaped with MTwo files, size 25/0.06 (VDW GmbH, Munich, Germany). After copious irrigation

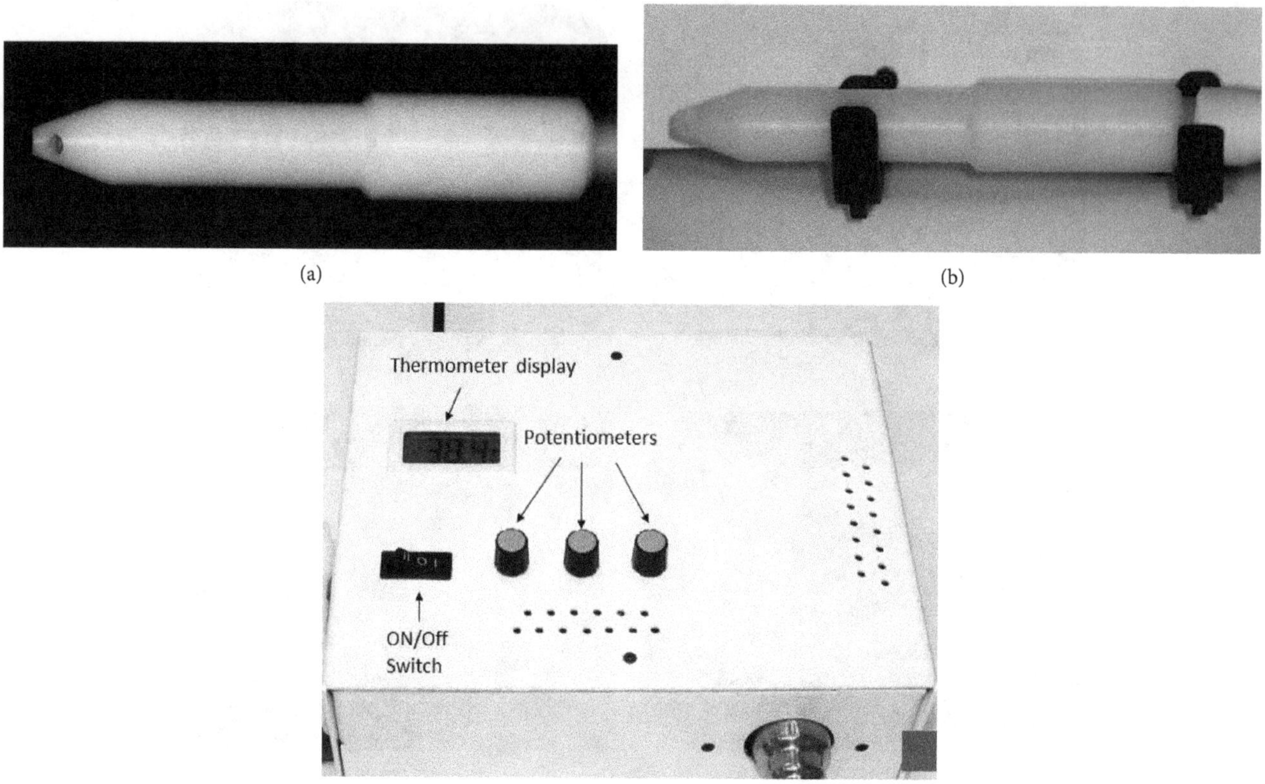

FIGURE 2: The custom-made air machine used in this study. Autoclavable handpiece made from polyacetate material (placed on the side wall of the device) (a, b). Front panel of the device and basic components (c).

with NaOCl solution (Chloraxid 2%, Cerkamed, Stalowa Wola, Poland), the final irrigation with EDTA solution (MD-Cleanser, Meta Biomed Europe GmbH, Mülheim an der Ruhr, Germany) and ethanol 95% (Chemax Pharma, Sofia, Bulgaria) was done before filling the canals with AH plus root canal sealer (Dentsply DeTrey, GmbH, Konstanz, Germany) and taper-matched gutta-percha cone (Sure Dent, Sagimakgol-ro, Jungwon-gu, Seongnam-si, Gyeonggi-do, South Korea) utilizing a single-cone technique (Figure 1).

Tooth preparation for the overlays was performed, and provisional acrylic restorations were placed (Unifast III, GC Corporation, Tokyo, Japan). Full-tray maxillary and mandibular impressions were taken on the next visit using VPS material (Variotime, Heraeus Kulzer GmbH, Hanau, Germany). Two LiS_2 overlays were fabricated from E.max Press, shade A 3.5 HT (Ivoclar Vivadent, Schaan, Liechtenstein).

The two ceramic overlays were air abraded with 50 μm Al_2O_3 at 1 bar. After the try-in procedures, the inner surfaces of the overlays were cleaned with ethanol and air-dried. A silane coupling agent (Monobond Plus, Ivoclar Vivadent, Schaan, Liechtenstein) was applied for 60 seconds. The key step in the protocol was the silane heat treatment performed with a custom-made hot air machine (Figure 2). The device is equipped with an autoclavable handpiece made from polyacetate material TECAFORM AH POM (Modern Plastics, Connecticut, USA). A thermocouple located in the working end of the handpiece measures the air temperature as near as possible to the treated surface. Temperature is measured to the first decimal place in degrees Celsius. The temperature range supported by the device is from 38°C to 140°C.

A constant 120°C airflow for 60 sec was applied, followed by dental adhesive OptiBond FL (Kerr Italia S.r.l., Scafati (SA), Italy). The steps are presented in Figure 3.

The tooth structures were etched with 37.5% phosphoric acid (LOT 6775164, Gel Etchant, Kerr Italia S.r.l., Scafati (SA), Italy), and an OptiBond FL dental adhesive was applied. A flowable composite (Gaeneal Universal Flow, GC Corporation, Tokyo, Japan) was used for the permanent fixation. Light curing for 60 sec on each tooth surface was performed with Elipar™ DeepCure-S LED Curing Light (3M ESPE, St. Paul, USA). Occlusal contact check and adjustments were done after the final polymerization with 40 μm articulating paper (Bausch Arti-Check, Dr. Jean Bausch GmbH & Co. KG, Koln, Germany). The final result is shown in Figure 4.

The FDI clinical criteria for the evaluation of direct and indirect restorations were used to evaluate the clinical appearance of the restorations after four years in use [22]. The appearance of the restorations could be assessed as clinically excellent/very good based on the aesthetic, functional, and biological properties. Lustre is comparable to that of enamel, and no surface staining, good color match, and ideal form preservation were observed. The absence of fractures, excellent marginal adaptation, normal contact points, and patient satisfaction correspond to clinical excellent/very good functional properties. The radiograph examination reveals a

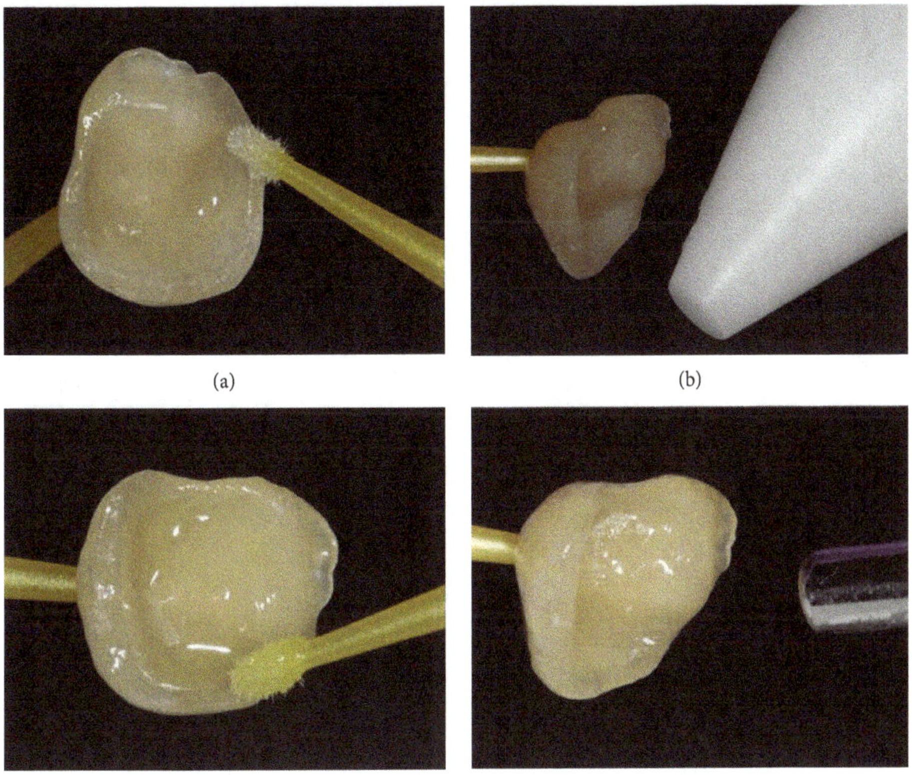

(a) (b) (c) (d)

FIGURE 3: Bonding procedure: silane application (a); postsilanization heat treatment with custom-made device (b); bonding agent application (c); bonding agent solvent evaporation (d).

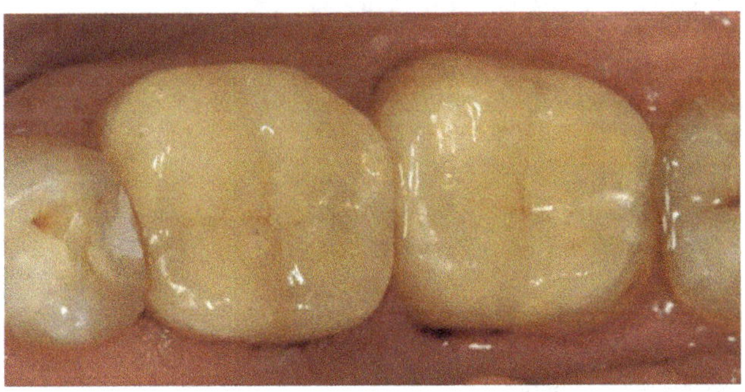

FIGURE 4: Postoperative view of the two overlays immediately after fixation and isolation removal.

harmonious transition between the restorations and the tooth structures. We observed no hypersensitivity, no secondary or primary caries, very good periodontal response, healthy mucosa, and no general oral symptoms (Figure 5).

3. Discussion

This clinical result supports many in vitro studies regarding the resin-ceramic bond strength and durability obtained through postsilanization heat treatment.

The adhesive bonding procedure is one of the most critical steps determining the success and durability of LiS_2 restorations. Proper tooth and ceramic preparation is mandatory. HF etching of the ceramic surface, followed by silane and dental adhesive application, is usually recommended for establishing a strong resin-ceramic bond. The HF etching dissolves partially the glassy phase of the silica-based ceramics, providing micromechanical retentions [23]. More undercuts and larger surface characterize etched ceramic compared to air-abraded ceramic; thus, a stronger resin-ceramic bond could be obtained [11, 24].

HF is a strong ceramic etching agent but potentially very harmful if it comes in contact with eyes, skin, or mouth tissues [16]. For this reason, some authors propose other etching agents, which are less effective, or to avoid the use of HF in the bonding procedure and use alternative protocols [25]. Despite the advantages of HF etching, it could weaken the material if the clinician exceeds the recommended etching time [26]. Overetching could also weaken the ceramic composite bond strength [27]. HF promotes selective dissolution of the glassy phase of silica-based ceramics. The etching process includes several chemical reactions that lead to the deposition of insoluble silica-fluoride salts on the surface that negatively affects the bond. Thus, proper postetching cleaning of the ceramic is mandatory [28]. One could avoid these possible complications of the bonding procedure by excluding the HF etching in the bonding protocol. If so, to enhance the bond strength, proper postsilanization heat treatment combined with an appropriate microbraided ceramic surface is mandatory. To obtain a more durable resin-ceramic bond in the presented case, we applied postsilanization heat treatment at 120°C and avoided HF etching.

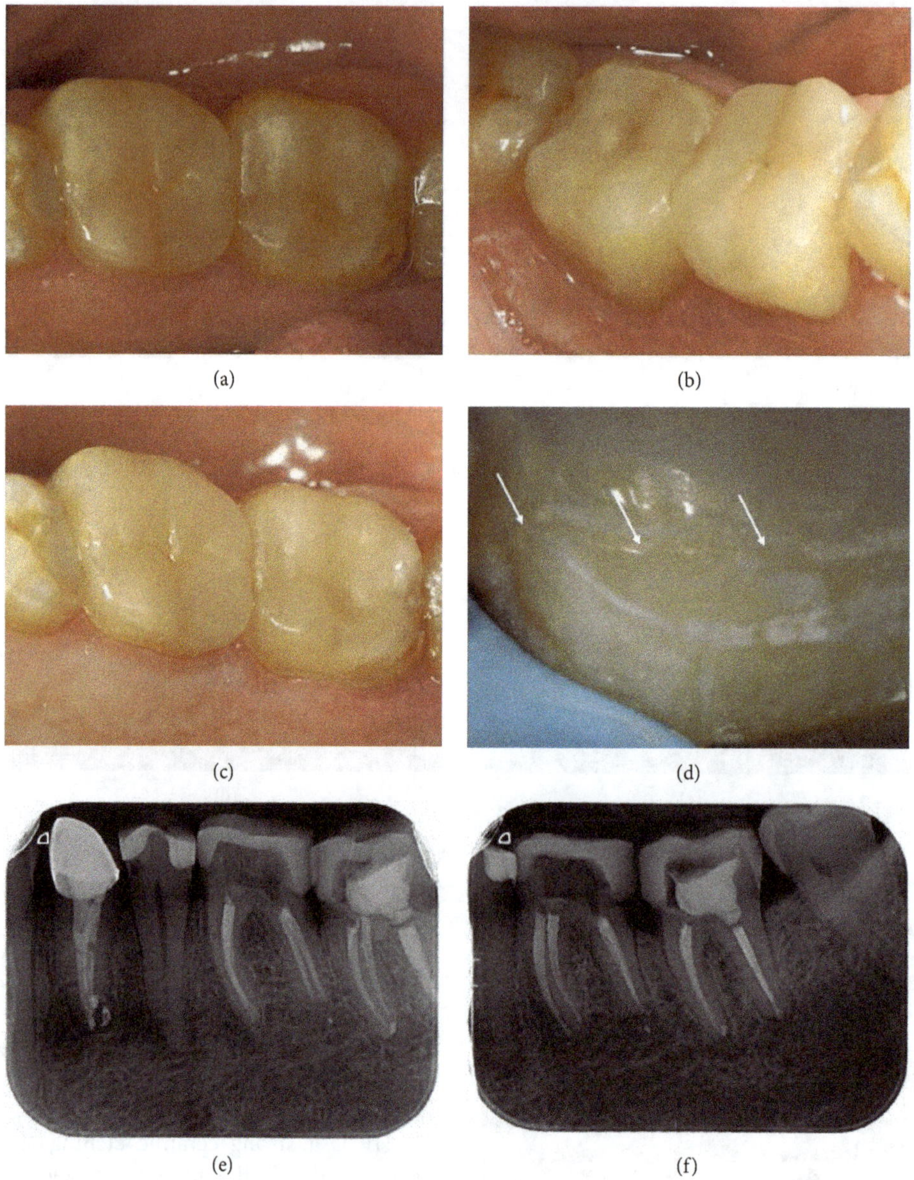

FIGURE 5: Four-year follow-up of the restorations: occlusal view (a); buccal view (b); lingual view (c); a close-up image of the overlay-tooth interface (d), white arrows pointing to the borders of the restorations; radiograph examination (e, f).

In addition to the micromechanical retentions, silane molecules can bond to both the functional groups of the silica phase of the ceramic and the resin material's organic matrix, thus providing chemical bonding between the two materials [29]. The efficacy of the chemical bonding depends on the type of the silane coupling agent, the material's application, and postsilanization treatment [30]. An interlayer is formed when a silane coupling agent is applied on the ceramic surface before resin application. Three different structures could be identified in the silane interlayer. The outermost layer comprises small oligomers, which could be easily eliminated by organic solvents and water at room temperature. The middle layer is formed by oligomers connected with stronger single siloxane bonds. In the inner layer, silane molecules form a network characterized by higher hydrolytic stability. Silane layer thickness should be as minimal as possible, and only the inner molecule layer is needed to obtain a strong and durable resin-ceramic bond. One of the most effective ways to obtain a highly condensed and stronger silane layer is postsilanization heat treatment [31].

Recommended temperatures vary among different authors. Fabianeli et al. and Roulet et al. propose 100°C heating temperature [17, 32]. Monticelli et al. use 38°C [33]. Hooshmand et al. tested three different temperatures—100°C (in oven), 80°C (boiled water), and 50°C (hot air) [34]. A recent study conducted a systematic comparison between different postsilanization heating temperatures. It showed the positive effect of higher temperatures on the bond strength between feldspathic ceramics and resin composite material [21]. The highest tensile bond strength was achieved among all groups when the bonding surface was treated with 120°C hot air. Since this was the most effective silane heat treatment method, we chose it appropriately in this clinical case. The 60 sec application of this temperature ensures a high condensation rate of the silane molecules; thus, a stronger chemical bond is achieved. It is harmless for both the patient and the clinician since the heating process is performed outside the mouth and the overlays are attached on a bonding stick.

Despite the very good outcome of the presented bonding method, there are some limitations. The follow-up period is relatively short (4 years). Different follow-up periods are reported in the literature—usually from 12 months to 15 years [2–4]. Thus, although the reported results are quite satisfactory, they should be considered preliminary. Since this case report presents only one patient and two overlays, it could not be accepted as scientific proof. Therefore, it could only be assumed as a promising result, and further randomized control trials should validate this approach and confirm the reliability of this method in vivo. Another limitation is the need for a specially designed hot air device, which is not supported by any manufacturer as far as we know.

4. Conclusion

The clinical appearance of the restorations could be defined as excellent/very good according to the FDI clinical criteria for the evaluation of direct and indirect restorations for the four-year follow-up period. Thus, it could be assumed that the bonding protocol used in this clinical case promotes a strong and durable ceramic-composite bond due to the combination of micromechanical retentions provided by air abrasion with AL_2O_3 and proper silane heat treatment. Although the results are promising, further studies should be conducted due to the limitations of this case report.

References

[1] M. Luciano, Z. Francesca, S. Michela, M. Tommaso, and A. Massimo, "Lithium disilicate posterior overlays: clinical and biomechanical features," *Clinical Oral Investigations*, vol. 24, no. 2, pp. 841–848, 2020.

[2] A. Moreira, F. Freitas, D. Marques, and J. Caramês, "Aesthetic rehabilitation of a patient with bruxism using ceramic veneers and overlays combined with four-point monolithic zirconia crowns for occlusal stabilization: a 4-year follow-up," *Case Reports in Dentistry*, vol. 2019, Article ID 1640563, 7 pages, 2019.

[3] C. van den Breemer, C. Vinkenborg, H. van Pelt, D. Edelhoff, and M. S. Cune, "The clinical performance of monolithic lithium disilicate posterior restorations after 5, 10, and 15 years: a retrospective case series," *The International Journal of Prosthodontics*, vol. 30, no. 1, pp. 62–65, 2017.

[4] G. Fabbri, F. Zarone, G. Dellificorelli et al., "Clinical evaluation of 860 anterior and posterior lithium disilicate restorations: retrospective study with a mean follow-up of 3 years and a maximum observational period of 6 years," *The International Journal of Periodontics & Restorative Dentistry*, vol. 34, no. 2, pp. 165–177, 2014.

[5] F. Zarone, M. I. di Mauro, P. Ausiello, G. Ruggiero, and R. Sorrentino, "Current status on lithium disilicate and zirconia: a narrative review," *BMC Oral Health*, vol. 19, no. 1, p. 134, 2019.

[6] G. T. Rocca and I. Krejci, "Crown and post-free adhesive restorations for endodontically treated posterior teeth: from direct composite to endocrowns," *The European Journal of Esthetic Dentistry*, vol. 8, no. 2, pp. 156–179, 2013.

[7] M. Ferrari, E. Ferrari Cagidiaco, C. Goracci et al., "Posterior partial crowns out of lithium disilicate (LS2) with or without posts: a randomized controlled prospective clinical trial with a 3-year follow up," *Journal of Dentistry*, vol. 83, pp. 12–17, 2019.

[8] G. Politano, B. Van Meerbeek, and M. Peumans, "Nonretentive bonded ceramic partial crowns: concept and simplified protocol for long-lasting dental restorations," *The Journal of Adhesive Dentistry*, vol. 20, no. 6, pp. 495–510, 2018.

[9] G. T. Rocca, R. Daher, C. M. Saratti et al., "Restoration of severely damaged endodontically treated premolars: the influence of the endo-core length on marginal integrity and fatigue resistance of lithium disilicate CAD-CAM ceramic endocrowns," *Journal of Dentistry*, vol. 68, pp. 41–50, 2018.

[10] R. Frankenberger, V. E. Hartmann, M. Krech et al., "Adhesive luting of new CAD/CAM materials," *International Journal of Computerized Dentistry*, vol. 18, no. 1, pp. 9–20, 2015.

[11] A. Della Bona and K. J. Anusavice, "Microstructure, composition, and etching topography of dental ceramics," *The International Journal of Prosthodontics*, vol. 15, no. 2, pp. 159–167, 2002.

[12] N. Mobilio, A. Fasiol, and S. Catapano, "Qualitative evaluation of the adhesive interface between lithium disilicate, luting composite and natural tooth," *Ann Stomatol (Roma)*, vol. 7, no. 1-2, pp. 1–3, 2016.

[13] W. J. Anderson and J. R. Anderson, "Hydrofluoric acid burns of the hand: mechanism of injury and treatment," *The Journal of Hand Surgery*, vol. 13, no. 1, pp. 52–57, 1988.

[14] F. Caliskan Tur and E. Aksay, "Hydrofluoric acid exposure," *Turk J Emerg Med*, vol. 15, no. 1, p. 1, 2015.

[15] T. L. Litovitz, W. Klein-Schwartz, K. S. Dyer, M. Shannon, S. Lee, and M. Powers, "1997 annual report of the American Association of Poison Control Centers Toxic Exposure Surveillance System," *The American Journal of Emergency Medicine*, vol. 16, no. 5, pp. 443–497, 1998.

[16] M. Ozcan, A. Allahbeickaraghi, and M. Dündar, "Possible hazardous effects of hydrofluoric acid and recommendations for treatment approach: a review," *Clinical Oral Investigations*, vol. 16, no. 1, pp. 15–23, 2012.

[17] A. Fabianelli, S. Pollington, F. Papacchini et al., "The effect of different surface treatments on bond strength between leucite reinforced feldspathic ceramic and composite resin," *Journal of Dentistry*, vol. 38, no. 1, pp. 39–43, 2010.

[18] C. Shen, W. S. Oh, and J. R. Williams, "Effect of post-silanization drying on the bond strength of composite to ceramic," *The Journal of Prosthetic Dentistry*, vol. 91, no. 5, pp. 453–458, 2004.

[19] C. Cotes, R. F. de Carvalho, E. T. Kimpara, F. P. Leite, and M. Ozcan, "Can heat treatment procedures of prehydrolyzed silane replace hydrofluoric acid in the adhesion of resin cement to feldspathic ceramic?," *The Journal of Adhesive Dentistry*, vol. 15, no. 6, pp. 569–574, 2013.

[20] R. F. de Carvalho, C. Cotes, E. T. Kimpara, F. P. Leite, and M. Özcan, "Heat treatment of pre-hydrolyzed silane increases adhesion of phosphate monomer-based resin cement to glass ceramic," *Brazilian Dental Journal*, vol. 26, no. 1, pp. 44–49, 2015.

[21] Medical College"Y Filaretova", Medical University - Sofia, Bulgaria, S. Yanakiev, B. Yordanov, and V. Dikov, "Influence of silane heat treatment on the tensile bond strength between EX-3 synthetic veneering porcelain and composite resin using five different activation temperatures," *Journal of IMAB - Annual Proceeding (Scientific Papers)*, vol. 23, no. 1, pp. 1456–1459, 2017.

[22] R. Hickel, A. Peschke, M. Tyas et al., "FDI World Dental Federation: clinical criteria for the evaluation of direct and indirect restorations-update and clinical examples," *Clinical Oral Investigations*, vol. 14, no. 4, pp. 349–366, 2010.

[23] M. C. Bottino, M. Özcan, P. G. Coelho, L. F. Valandro, J. C. Bressiani, and A. H. Bressiani, "Micro-morphological changes prior to adhesive bonding: high-alumina and glassy-matrix ceramics," *Brazilian Oral Research*, vol. 22, no. 2, pp. 158–163, 2008.

[24] S. Canay, N. Hersek, and A. Ertan, "Effect of different acid treatments on a porcelain surface," *Journal of Oral Rehabilitation*, vol. 281, pp. 95–101, 2001.

[25] M. Ozcan, "Evaluation of alternative intra-oral repair techniques for fractured ceramic-fused-to-metal restorations," *Journal of Oral Rehabilitation*, vol. 30, no. 2, pp. 194–203, 2003.

[26] T. Hooshmand, S. Parvizi, and A. Keshvad, "Effect of surface acid etching on the biaxial flexural strength of two hot-pressed glass ceramics," *Journal of Prosthodontics*, vol. 17, no. 5, pp. 415–419, 2008.

[27] J. H. Chen, H. Matsumura, and M. Atsuta, "Effect of etchant, etching period, and silane priming on bond strength to porcelain of composite resin," *Operative Dentistry*, vol. 23, no. 5, pp. 250–257, 1998.

[28] G. Bruzi, A. O. Carvalho, M. Giannini, H. P. Maia, and P. Magne, "Post-etching cleaning influences the resin shear bond strength to CAD/CAM lithium-disilicate ceramics," *Appl Adhes Sci*, vol. 5, no. 1, 2017.

[29] R. Li, S. Q. Ma, C. C. Zang et al., "Enhanced bonding strength between lithium disilicate ceramics and resin cement by multiple surface treatments after thermal cycling," *PLoS One*, vol. 14, no. 7, article e0220466, 2019.

[30] J. P. Matinlinna, L. V. Lassila, M. Ozcan, A. Yli-Urpo, and P. K. Vallittu, "An introduction to silanes and their clinical applications in dentistry," *The International Journal of Prosthodontics*, vol. 17, no. 2, pp. 155–164, 2004.

[31] E. Metwalli, D. Haines, O. Becker, S. Conzone, and C. G. Pantano, "Surface characterizations of mono-, di-, and tri-aminosilane treated glass substrates," *Journal of Colloid and Interface Science*, vol. 298, no. 2, pp. 825–831, 2006.

[32] J. F. Roulet, K. J. M. Söderholm, and J. Longmate, "Effects of treatment and storage conditions on ceramic/composite bond strength," *Journal of Dental Research*, vol. 74, no. 1, pp. 381–387, 1995.

[33] F. Monticelli, M. Toledano, R. Osorio, and M. Ferrari, "Effect of temperature on the silane coupling agents when bonding core resin to quartz fiber posts," *Dental Materials*, vol. 22, no. 11, pp. 1024–1028, 2006.

[34] T. Hooshmand, R. van Noort, and A. Keshvad, "Bond durability of the resin-bonded and silane treated ceramic surface," *Dental Materials*, vol. 18, no. 2, pp. 179–188, 2002.

31

Isolated Bone Lesions in the Mandible and Maxilla of Langerhans Cell Histiocytosis Treated with Fractionated Stereotactic Low-Dose Radiotherapy: Case Report and 5-Year Follow-Up

Antoine Berberi,[1] Georges Aoun,[2] Georges Aad,[2] and Elie Azar[3]

[1]*Department of Oral and Maxillofacial Surgery, Faculty of Dental Medicine, Lebanese University, Lebanon*
[2]*Department of Oral Medicine and Maxillofacial Radiology, Faculty of Dental Medicine, Lebanese University, Lebanon*
[3]*Department of ENT, Faculty of Medicine, Lebanese University, Lebanon*

Correspondence should be addressed to Antoine Berberi; aberberi@ul.edu.lb

Academic Editor: Tommaso Lombardi

Langerhans cell histiocytosis is a benign histiocytic disorder touching both genders and can occur at any age. It is currently classified by the Histiocyte Society as an inflammatory myeloid neoplasm of mixed cellularity. Clinically, it is illustrated by single or multiple osteolytic bone lesions associated with ulceration of the skin and soft tissues. Disease outcome is highly variable, depending on the degree of involvement. Bone pathologies are observed in 60% of cases as uni- or multifocal lesions. Several treatment modalities have been proposed and include surgical excision, intralesion steroid injection, chemotherapy, and low-dose radiotherapy. In this paper, we report a case of a 42-year-old male suffering from gingival swelling in the left side of his mandible and the right side of the maxilla. Clinical, radiological, and histological examinations confirm the diagnosis of Langerhans cell histiocytosis. Hematological investigation, entire body CT scan, and bone scintigraphy confirmed the limitation of the lesions in the right maxilla and on the left mandible. The lesions were treated with fractionated stereotactic low-dose radiotherapy, 24 Gy in 16 fractions, by using a linear accelerator with a custom-made rigid mask for accurate immobilization of the head with confirmed precision, which allows noninvasive approaches. Complete remission was achieved clinically and radiologically after one year, and a panoramic X-ray after 5 years confirms the bone healing process. Fractionated stereotactic low-dose RT could be adopted as an effective treatment.

1. Introduction

Langerhans cell histiocytosis (LCH), named by the Histiocyte Society (HS) in 1987, previously identified as histiocytosis X (HX), is a hyperplastic cellular disease of undetermined causes [1]. LCH is categorized by an uncontrolled clonal proliferation of Langerhans cells, which is a part of the human mononuclear phagocytic system [2].

Usually characterized by single (monostotic) or multiple (polyostotic) osteolytic bone lesions, solitary or multiple lymph node involvements associated to ulcerations of skin and soft tissues, and involvement of the central nervous system (CNS) [3].

Bones, excluding hands and feet, are the most commonly affected organs (80%) with 75% unifocal lesions and painful soft tissue swelling [3–5]. LCH is divided into 3 types: acute, disseminated, chronic, multifocal, and chronic focal [6]. Subdivisions for localized and disseminated LCH are reported by the blood group in 2016 [2]. Treatment modalities for adults have never been clarified by a clinical trial and the clinical reports deliver minimal data on the efficiency of various adopted treatments, which include surgery/curettage, steroids, low-dose radiotherapy (RT), and various chemotherapy regimens [7–14].

In this manuscript, we reported a case of isolated osteolytic lesions related to HLC observed in both jaws and treated with fractionated stereotactic low-dose RT with a 5-year follow-up period.

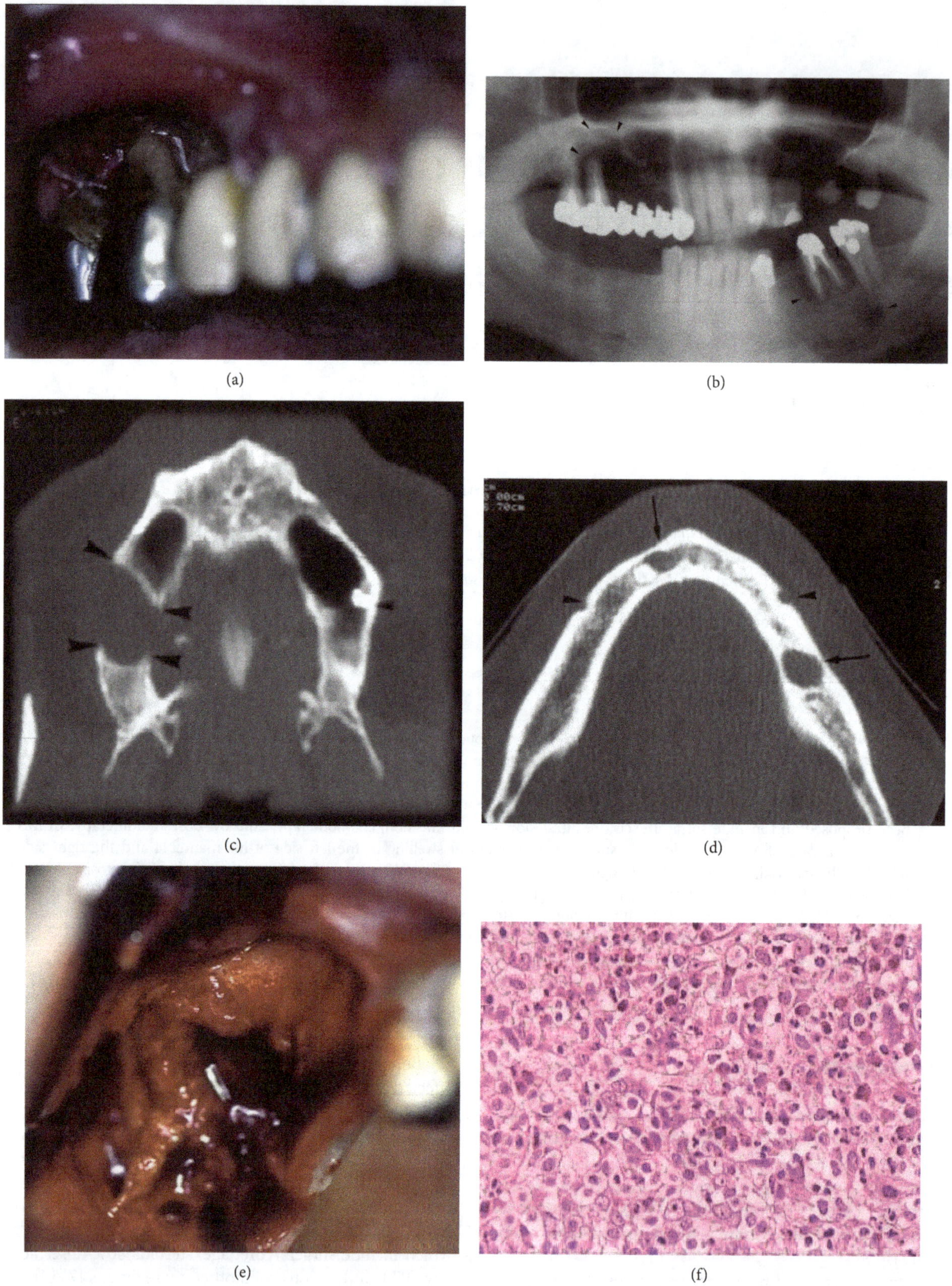

FIGURE 1: (a) Gingival ulcer proliferative growth in relation with the restored right maxillary molars. (b) 2D panoramic radiograph showing the unilocular radiolucency in the maxilla and the mandible. (1) Axial images of the CT scan exposed the presence of radiolucency in the maxilla with cortical bone deterioration. (d) axial images of the CT scan displaying a well-defined localized radiolucency in the body of the mandible. (e) The excised tissue after tooth extraction. (f) Histopathology of Langerhans cell histiocytosis: prominent histiocytes with abundant cytoplasm against the background of mixed population of eosinophils and multinucleated giant cells (HE ×10).

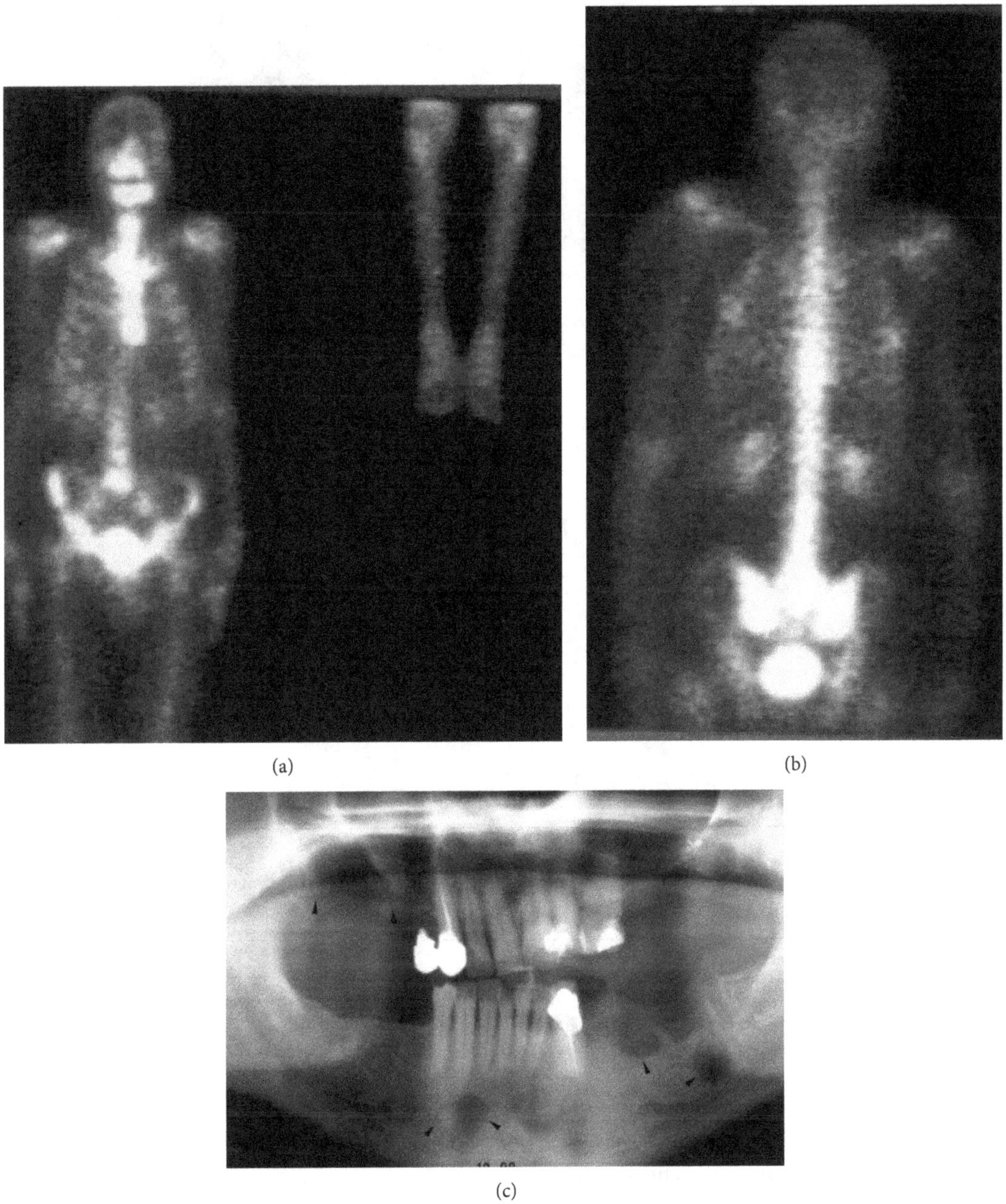

FIGURE 2: (a, b) Complete body scintigraphy with Te 99 revealing the only localization of LCH lesions in the jaws. (c) Panoramic radiograph after teeth extractions.

2. Case Report

A 42-year-old male has been oriented to our department, complaining of unilateral facial swelling with persistent pain, one year after extraction of the left mandibular premolars.

Additionally, he presented a gingiva swelling in the right maxilla related to a fixed bridge.

The clinical exam showed palpable lymph node, nontender, freely movable on the left submandibular area, and intraoral examination revealed a painful buccal cortical expansion in relation to the first and second mandibular molars. In the maxilla, a gingival ulcer proliferative growth in relation to the restored right molars was observed with a mobility type II (Figure 1(a)). A 2D panoramic radiograph was taken and showed a well-defined unilocular radiolucency in the apical area of the second maxillary molar with no extension to the maxillary sinus. In the left side of the mandible, two well-defined radiolucencies were noted, the first in relation to the mesial root of the first molar and the second on the mandibular body apically to the second molar (Figure 1(b)).

The axial images of the CT scan revealed the presence of radiolucency in the maxilla with cortical bone deterioration buccally and palatally and in the mandible and a well-defined localized radiolucency in the body of the mandible (Figures 1(c) and 1(d)).

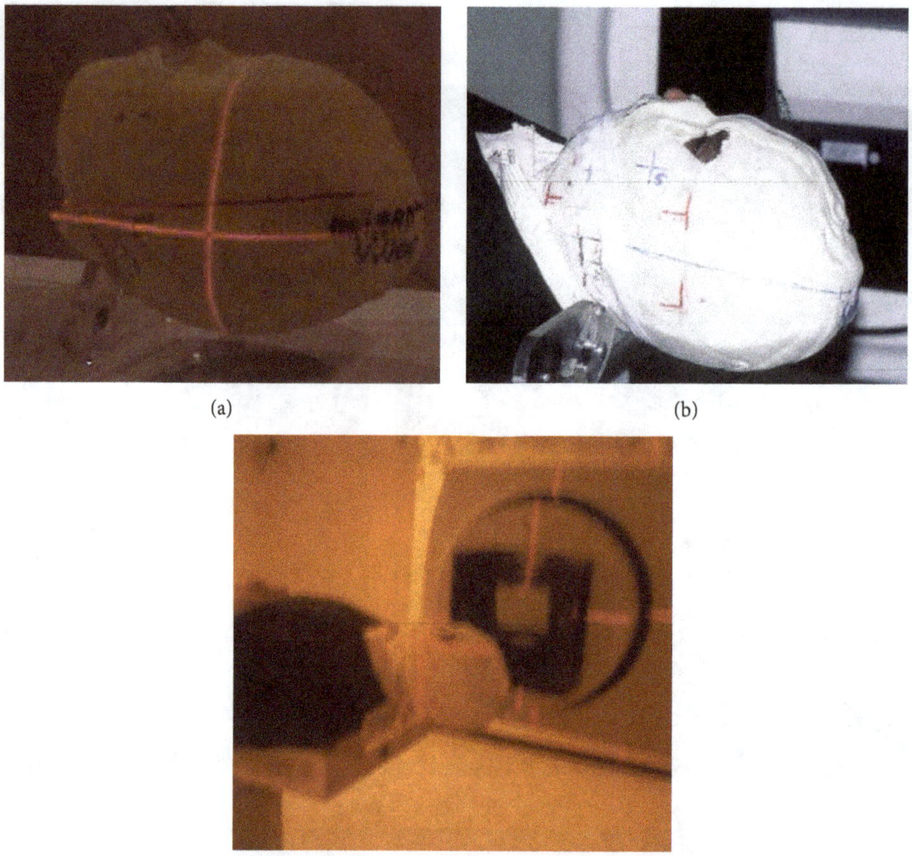

(a) (b) (c)

Figure 3: (a) Custom-made rigid mask. (b) Patient wearing the stabilisation mask. (c) 3D treatment planning is done using the CT scan images.

Based on clinical and radiological findings, the differential diagnosis suggested was a radicular cyst, osteomyelitis, primary bone tumor, lymphoma, and LCH.

The extraction of the maxillary molars was proposed by us and approved by the patient. Under loco-regional analgesia, the two teeth were extracted, and the excised tissue was sent for histological evaluation (Figure 1(e)). The result came out with an LCH diagnosis (Figure 1(f)).

Histological examination exposed cellular proliferation characterized by unique reniform nuclei with eosinophilic cytoplasm representing Langerhans cells, in a stroma with numerous acute and chronic inflammatory infiltrate cells.

The patient was oriented to the internal medicine department to determine the degree of the disorder and to discuss the appropriate treatment protocol.

Hematological explorations displayed a significant increase in eosinophil count by 12%.

An entire body CT scan was accomplished which showed no evidence of lesions in other organs. Bone scintigraphy was completed and confirms that the lesions are limited in the right maxilla and on the left mandible (Figures 2(a) and 2(b)).

The treatment plan we proposed and accepted by the patient was the extraction of all the teeth in the affected region followed by fractionated stereotactic low-dose RT after two months (Figure 2(c)).

2.1. Radiation Therapy. A 6-megavolt linear accelerator was used with a 0.5 mm precision of its isocenter.

A custom-made rigid mask was fabricated and used for accurate immobilization of the head as described by Al Salah and El Hajj [15]. The objective of the custom-made rigid mask is to stabilize the head during the radiotherapy sessions (Figures 3(a) and 3(b)).

3D treatment planning is prepared using the CT scan images fed into the planning system (Figure 3(c)). The target volume is determinate and verified by the radiation oncologist. Dosimetry planning is organized around three isocenters for the mandible and a single isocenter for the right maxillary sinus. Planning has been done to avoid the parotid glands.

Each of the right maxilla and the left mandible received 24 Gy in 16 fractions (1.5 Gy in each session) during 32 days.

Preventive and palliative treatments included dexamethasone cream applied twice daily to the irradiated skin and mouth baths of a mixture of bicarbonate, antifungal gel, and local anesthetic application 3 times per day. Moreover, customized tooth adapted aligners were fabricated before the RT sessions for fluoride gel application for 5 minutes every day before, during, and after the end of RT treatment for 3 months. The patient presented a

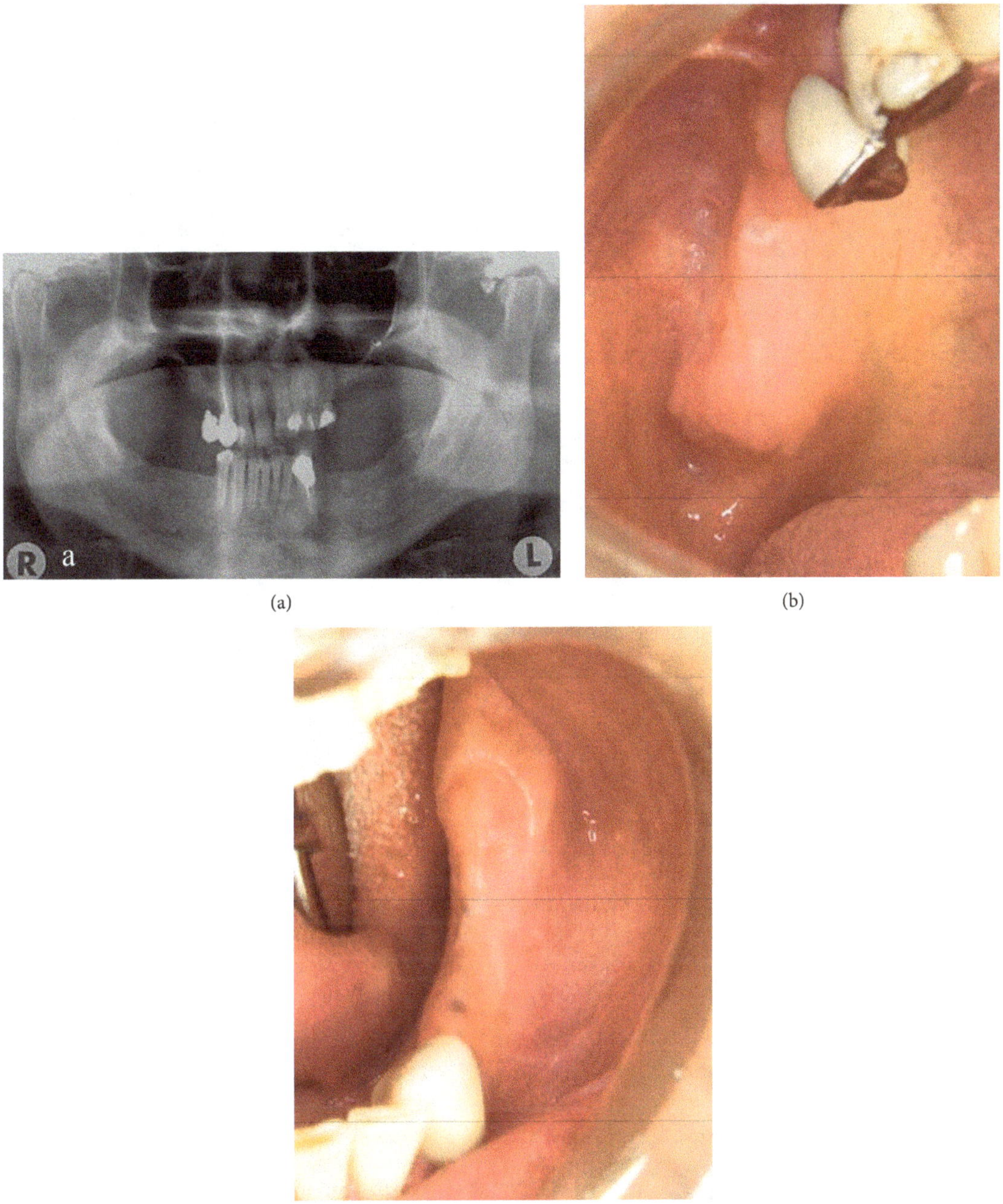

(a) (b) (c)

Figure 4: One-year follow-up after the end of RT treatment: (a) panoramic radiograph; (b) maxillary soft tissue healing; (c) mandibular soft tissue healing.

grade two mucositis during the treatment and was treated with corticosteroid oral rinses beside the good oral hygiene.

Xerostomia grade two has been experienced during the last two weeks of irradiation, but complete recovery has been reached one month after the treatment.

The patient was followed up in the beginning, every 6 months yearly. Complete remission was achieved clinically and radiologically after one year (Figures 4(a)–4(c)).

The panoramic X-ray and CBCT after 5 years confirm the complete bone healing process (Figures 5(a)–5(c)).

3. Discussion

Several treatment modalities have been reported for solitary and polyostotic bone lesions such as curettage or excision [7, 9], intralesion steroid injection [10], chemotherapy treatment with vinblastine, and prednisone [9] or cytosine arabinoside [8], and low-dose RT [11–14]. The effectivity of RT in LCH has been widely reported, but several elements should be respected such as the age of patients, the possibility of radiogenic malignancies, and the semibenign character of the disease [11–14].

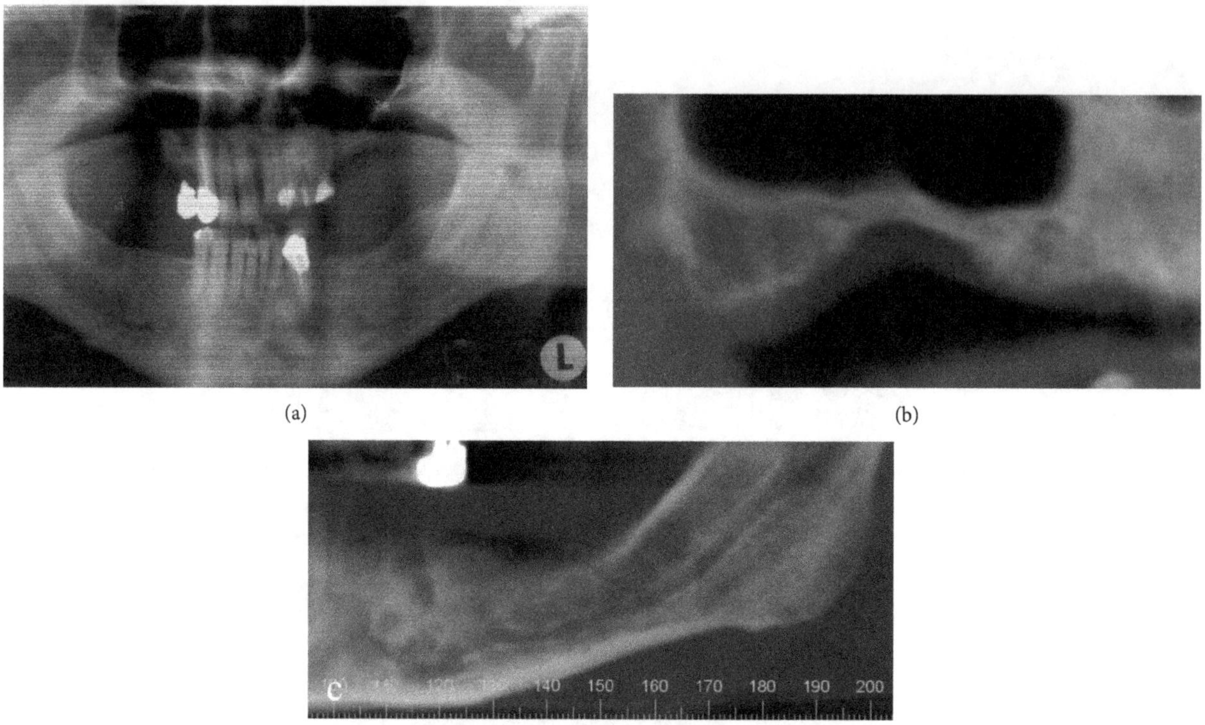

(a) (b) (c)

Figure 5: 5-year follow-up radiographs: (a) panoramic radiograph; (b) sagittal CBCT image showing complete bone healing in the maxilla; (c) sagittal CBCT image showing complete bone healing in the mandible.

It is used as a single treatment option or in combination with chemotherapy, surgery, or steroid injections [7–14].

The mechanism of action induced by ionizing radiation on target cells remains unclear [12, 13].

In adults, the recommended doses range between 10 and 45 Gy and should be supplied in fractions of 1–2 Gy by session to respect the capacity for tissue repair mechanisms [11–13].

Olschewski and Seegenschmiedt (2006), evaluated 89 LCH patients treated by RT with fractionation and 2 Gy as a median single dose and 24 Gy as median total, 91% got a local remission of the treated lesions, 77.5% had a complete remission, and only 9% developed recurrence [11].

Kriz et al. (2013) published the results of a retrospective analysis performed by the German Cooperative Group for Benign Diseases where 80 patients suffering from LCH were treated with RT during the last past 45 years and found that 77% achieved a complete remission with a median follow-up period of 54 months. They used RT with fractionation of a median total dose of 15 Gy, and the median single fraction was 2 Gy [12].

The treatment protocol proposed to our patient was very mild toxicity.

Healing of soft tissue and bone was observed over the 5-year follow-up.

4. Conclusion

LCH is an idiopathic benign disorder touching both genders at any age and can affect one or more organs. It is usually characterized by monostotic or polyostotic osteolytic bone lesions.

There is no consensus treatment for the management of these lesions. Fractionated stereotactic low-dose RT is deemed to be an efficient option for LCH treatment alone or combined with other treatment modalities.

Consent

Patient signed the consent.

Acknowledgments

The author thanks Pr. Saad Khairalah, Pr. Labib, el Hajj, and Pr. Dani Gergis for their valuable help and assistance.

References

[1] T. Chu, G. J. D'Angio, B. E. Favara, S. Ladisch, M. Nesbit, and J. Pritchard, "Histiocytosis syndromes in children. Writing Group of the Histiocyte Society," *Lancet*, vol. 2, no. 8549, pp. 41-42, 1987.

[2] J. F. Emile, O. Abla, S. Fraitag et al., "Revised classification of histiocytoses and neoplasms of the macrophage-dendritic cell lineages," *Blood*, vol. 127, no. 22, pp. 2672–2681, 2016.

[3] J. Krooks, M. Minkov, and A. G. Weatherall, "Langerhans cell histiocytosis in children: history, classification, pathobiology, clinical manifestations, and prognosis," *Journal of the American Academy of Dermatology*, vol. 78, no. 6, pp. 1035–1044, 2018.

[4] M. Aricò, I. Astigarraga, J. Braier et al., "Lack of bone lesions at diagnosis is associated with inferior outcome in multisystem langerhans cell histiocytosis of childhood," *British Journal of Haematology*, vol. 169, no. 2, pp. 241–248, 2015.

[5] S. Khung, J. F. Budzik, E. Amzallag-Bellenger et al., "Skeletal involvement in Langerhans cell histiocytosis," *Insights Into Imaging*, vol. 4, no. 5, pp. 569–579, 2013.

[6] C. Lian, Y. Lu, and S. Shen, "Langerhans cell histiocytosis in adults: a case report and review of the literature," *Oncotarget*, vol. 7, no. 14, pp. 18678–18683, 2016.

[7] M. Kobayashi and A. Tojo, "Langerhans cell histiocytosis in adults: advances in pathophysiology and treatment," *Cancer Science*, vol. 109, no. 12, pp. 3707–3713, 2018.

[8] M. A. Cantu, P. J. Lupo, M. Bilgi, M. J. Hicks, C. E. Allen, and K. L. McClain, "Optimal therapy for adults with Langerhans cell histiocytosis bone lesions," *PLoS One*, vol. 7, no. 8, article e43257, 2012.

[9] F. Gargano, J. J. Welch, P. M. Klinge, S. R. Sullivan, and H. O. Taylor, "Langerhans cell histiocytosis in the pediatric population," *The Journal of Craniofacial Surgery*, vol. 30, no. 4, pp. 1191–1193, 2019.

[10] T. F. Putters, J. G. de Visscher, A. van Veen, and F. K. Spijkervet, "Intralesional infiltration of corticosteroids in the treatment of localised langerhans' cell histiocytosis of the mandible: Report of known cases and three new cases," *International Journal of Oral and Maxillofacial Surgery*, vol. 34, no. 5, pp. 571–575, 2005.

[11] T. Olschewski and M. H. Seegenschmiedt, "Radiotherapy for bony manifestations of Langerhans cell histiocytosis. Review and proposal for an international registry," *Strahlentherapie und Onkologie*, vol. 182, no. 2, pp. 72–79, 2006.

[12] J. Kriz, H. T. Eich, F. Bruns et al., "Radiotherapy in langerhans cell histiocytosis - a rare indication in a rare disease," *Radiation Oncology*, vol. 8, no. 1, p. 233, 2013.

[13] R. Kotecha, R. Venkatramani, R. F. Jubran, A. Arkader, A. J. Olch, and K. Wong, "Clinical outcomes of radiation therapy in the management of Langerhans cell histiocytosis," *American journal of clinical oncology*, vol. 37, no. 6, pp. 592–596, 2014.

[14] J. Laird, J. Ma, K. Chau et al., "Outcome after radiation therapy for langerhans cell histiocytosis is dependent on site of involvement," *International Journal of Radiation Oncology • Biology • Physics*, vol. 100, no. 3, pp. 670–678, 2018.

[15] A. Al Salah and L. El Hajj, "The use of custom- made masks in stereotactic radiation therapy," *Physica Medica*, vol. 17, no. 2, p. 111, 2001.

32

Oral Surgery Procedures in a Patient Affected by Hereditary Angioedema Type I

Chiara Cinquini, Simonetta Santarelli, Alberto Marianelli, Marco Nisi, Mario Gabriele, and Antonio Barone

Department of Surgical, Medical, Molecular and of Critical Area Pathologies, Complex Operative Unit of Stomatology and Oral Surgery, University-Hospital of Pisa, University of Pisa, 56126 Pisa, Italy

Correspondence should be addressed to Antonio Barone; barosurg@gmail.com

Academic Editor: Vlaho Brailo

Hereditary Angioedema (HAE) is a rare disease characterized by a deficiency or a reduced function of the plasma protein C1 esterase inhibitor (C1-INH), which is involved in the downregulation of several inflammatory pathways. Patients affected by HAE suffer from episodic swellings of subcutaneous or submucosal tissues. Swellings can be caused by stress or dental and surgical procedures and can be life-threatening if the airways are involved. We have reported a clinical case of a patient affected by HAE type I who underwent oral surgery procedures under a short-term prophylaxis with C1-INH plasma-derived concentrate. The patient underwent a cyst removal, multiple tooth extractions, and an excisional biopsy with a prophylaxis with C1-INH plasma-derived concentrate and was hospitalized for 36 hours after the surgery to be monitored for possible HAE attacks. During the hospitalization, the patient did not show signs of swelling nor of HAE attacks. At 14 and 28 days after the surgery, the patient presented a good surgical healing. The prophylactic intravenous infusion of C1-INH concentrate was successful in preventing acute HAE attacks after oral surgery procedures.

1. Introduction

Hereditary angioedema (HAE) is a rare autosomal dominant disease characterized by a deficiency or a reduced function of the C1 esterase inhibitor (C1-INH) [1], a plasma protein belonging to the serine protease inhibitors encoded by the SERPING 1 gene [2]. Its incidence ranges from 1/50.000 to 1/100.000, with no distinction of race and sex [3]. Three variants of HAE are portrayed in scientific literature: type I affects 85% of patients and presents low plasma levels of C1-INH, and type II affects 15% of patients and is characterized by inactive C1-INH with normal plasma levels [4]. HAE with normal C1-INH (HAE-nC1INH) is rare and is characterized by normal C1-INH level and function and may be associated with mutations in the coagulation factor XII gene or in other known and unknown genes [5, 6].

C1 esterase inhibitor (C1-INH) is involved in the regulation of several inflammatory pathways [1]. Mutations in the gene encoding for the protein C1-INH (SERPING 1 gene) might prevent the synthesis of the protein (HAE type I) or produce a nonfunctioning protein (HAE type II) and both mutations lead to the failure to control the local production of bradykinin. The massive release of this inflammatory mediator increases vascular permeability, thus causing consequent edema of the anatomical areas involved [7]. HAE diagnosis may be suggested by recurrent episodes of swelling and by the presence of abdominal pain [8], even though the final diagnosis can be confirmed only through serological tests [9].

HAE type I is characterized by low plasma levels of C1-INH associated with a reduced function and reduced levels of a protein, called complement component 4 (C4), which is a protein belonging to the complement system [10].

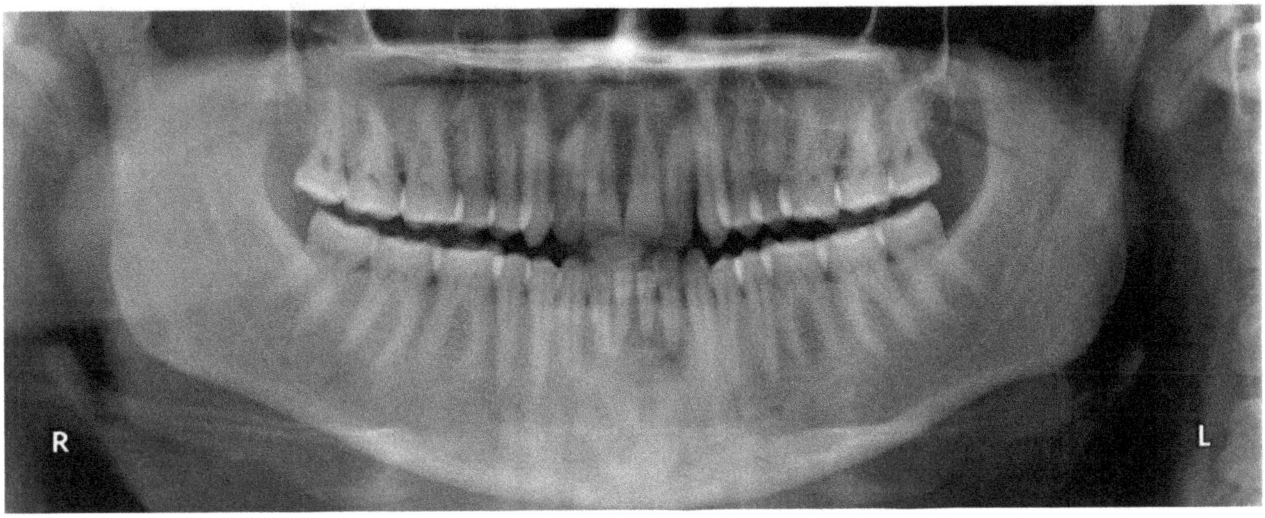

FIGURE 1: Orthopantomogram showing the mandibular radiolucent area.

Some authors showed that the key factors indicating high clinical suspicion for hereditary angioedema are family history and early age in onset of symptoms [8].

Patients affected by HAE suffer from episodic swellings affecting the subcutaneous and submucosal tissues of hands, feet, face, genitals, or gastrointestinal tract [11]; these acute onsets can be life-threatening when the upper airways are involved, especially the larynx, which can cause asphyxia. HAE attacks can be triggered by physical or psychological stress or can arise spontaneously; local trauma such as dental treatments and routine oral surgery procedures may increase the risk of HAE attacks within 4-48 hours from the intervention [12], typically starting near the area of trauma [9]. Several cases of patients' death after dental procedures are described in literature, involving not exclusively patients with recurrent HAE attacks. The mortality rate after oral surgery procedures without adequate prophylaxis was set at 30-40% in the past decades [13]; at the present time, short-term prophylaxis is used to prevent possible HAE attacks following surgical procedures or other possible triggers [14]. Throughout the years, a considerable number of drugs have been used for prophylaxis before surgical procedures such as C1-INH concentrate, attenuated androgenic hormone therapy, episolon aminocaproic acid, and fresh frozen plasma [12]; C1-INH concentrate has been the most efficient medication because it was developed focusing on the origins of HAE [7].

C1-INH concentrate (plasma-derived or recombinant) has been successfully used to treat acute HAE attacks for many years and, from 2013, has been approved in Europe for short-term prophylaxis before dental or surgical procedures in patients affected by HAE type I [14]. C1-INH concentrate has a long half-life and can persist in the blood stream for 1-2 days after the intravenous infusion administration [13].

Other medications approved for the treatment of acute HAE attacks are the kallikrein inhibitors (Ecallantide) and the bradykinin B2 receptor antagonists (Icatibant) [15, 16].

Hereditary angioedema is a rare disease that requires special precautions even for common dental or surgical procedures because the consequences might be fatal.

An adjunctive issue is the frequent delayed diagnosis of HAE [17], leading to the effective possibility of having to deal with patients affected by HAE and without being aware of the disease.

This report describes the management of oral surgical intervention in a patient affected by HAE type I.

2. Case Report

A 37-year-old man referred to the Unit of Oral Surgery because of episodic swellings in the inferior incisive area. The patient received a complete intraoral examination, showing a complete dentition and a pedunculate lesion of the right buccal mucosa.

During the clinical examination, a diffuse mild swelling was detected at the mandibular buccal incisive area; an orthopantomogram was then prescribed to further investigate the possible origin of the swelling. The radiographic examination revealed a unilocular radiolucency with thin sclerotic margins adjacent to the apical area of mandibular incisors (Figure 1).

Pulp vitality test was negative for teeth 3.1 and 3.2 (lower left incisors), and the teeth were sensitive to percussion. Moreover, teeth 4.1, 3.1, and 3.2 showed a grade III mobility. The suspected diagnosis was inflammatory odontogenic cyst, and the planned surgical intervention was the enucleation of the osteolytic lesion and the evaluation of the involved teeth. Moreover, the biopsy of the pedunculate lesion of the right buccal mucosa was scheduled.

The patient's medical history was collected: since the age of 14, he suffered from four episodes of swelling per year, localized in the hands, feet, face, and genitals. During these episodes, the swelling occurred slowly, involving only one anatomical site. It was associated with a nonpruritic rash and absence of fever, which gradually reduced during the

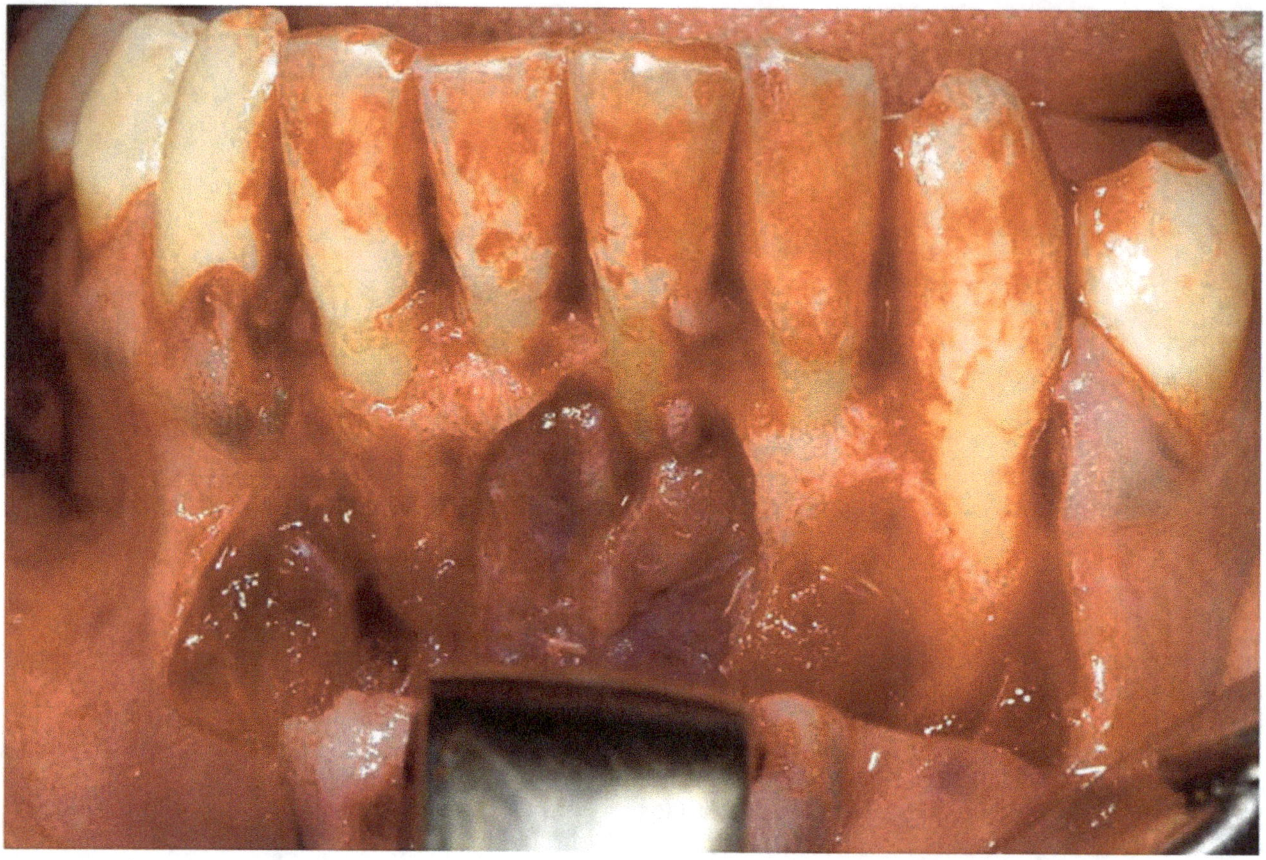

FIGURE 2: Flap elevation and cyst exposure.

following 3-4 days. In the past years, the patient had been hospitalized many times for episodes of abdominal pain and diarrhea. The hematologic analysis for suspected HAE was performed in December 2018: the C1-INH plasmatic concentration was 7.8 mg/dl (with a normal range between 12 and 30), the functional C1-INH was 34% (with a normal range between 30 and 130), and C4 was 7.7 mg/dl (with a normal range between 10 and 40), confirming the diagnosis of HAE type I.

The medical family history was positive; indeed, his brother, diagnosed with HAE type I, had died from asphyxia due to an HAE attack which occurred after a dental extraction. Complete hematologic analysis was requested a few days before the surgical procedure; erythrocyte, leucocyte, platelet count, prothrombin activity, aPTT and fibrinogen, and coagulation factors were within a normal range.

In agreement with the Immuno-allergology Department, the patient underwent the surgical procedure with a prophylaxis with C1-INH plasma-derived concentrate (Berinert). Berinert is a C1-INH plasma-derived concentrate, usually administered for the short-term prophylaxis of HAE attacks before surgical procedures. The recommended dose of Berinert is 20 IU/kg (international unit/kilogram), depending on the body weight. On the basis of the patient's weight, 1500 IU were slowly infused intravenously 1 hour before the surgery.

All the surgical procedures were performed under local anesthesia with lidocaine, while monitoring the vital signs (electrocardiography, hearth-rate, blood pressure, and SpO_2). A mucoperiosteal flap was elevated in the central area of the mandible, revealing a mandibular cyst of approximately 1.5 × 1.2 cm. The cyst was surgically excised, and three mandibular incisors (4.1, 3.1, and 3.2) were extracted due to the extensive bone loss and high mobility (Figures 2 and 3); in fact, both lingual and buccal cortical plates were completely absent once the cyst was removed and the teeth showed a grade III mobility, resulting in an endodontic-periodontal lesion with a hopeless prognosis. The preservation of these teeth could have been resulted in the persistent presence of infection and inflammation, which should be avoided in a HAE patient [4]. An excisional biopsy was also performed to remove and analyze the pedunculate lesion of the right buccal mucosa.

Absorbable sutures were placed to avoid postsurgical removal (Figure 4). Moreover, these sutures made of copolymers of glycolide and lactide are broken down by hydrolysis processes and are not associated with a strong inflammatory reaction [18]. Both surgical specimens were delivered to the Pathological Anatomy Laboratory for the histopathological evaluation. Ropivacaine was instilled in the surgical wound immediately after the surgery to reduce postoperative pain and the consequent stress for the patient.

After the surgery, the patient was asked to report pain using the Numeric Rating Score (NRS) from 0 (no pain at all) to 10 (worst imaginable pain); the NRS value assessed was 6, and the patient was provided with Tramadol 100 mg

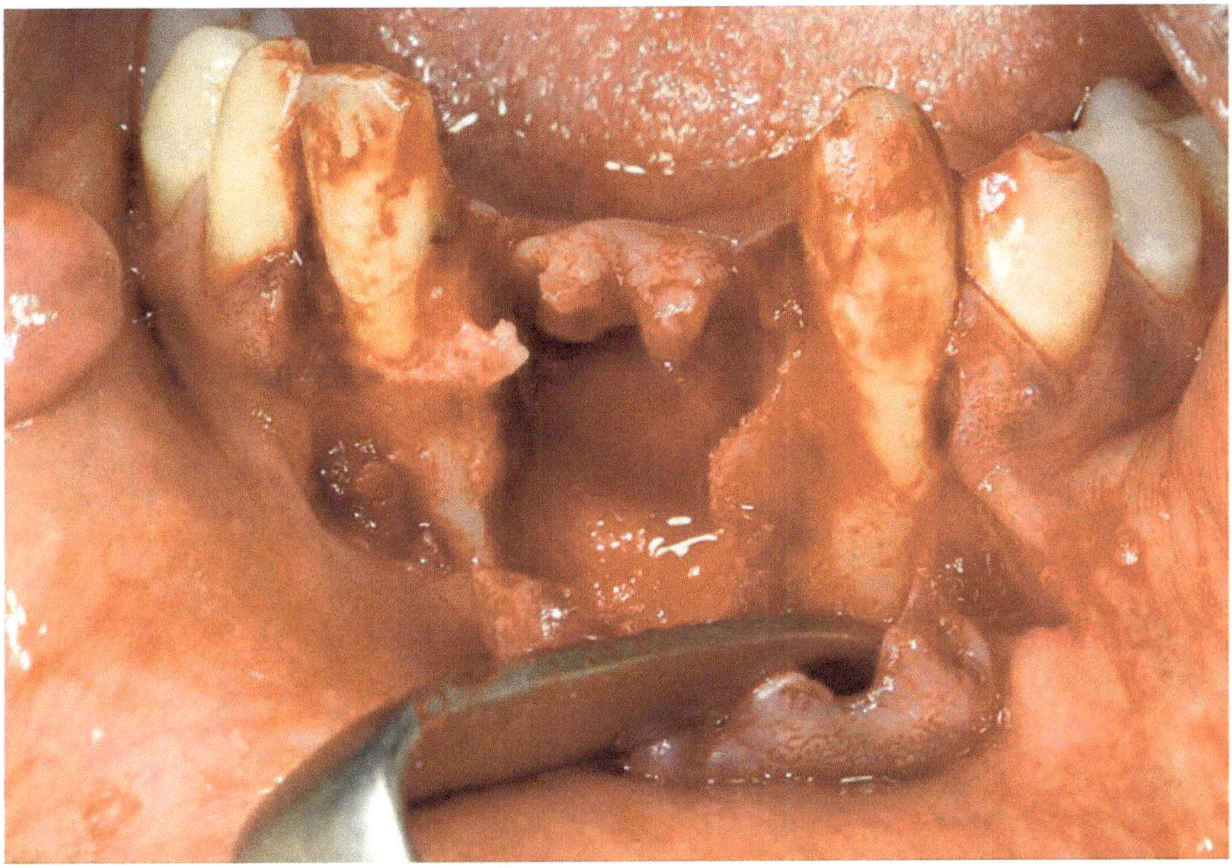

FIGURE 3: Bone defect after tooth extractions and cyst removal.

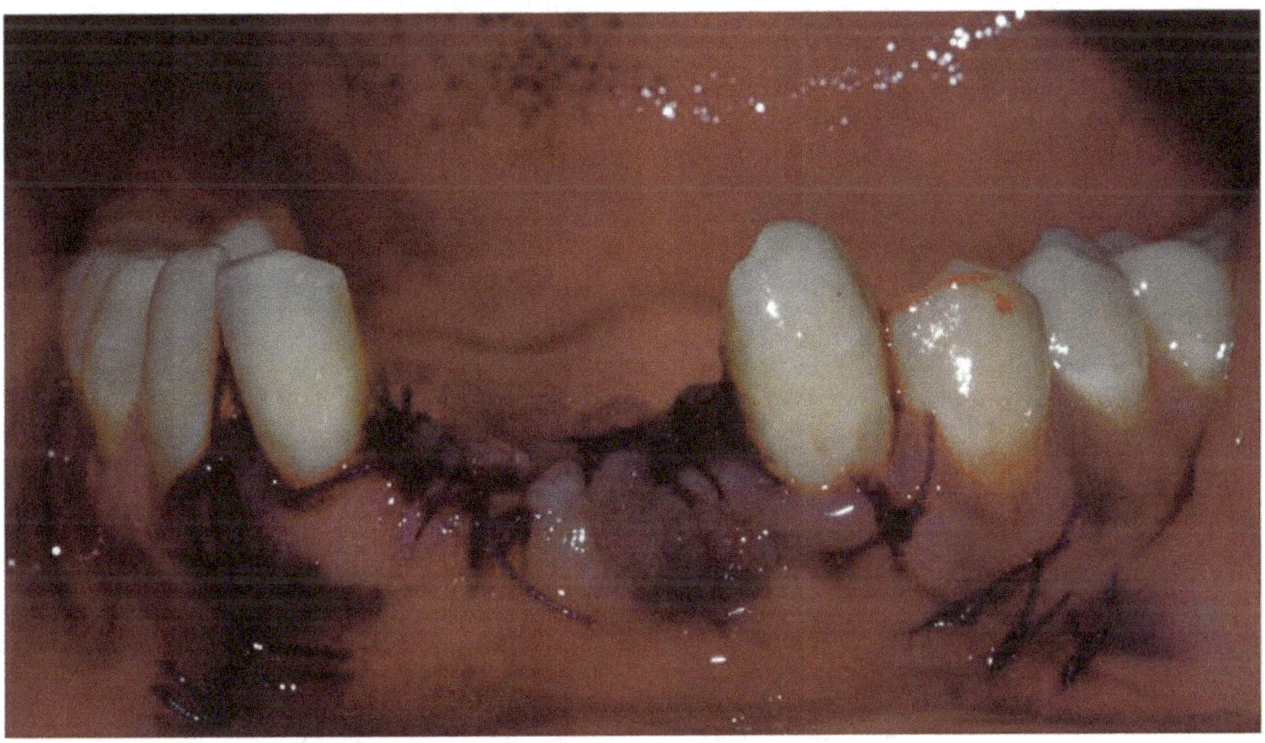

FIGURE 4: Clinical image immediately after the surgery.

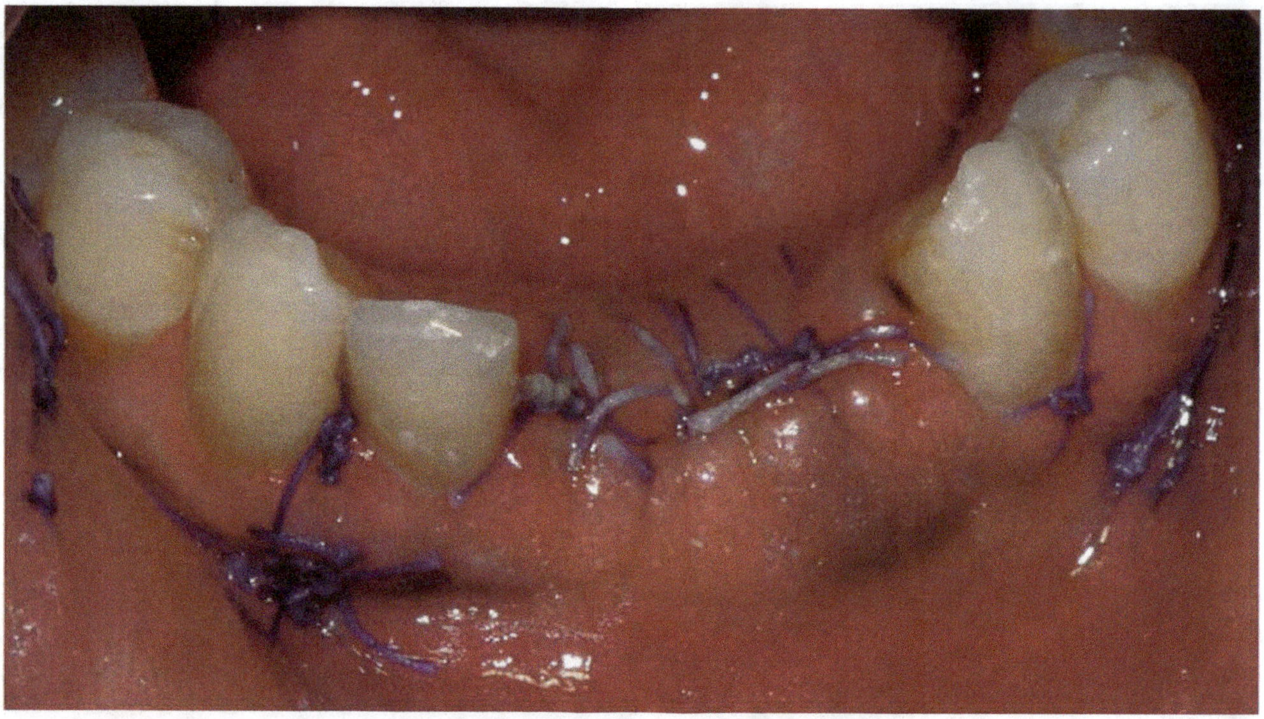

Figure 5: Clinical image after 14 days from the surgery.

administered intravenously. A postsurgical antibiotic prophylaxis with Clarithromycin was prescribed at the dosage of 500 mg (one tablet) every 12 hours for seven days. Betalactam antibiotics such as amoxicillin were avoided since they may cause drug-induced angioedema [19].

The patient was hospitalized for 36 hours after the surgery to be monitored for possible HAE attacks.

After 36 hours of hospitalization, the patient showed absence of acute HAE episode and he was discharged. He was given exhaustive postsurgical instructions and provided with Icatibant (Firazyr), an antagonist of bradykinin B2 receptors, to be administered subcutaneously by the patient himself in case of an acute attack after the hospitalization period. He was also given the recommendation to go to the emergency department in case of any suspected HAE attacks.

The patient was reevaluated 7 days after the surgery. He had had no occurrence of swelling in the past days and had not required to access the emergency department.

No relevant surgical-related edema was observed. The patient reported no pain (NRS = 0) and no reduction in mouth opening. At the clinical examination, no suppuration or local signs of inflammation were evident.

At 14 (Figure 5) and 28 days after the surgery, the patient presented a good surgical healing and an excellent oral hygiene.

The histopathological findings of the intrabony lesion showed the presence of a fibrous wall with a lymphoplasmacytic and monocytic infiltrate, and a lining epithelium, confirming the clinical diagnosis of inflammatory odontogenic cyst (radicular cyst). With regard to the pedunculate lesion of the buccal mucosa, the presence of sclerotic connective tissue with signs of acanthosis and parakeratosis was compatible with a local fibrous hyperplasia on an irritative basis.

Special attention will be paid for future prosthetic rehabilitation since in literature; there are described acute HAE attacks following impressions for prosthetic rehabilitations [20].

3. Discussion

In the past years, the administration of preoperative fresh frozen plasma (FFP) has been an effective method to prevent HAE attacks following dental or surgical procedures [21].

The use of C1-INH concentrate was approved in 2009 in Europe and in 2010 in the USA for the treatment of acute HAE attacks, while its use as prophylactic treatment was finally approved in Europe in 2013.

Many studies in literature reported the use of C1-INH concentrate as prophylaxis before surgical procedures, showing good outcomes.

Maeda et al. [7] described a case report of a patient affected by HAE type I who suffered from swellings after the injection of local anesthetics for routinary dental treatments. The patient required the extraction of a lower third molar, and he was treated under local anesthesia; the infusion of C1-INH was performed just after the surgical procedure. In this case, no postprocedural swelling was observed.

Sanuki et al. [22] reported a successful management of multiple tooth extractions in a patient affected by HAE with the preprocedural administration of the C1-INH concentrate. The postoperative period was uneventful, and the patient was discharged home 3 days after the surgery.

A retrospective study on the efficacy of C1-INH concentrate prophylaxis in preventing HAE attacks showed that out of 24 patients who underwent invasive surgical procedures (varying from dental extractions to aortic aneurysm repair), none of them had a HAE attack [14].

Another retrospective study performed on 24 HAE patients who underwent 66 dental procedures (ranging from dental extraction to orthodontic treatment) showed the efficacy of a preprocedural prophylaxis with C1-INH concentrate or treatment with attenuated androgens (AAs) [11]. According to the authors, only 3 patients experienced a mild upper airway edema; none of these patients received a preprocedural prophylaxis with C1-INH or a maintenance treatment with AAs.

A larger study including 91 patients suffering from HAE showed that 98% of the patients, who were treated with C1-INH concentrate as prophylaxis, had an uneventful healing period after surgical procedures [23].

The International WAO/EAACI (World Allergy Organization and the European Academy of Allergy and Clinical Immunology) guidelines suggest the use of the C1-INH concentrate as presurgical prophylaxis in patients affected by HAE [10].

The importance of presurgical prophylaxis is confirmed by the fact that HAE attacks do not respond to many antiedema treatments such as antihistamines, corticosteroids, and adrenaline [24].

The prevention of acute attacks is the best course of action in cases of surgical procedures for patients affected by HAE, especially considering the fact that the treatment of acute attacks may be difficult and a potentially life-threatening complication. However, it should be remembered that acute HAE attacks may occur after relatively minor surgical procedures despite the presurgical prophylaxis [25]; for this reason, patients should be carefully monitored and instructed on what to do at home in case of an acute attack, according to what is reported in the case report section.

In the present case, a presurgical prophylaxis with C1-INH concentrate was effective in preventing acute HAE attacks and the postsurgical period was uneventful.

Consent

The authors declare that the patient has been informed of the publication of this Case Report and signed an appropriate consent form. The patient has given his consent for the publication of anonymized clinical information and radiographic/photographic reports.

Authors' Contributions

All the authors approved the final version of the manuscript and agreed to be accountable for all aspects of the work.

Acknowledgments

The authors declare that they have no conflict of interest.

References

[1] H. Longhurst and M. Cicardi, "Hereditary angio-oedema," *Lancet*, vol. 379, no. 9814, pp. 474–481, 2012.

[2] A. E. Germenis and M. Speletas, "Genetics of hereditary angioedema revisited," *Clinical reviews in allergy & immunology*, vol. 51, no. 2, pp. 170–182, 2016.

[3] M. S. Gakhal, G. Marcotte, and v., "Hereditary angioedema: imaging manifestations and clinical management," *Emergency radiology*, vol. 22, no. 1, pp. 83–90, 2015.

[4] T. Caballero, M. L. Baeza, R. Cabañas et al., "Consensus statement on the diagnosis, management, and treatment of angioedema mediated by bradykinin. Part II. Treatment, follow-up, and special situations," *Journal of investigational allergology & clinical immunology*, vol. 21, no. 6, pp. 422-423, 2011.

[5] B. L. Zuraw, "Clinical practice. Hereditary angioedema," *The New England journal of medicine*, vol. 359, no. 10, pp. 1027–1036, 2008.

[6] B. L. Zuraw, K. Bork, K. E. Binkley et al., "Hereditary angioedema with normal C1 inhibitor function: consensus of an international expert panel," *Allergy and Asthma Proceedings*, vol. 33, no. 6, 2012.

[7] S. Maeda, T. Miyawaki, S. Nomura, T. Yagi, and M. Shimada, "Management of oral surgery in patients with hereditary or acquired angioedemas: review and case report," *Oral surgery, oral medicine, oral pathology, oral radiology, and endodontics*, vol. 96, no. 5, pp. 540–543, 2003.

[8] M. M. Gompels, R. J. Lock, D. J. Unsworth et al., "Misdiagnosis of hereditary angio-oedema type 1 and type 2," *The British journal of dermatology*, vol. 148, no. 4, pp. 719–723, 2003.

[9] M. Kunschak, W. Engl, F. Maritsch et al., "A randomized, controlled trial to study the efficacy and safety of C1 inhibitor concentrate in treating hereditary angioedema," *Transfusion*, vol. 38, no. 6, pp. 540–549, 1998.

[10] M. Maurer, M. Magerl, I. Ansotegui et al., "The international WAO/EAACI guideline for the management of hereditary angioedema-the 2017 revision and update," *Allergy*, vol. 73, no. 8, pp. 1575–1596, 2018.

[11] J. Jurado-Palomo, J. M. Muñoz-Caro, M. C. López-Serrano et al., "Management of dental-oral procedures in patients with hereditary angioedema due to C1 inhibitor deficiency," *Journal of investigational allergology & clinical immunology*, vol. 23, no. 1, pp. 1 6, 2013.

[12] N. J. van Sickels, R. B. Hunsaker, and J. E. van Sickels, "Hereditary angioedema: treatment, management, and precautions in patients presenting for dental care," *Oral surgery, oral medicine, oral pathology, oral radiology, and endodontics*, vol. 109, no. 2, pp. 168–172, 2010.

[13] K. Bork and S.-E. Barnstedt, "Laryngeal edema and death from asphyxiation after tooth extraction in four patients with hereditary angioedema," *Journal of the American Dental Association*, vol. 134, no. 8, pp. 1088–1094, 1939.

[14] G. Gavigan, W. H. Yang, S. Santucci, R. Harrison, and J. Karsh, "The prophylactic use of C1 inhibitor in hereditary angioedema patients undergoing invasive surgical procedures: a ret-

rospective study," *Allergy, asthma, and clinical immunology : official journal of the Canadian Society of Allergy and Clinical Immunology*, vol. 10, no. 1, p. 17, 2014.

[15] G. Hwang, A. Johri, S. Ng, and T. Craig, "A review of kallikrein inhibitor lanadelumab in hereditary angioedema," *Immunotherapy*, vol. 11, no. 11, pp. 937–944, 2019.

[16] M. Cicardi, A. Banerji, F. Bracho et al., "Icatibant, a new bradykinin-receptor antagonist, in hereditary angioedema," *The New England journal of medicine*, vol. 363, no. 6, pp. 532–541, 2010.

[17] M. D. Guarino, C. Perricone, S. Guarino et al., "Denaturing HPLC in laboratory diagnosis of hereditary angioedema," *The Journal of allergy and clinical immunology*, vol. 120, no. 4, pp. 962–965, 2007.

[18] M. Byrne and A. Aly, "The surgical suture," *Aesthetic surgery journal*, vol. 39, Supplement_2, pp. S67–S72, 2019.

[19] N. Inomata, "Recent advances in drug-induced angioedema," *Allergology International*, vol. 61, pp. 545–557, 2012.

[20] S. R. Aziz and P. Tin, "Spontaneous angioedema of oral cavity after dental impressions," *The New York state dental journal*, vol. 68, no. 2, pp. 42–45, 2002.

[21] J. C. Atkinson and M. M. Frank, "Oral manifestations and dental management of patients with hereditary angioedema," *Journal of Oral Pathology & Medicine*, vol. 20, no. 3, pp. 139–142, 1991.

[22] T. Sanuki, T. Watanabe, S. Kurata, and T. Ayuse, "Perioperative management of tooth extractions for a patient with hereditary angioedema," *Journal of Oral and Maxillofacial Surgery*, vol. 72, no. 2421, pp. e1–2421.e24213, 2014.

[23] J. A. Grant, M. White, H. H. Li et al., "Preprocedural administration of nanofiltered C1 esterase inhibitor to prevent hereditary angioedema attacks," *Allergy and asthma proceedings*, vol. 33, no. 4, pp. 348–353, 2012.

[24] B. L. Zuraw, "Current and future therapy for hereditary angioedema," *Clinical immunology (Orlando, Fla).*, vol. 114, no. 1, pp. 10–16, 2005.

[25] E. Aygören-Pürsün, I. Martinez Saguer, W. Kreuz, T. Klingebiel, and D. Schwabe, "Risk of angioedema following invasive or surgical procedures in HAE type I and II– the natural history," *Allergy*, vol. 68, no. 8, 2013.

Permissions

All chapters in this book were first published by Hindawi Publishing Corporation; hereby published with permission under the Creative Commons Attribution License or equivalent. Every chapter published in this book has been scrutinized by our experts. Their significance has been extensively debated. The topics covered herein carry significant findings which will fuel the growth of the discipline. They may even be implemented as practical applications or may be referred to as a beginning point for another development.

The contributors of this book come from diverse backgrounds, making this book a truly international effort. This book will bring forth new frontiers with its revolutionizing research information and detailed analysis of the nascent developments around the world.

We would like to thank all the contributing authors for lending their expertise to make the book truly unique. They have played a crucial role in the development of this book. Without their invaluable contributions this book wouldn't have been possible. They have made vital efforts to compile up to date information on the varied aspects of this subject to make this book a valuable addition to the collection of many professionals and students.

This book was conceptualized with the vision of imparting up-to-date information and advanced data in this field. To ensure the same, a matchless editorial board was set up. Every individual on the board went through rigorous rounds of assessment to prove their worth. After which they invested a large part of their time researching and compiling the most relevant data for our readers.

The editorial board has been involved in producing this book since its inception. They have spent rigorous hours researching and exploring the diverse topics which have resulted in the successful publishing of this book. They have passed on their knowledge of decades through this book. To expedite this challenging task, the publisher supported the team at every step. A small team of assistant editors was also appointed to further simplify the editing procedure and attain best results for the readers.

Apart from the editorial board, the designing team has also invested a significant amount of their time in understanding the subject and creating the most relevant covers. They scrutinized every image to scout for the most suitable representation of the subject and create an appropriate cover for the book.

The publishing team has been an ardent support to the editorial, designing and production team. Their endless efforts to recruit the best for this project, has resulted in the accomplishment of this book. They are a veteran in the field of academics and their pool of knowledge is as vast as their experience in printing. Their expertise and guidance has proved useful at every step. Their uncompromising quality standards have made this book an exceptional effort. Their encouragement from time to time has been an inspiration for everyone.

The publisher and the editorial board hope that this book will prove to be a valuable piece of knowledge for researchers, students, practitioners and scholars across the globe.

List of Contributors

Hung-Yi Liao, Ya-Fen Yang and Pei-Bang Liao
Division of Prosthodontics, Department of Dentistry, Taipei Medical University Hospital, Taipei, Taiwan

May-Show Chen, Sheng-Wei Feng and Po-kai Juan
School of Dentistry, College of Oral Medicine, Taipei Medical University, Taipei, Taiwan

Jagadish Chandra
Dept. of Oral Surgery, Yenepoya Dental College, Yenepoya University, Deralakatte, India

Junaid Ahmed, Nandita Shenoy and Nanditha Sujir
Dept. of Oral Medicine and Radiology, Manipal College of Dental Sciences, Mangalore, Manipal Academy of Higher Education (MAHE), Manipal, Karnataka 576104, India

K. M. Veena
Dept. of Oral Medicine and Radiology, Yenepoya Dental College, Yenepoya University, Deralakatte, Karnataka, India

M. Vijayakumar
Department of Surgical Oncology, Yenepoya Medical College, Yenepoya University, Deralakatte, Mangalore, India

Igor Smojver
St. Catherine Specialty Hospital, Zagreb, Croatia

Marko Vuletić and Dragana Gabrić
Department of Oral Surgery, School of Dental Medicine, University of Zagreb, Croatia
Croatian Society for Hospital Dentistry / Dentistry of Special Care of the Croatian Medical Association, Zagreb, Croatia

Spomenka Manojlović
Department of Pathology, School of Medicine, University of Zagreb, Croatia

Guilherme Augusto Alves de Oliveira, Rafael Pereira da Mata Santos and Flávio Ricardo Manzi
Department of Dentistry of the Pontifical Catholic University of Minas Gerais (PUC-MG), Belo Horizonte, Minas Gerais, Brazil

Cleiterson Rezende de Sá and Omar Ribeiro Santos Junior
Preventive Cardiology Department of Núcleo Cardiológico Integrado Ltda., Mateus Leme, Minas Gerais, Brazil

Ekaterina Diachkova, Elena Morozova, Natalia Blagushina and Svetlana Tarasenko
Department of Dental Surgery of Borovsky Institute of Dentistry, Sechenov First Moscow State Medical University (Sechenov University), Russia

Jian-tong Cui, Shao-qing Zhang and Hui-xia He
Department of Stomatology, The First Medical Center, Chinese PLA General Hospital, Beijing, 100853, China

Hassan Sartawi
Department of Dentistry, Al-Haramain Medical Complex, Riyadh, Ahad Rufaidah, Saudi Arabia

Hana Bougatef, Eya Moussaoui, Ines Kallel, Mahmoud Smaoui, Lamia Oualha and Nabiha Douki
Department of Dental Medicine, EPS Sahloul, Sousse, Tunisia
Faculty of Dental Medicine, Oral Health and Oro-Facial Rehabilitation Laboratory Research (LR12ES11), University of Monastir, 5019 Monastir, Tunisia

Nur Hafizah Kamar Affendi and Rohana Ahmad
Unit of Prosthodontics, Centre of Restorative Dentistry Studies, Faculty of Dentistry, Universiti Teknologi MARA, Sungai Buloh Campus, Jalan Hospital, 47000 Sungai Buloh, Selangor, Malaysia

Farhad Vahidi
Department of Prosthodontics, New York University, College of Dentistry, 205 E. 64th St., Ste 403, New York, NY 10065, USA

Mohd Zulkifli Hassan
Universiti Kebangsaan Malaysia, Jalan Raja Muda Abdul Aziz, 50300 Kuala Lumpur, Federal Territory of Kuala Lumpur, Malaysia

Siti Nadia Rahimi
Faculty of Dentistry, Islamic Science University of Malaysia (USIM), Malaysia

Pablo Glera-Suarez and David Peñarrocha-Oltra
Department of Stomatology, Faculty of Medicine and Dentistry, University of Valencia, Spain

Blanca Serra-Pastor
Prosthodontics Unit, Department of Stomatology, Faculty of Medicine and Dentistry, University of Valencia, Spain

Miguel Peñarrocha-Diago
Department of Stomatology, Faculty of Medicine and Dentistry, University of Valencia, Spain
IDIBELL Institute, Barcelona, Spain

Cosme Gay-Escoda
IDIBELL Institute, Barcelona, Spain
Oral and Maxillofacial Surgery Department, Faculty of Medicine and Health Sciences (School of Dentistry), University of Barcelona, Spain

Kun-Hwa Sung, Ho-Keel Hwang and Hyoung-Hoon Jo
Department of Conservative Dentistry, School of Dentistry, Chosun University, Gwangju, Republic of Korea

Rym Mabrouk and Afef Oueslati
Endodontics and Restorative Dentistry, Department of Dental Medicine, Hospital of Charles Nicolle, Tunis, Tunisia

Souha Yahia
Endodontics and Restorative Dentistry, Service of Dental Medicine, Military Principal Hospital of Instruction, Tunis, Tunisia

Nadia Frih
Forensic Dentistry and Head of Service, Department of Dental Medicine, Hospital of Charles Nicolle, Tunis, Tunisia

Yosra Mabrouk, Sinda Ammar, Amel Labidi and Lamia Mansour
Removable Prosthetics Department, ABCDF Laboratory (LR12ES10), Faculty of Dental Medicine, University of Monastir, Tunisia

Sonia Ghoul
ABCDF Laboratory (LR12ES10), Faculty of Dental Medicine, University of Monastir, Tunisia

Hui Li, Qiang Wang and Mingwen Fan
Department of Operative Dentistry and Endodontics, Wuhan First Stomatological Hospital, No. 675 Jianshe Avenue, Jianghan District, Wuhan 430000, China

Qingan Xu
Department of Operative Dentistry and Endodontics, Wuhan First Stomatological Hospital, No. 675 Jianshe Avenue, Jianghan District, Wuhan 430000, China
Department of Stomatology, School of Medicine, Jianghan University, No. 8 SanJiao Lake Road, Economic and Technological Development District, Wuhan 430000, China

Satoshi Nakamura, Miki Yamada, Yosuke Iijima, Shunsuke Hino, Takahiro Kaneko and Norio Horie
Department of Oral and Maxillofacial Surgery, Saitama Medical Center, Saitama Medical University, Saitama, Japan

Keisuke Sawada
Department of Pathology, Saitama Medical Center, Saitama Medical University, Saitama, Japan

Snehashish Ghosh
Department of Oral Pathology, College of Medical Sciences, Bharatpur, Nepal

Safal Dhungel
Department of Oral and Maxillofacial Surgery, College of Medical Sciences, Bharatpur, Nepal

Bhawana Subedi
Department of Oral Medicine and Radiology, College of Medical Sciences, Bharatpur, Nepal

Subi Pradhan
College of Medical Sciences, Bharatpur, Nepal

Rana A. Alamoudi and Sara M. Bagher
Pediatric Dentistry Department, Faculty of Dentistry, King Abdulaziz University, Jeddah 21589, Saudi Arabia

Asmaa A. Yaseen
Pediatric Dentistry Resident, Department of Pediatric Dentistry, King Salman Armed Forces Hospital, Tabuk, Saudi Arabia

Amjad S. Alharthi
Pediatric Dentistry Resident, Department of Pediatric Dentistry, King Abdulaziz University, Jeddah, Saudi Arabia

Kenji Yamagata, Naomi Ishibashi-Kanno, Fumihiko Uchida, Satoshi Fukuzawa and Hiroki Bukawa
Department of Oral and Maxillofacial Surgery, Institute of Clinical Medicine, Faculty of Medicine, University of Tsukuba, Japan

Ryota Matsuoka
Department of Diagnostic Pathology, Institute of Clinical Medicine, Faculty of Medicine, University of Tsukuba, Japan

Hamid Kermanshah and Elmira Najafrad
Dental Research Center, Dentistry Research Institute, Tehran University of Medical Sciences, Tehran, Iran
Restorative Dentistry Department, School of Dentistry, Tehran University of Medical Sciences, Tehran, Iran

Sara Valizadeh
Dental Research Center, Dentistry Research Institute, Tehran University of Medical Sciences, Tehran, Iran
Restorative Dentistry Department, School of Dentistry, Tehran University of Medical Sciences, Tehran, Iran
Oral Biological and Medical Sciences Department, University of British Columbia, Faculty of Dentistry, Vancouver, BC, Canada

Oumaima Tayari, Jamila Jaouadi, Safa Jemli, Hela Haloui and Ali Ben Rahma
Complete Removable Prosthodontic Department, Research Laboratory LR12ES11, Faculty of Dental Medicine, University of Monastir, Monastir, Tunisia

Takumi Takahashi, Miki Yamada, Nami Nakayama, Yosuke Iijima, Shunsuke Hino, Takahiro Kaneko and Norio Horie
Department of Oral and Maxillofacial Surgery, Saitama Medical Center, Saitama Medical University, Saitama, Japan

Keisuke Sawada
Department of Pathology, Saitama Medical Center, Saitama Medical University, Saitama, Japan

Sara Valizadeh and Ladan Ranjbar Omrani
Restorative Dentistry Department, School of Dentistry, Tehran University of Medical Sciences, Tehran, Iran

Simone Deliperi
Tufts University School of Dental Medicine, Boston, MA, USA
Private Practice, Cagliari, Italy

Farzaneh Sadeghi Mahounak
Restorative Dentistry Department, School of Dentistry, Shahid beheshti University of Medical Sciences, Tehran, Iran

Riccardo Aiuto and Dino Re
Department of Biomedical, Surgical and Dental Sciences, Istituto Stomatologico Italiano, University of Milan, Milan, Italy

Gianluca Fumei
Department of Restorative Dentistry and Endodontics, University of Insubria, Varese, Italy

Erica Lipani and Daniele Garcovich
Department of Dentistry, Universidad Europea de Valencia, Valencia, Spain

Mario Dioguardi
Department of Clinical and Experimental Medicine, University of Foggia, Foggia, Italy

Kazuhiro Terada
Department of Oral and Maxillofacial Surgery, Faculty of Medicine, University of Tsukuba, Tsukuba, Japan
Department of Oral and Maxillofacial Surgery, Tsukuba Medical Center Hospital, Tsukuba, Japan

Kenji Yamagata, Fumihiko Uchida, Satoshi Fukuzawa, Naomi Ishibashi-Kanno and Hiroki Bukawa
Department of Oral and Maxillofacial Surgery, Faculty of Medicine, University of Tsukuba, Tsukuba, Japan

Marcio Augusto de Oliveira
Department of Stomatology, School of Dentistry, University of São Paulo, Av Prof. Lineu Prestes 2227, 05508-000 São Paulo, Brazil

Bruna Reis, Debora Pallos, Yeon Jung Kim and Fabiana Martins
Dental School, University of Santo Amaro, R. Prof. Eneas de Siqueia Neto 340, 04829-300 São Paulo, Brazil

Paulo Henrique Braz-Silva
Department of Stomatology, School of Dentistry, University of São Paulo, Av Prof. Lineu Prestes 2227, 05508-000 São Paulo, Brazil
Laboratory of Virology, Institute of Tropical Medicine of São Paulo, University of São Paulo, v. Dr. Enéas Carvalho de Aguiar 470, 05403-000 São Paulo, Brazil

Bandar Alyami
Department of Preventive Dentistry, Faculty of Dentistry, Najran University, Najran, Saudi Arabia

Eleonora Ortu, Davide Pietropaoli, Alessandra Mummolo, Mario Giannoni and Annalisa Monaco
MeSVA Department, Division of Dentistry, University of L'Aquila, P.le Salvatore Tommasi, 67100 L'Aquila, Italy

Kasumi Shimizu, Miho Hayashi, Nozomi Ito, Kokoro Hamada, Gaku Koizumi, Kazuto Kurohara and Naoya Arai
Department of Oral and Maxillofacial Surgery, Department of Clinical Sciences, Medical Life Science, Mie University Graduate School of Medicine, Tsu, Mie 514-8507, Japan

Mohammad Jafarian
Department of Oral and Maxillofacial Surgery, School of Dentistry, Shahid Beheshti University of Medical Sciences, Tehran, Iran

Fatemeh Mashhadi Abbas and Homeira Saebnoori
Department of Oral and Maxillofacial Pathology, School of Dentistry, Shahid Beheshti University of Medical Sciences, Tehran, Iran

Mitra Ghazizadeh Ahsaie
Department of Oral and Maxillofacial Radiology, School of Dentistry, Shahid Beheshti University of Medical Sciences, Tehran, Iran

Spartak Spasov Yanakiev
Medical College, Medical University of Sofia, Yordanka Filaretova Str. No. 3, Sofia, Bulgaria

Mirela Borislavova Marinova-Takorova
Department of Conservative Dentistry, Faculty of Dental Medicine, Medical University of Sofia, Georgi Sofiiski 3 Str., Sofia, Bulgaria

Antoine Berberi
Department of Oral and Maxillofacial Surgery, Faculty of Dental Medicine, Lebanese University, Lebanon

Georges Aoun and Georges Aad
Department of Oral Medicine and Maxillofacial Radiology, Faculty of Dental Medicine, Lebanese University, Lebanon

Elie Azar
Department of ENT, Faculty of Medicine, Lebanese University, Lebanon

Chiara Cinquini, Simonetta Santarelli, Alberto Marianelli, Marco Nisi, Mario Gabriele and Antonio Barone
Department of Surgical, Medical, Molecular and of Critical Area Pathologies, Complex Operative Unit of Stomatology and Oral Surgery, University-Hospital of Pisa, University of Pisa, 56126 Pisa, Italy

Index

www.ingramcontent.com/pod-product-compliance
Lightning Source LLC
LaVergne TN
LVHW082230200926
848484LV00008B/2326